Mast Cells,
Mediators and
Disease

IMMUNOLOGY AND MEDICINE SERIES

_____IMMUNOLOGY_____
· SERIES · SERIES · SERIES · SERIES **AND** SERIES · SERIES · SERIES · SERIES ·
MEDICINE

Mast Cells, Mediators and Disease

Edited by
S. T. Holgate
MRC Clinical Research Professor of Immunopharmacology
University of Southampton

Series Editor: W. G. Reeves

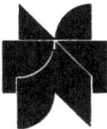

KLUWER ACADEMIC PUBLISHERS
DORDRECHT / BOSTON / LONDON

Distributors

for the United States and Canada: Kluwer Academic Publishers, PO Box 358, Accord Station, Hingham, MA 02018-0358, USA
for all other countries: Kluwer Academic Publishers Group, Distribution Center, PO Box 322, 3300 AH Dordrecht, The Netherlands

British Library Cataloguing in Publication Data

Mast cell, mediators and disease.
  1. Man. Diseases. Role of mast cells
  I. Holgate, Stephen T. II. Series
  616.07′1
  ISBN-13: 978-94-010-7072-0

Library of Congress Cataloging-in-Publication Data

Mast cells, mediators, and disease/edited by S. T. Holgate.
      p. cm. — (Immunology and medicine series)
    Includes bibliographies and index.

    1. Mast cells—Immunology. 2. Mast cells—Physiology.
  3. Allergy—Pathogenesis. I. Holgate, S. T. II. Series.
    [DNLM: 1. Mast Cells—Immunology. QS 532.5.C7 M4235]
  QR185.8.M35M37 1988
  616.07′9—dc 19
  DNLM/DLC
  for Library of Congress   88-21568 CIP
  ISBN-13: 978-94-010-7072-0   e-ISBN-13: 978-94-009-1287-8
  DOI: 10.1007/978-94-009-1287-8

Copyright

Published in the United Kingdom by Kluwer Academic Publishers, PO Box 55, Lancaster, UK.

Kluwer Academic Publishers BV incorporates the publishing programmes of D. Reidel, Martinus Nijhoff, Dr W. Junk and MTP Press.

Typeset by Blackpool Typesetting Services Ltd., Blackpool, UK.

Contents

Preface

In 1879 Paul Ehrlich first described the mast cell as a tissue fixed cell containing many granules which, when stained with basic dyes, such as toluidine blue, changed the colour spectrum of the dye in a process called metachromasia. Since this early description, pathologists, physicians and pharmacologists have been fascinated by this cell on account of its central involvement in human allergic diseases. Approximately four decades after Ehrlich's first description of the mast cell, Prausnitz and Küstner reported their pioneer experiment, demonstrating that the immediate skin wheal response to allergen could be passively transferred with serum. They named the antigen-specific serum factor reagin. A further four and one half decades had to pass before the connection between the mast cell and reagin could be made with the identification of reagin as an immunoglobulin E by Johansson and Ishizaka and its unique property to bind with high affinity to specific receptors on mast cells and basophils.

Meanwhile in the 1920s Coca published a series of papers in which he described the clinical features of acute allergic responses and first used the term atopy. This, together with the fundamental pharmacological studies of Sir Henry Dale in identifying histamine as one mediator of the acute anaphylactic reaction, provided the second approach which eventually linked the mast cell to allergic tissue reactions. Indeed, it was Best, working in Dale's group who first showed that histamine was a chemical stored in mast cells.

The advent of the eras of biochemistry and molecular biology has opened the door for the detailed dissection of the mast cell as a mediator secreting cell and its contribution to the pathogenesis of allergic diseases. The last decade has witnessed an enormous effort in defining the biochemical pathways of mast cell activation, the plethora of chemical mediators that they secrete and the pharmacological agents that may inhibit secretation. The discovery of mast cell growth factors from lymphocytes and fibroblasts and the existence of morphological and functional heterogeneity of mast cells, both between animal species and between individual tissues within a single species, has served to promote further interest in this unique cell.

So rapid have been the developments relating to mast cells that many of those not actively involved in one of the advancing research fronts may easily become out of date and confused. It is the purpose of this short volume to describe some of the new and exciting discoveries regarding the structure and function of mast cells and to put into perspective their ontogony and function. The authors that have contributed to this volume are leaders in their field and I am grateful to them for presenting an overview of their area of interest with precision and clarity. I hope those who read this book discover what a fascinating cell the mast cell is and why for almost a century it has stolen the enthusiasm for so many investigators.

S. T. Holgate

Series Editor's Note

The modern clinician is expected to be the fount of all wisdom concerning conventional diagnosis and management relevant to his sphere of practice. In addition, he or she has the daunting task of comprehending and keeping pace with advances in basic science relevant to the pathogenesis of disease and ways in which these processes can be regulated or prevented. Immunology has grown from the era of anti-toxins and serum sickness to a state where the study of many diverse cells and molecules has become integrated into a coherent scientific discipline with major implications for many common and crippling diseases prevalent throughout the world.

Many of today's practitioners received little or no specific training in immunology and what was taught is very likely to have been overtaken by subsequent developments. This series of titles on IMMUNOLOGY AND MEDICINE is designed to rectify this deficiency in the form of distilled packages of information which the busy clinician, pathologist or other health care professional will be able to open and enjoy.

Professor W. G. Reeves, FRCP, FRCPath
Department of Immunology
University Hospital, Queen's Medical Centre
Nottingham

List of Contributors

R. C. BENYON
Immunopharmacology Group
Clinical Pharmacology
University of Southampton
Faculty of Medicine
Level F, Centre Block
Southampton General Hospital
Southampton SO9 4XY
UK

M. K. CHURCH
Department of Clinical Pharmacology
University of Southampton
Faculty of Medicine
Centre Block
Southampton General Hospital
Southampton SO9 4XY
UK

D. H. CONRAD
Subdepartment of Immunology
The Johns Hopkins University
School of Medicine
725 N. Wolfe Street
Baltimore, MD 21205
USA

J. A. DENBURG
Department of Medicine
McMaster University Medical Center
1200 Main Street West
Hamilton, Ontario L8N 3Z5
Canada

A. M. DVORAK
Department of Pathology
Beth Israel Hospital
330 Brookline Avenue
Boston, MA 02215
USA

R. FULLER
Department of Clinical Pharmacology
Royal Postgraduate Medical School
Du Cane Road
London W12 0HS
UK

S. T. HOLGATE
Immunopharmacology Group
Clinical Pharmacology
University of Southampton
Faculty of Medicine
Level D, Centre Block
Southampton General Hospital
Southampton SO9 4XY
UK

A. B. KAY
Department of Allergy and Clinical
    Immunology
Cardiothoracic Institute
Dovehouse Street
London SW3 6LY
UK

F. L. PEARCE
Department of Chemistry
University College London
20 Gordon Street
London WC1H 0AJ
UK

C. ROBINSON
Department of Clinical Pharmacology
University of Southampton
Centre Block
Southampton General Hospital
Southampton SO9 4XY
UK

L. B. SCHWARTZ
Departments of Internal Medicine,
Microbiology and Immunology and
Pathology
Medical College of Virginia
Virginia and Commonwealth
University
Box 263, Richmond, VI 23298
USA

1
Phylogeny and Ontogeny of Basophils, Mast Cells and Eosinophils

J. A. DENBURG

INTRODUCTION

Postulated origins of basophils, mast cells and eosinophils

Basophils and eosinophils: progenitors

It has been traditionally assumed that basophils, eosinophils and neutrophils are derived from a common, myeloid bone marrow progenitor, by analogy to erythroid and megakaryocytic lineages. However, the hypothesis of a fixed, common granulocyte progenitor, present in the bone marrow and giving rise to all lineages of granulated (myeloid) cells, has only been partly supported by *in vivo* and *in vitro* observations.

First, there exist *in vivo* deficiencies or granular anomalies of polymorphonuclear leukocytes which can involve all three, two or even only one of the neutrophilic, eosinophilic or basophilic lineages[1,2]. This implies that at some level there must exist separate control (i.e. progenitors or growth factors or differentiation sequences) of the ontogeny of each lineage. Second, and in support of the above, recent studies of *in vitro* bone marrow and peripheral blood progenitor growth and differentiation in both mouse and man have demonstrated that single bone marrow progenitors express random ('stochastic') combinations of differentiative potential[3,4]; i.e. one can identify, among others, basophil–eosinophil–neutrophil, basophil–eosinophil, eosinophil–neutrophil progenitors, as well as progenitors giving rise to only one myeloid lineage. This confirms the validity of inferences made concerning bone marrow progenitors specific for basophils or eosinophils from morphologic and cytochemical analyses[1,2]. The findings imply that haemopoietic processes follow, in general, a pattern more analogous to the 'clonal selection' model of specific immunocompetence rather than the now untenable 'instructive' model. The corollary of this is that specific growth

1

and differentiation factors for each haemopoietic lineage 'select' specific progenitors, which randomly express lineage- or even differentiation stage-specific receptors for these factors, resulting in specific haemopoietic clonal expansion or suppression. It is important to note, however, that basophils and eosinophils appear to share with each other more specific pathways of differentiation, as evidenced by common congenital anomalies and cellular protein content, than do either of these with neutrophils. Until the genetic sequences underlying myeloid differentiative processes are unraveled, it can only be speculated that the basophil and eosinophil lineages are closely linked at the level of structural and regulatory genes involved in their ontogeny.

Basophils and eosinophils: numbers

All three polymorphonuclear leukocytes circulate (with varying halflives)[2] in the peripheral blood, are stored and/or mature in the bone marrow, and are present along blood vessel walls from which they may demarginate. Both basophils and eosinophils can be found to fluctuate in numbers in response to several stimuli or in certain conditions[1]: e.g. in myeloproliferative disorders or aplastic anaemias, both may be increased or decreased, respectively, in the circulation. However, in some conditions there are preferential increases or decreases in one, but not the other (e.g. increases in eosinophils only in hyper-eosinophilic syndromes, increases in basophils primarily in the rare baso-philic leukaemia); in some leukopoenias or immunodeficiencies, decreases in neutrophils only are observed, in the presence of a relative basophilia or eosinophilia. Conversely, in certain haematologic disorders or endocrino-pathies there appear to be selective changes in basophils and eosinophils, sparing neutrophils; these can be due to specific changes in bone marrow pro-genitor numbers or to fluctuations in kinetics (which are altered in states of excess or deficiency). The tissue compartment of eosinophils, for example, is much more extensive than that of the neutrophil – in fact, it has been estimated that for rodent eosinophils there is a 500 : 1 ratio between tissue and circulating compartments[2]. It cannot, however, be excluded that some hor-monally induced changes in peripheral blood basophils or eosinophils (e.g. mild to moderate decreases in hyperadrenalism or increases in hypo-adrenalism) may be due, at least in part, to effects at the level of progenitors in the bone marrow. Recent studies of T-cell dependent and independent effects of corticosteroids on granulopoiesis have highlighted the complexity of the physiological regulation of basophil and eosinophil numbers in blood and tissues. In fact, the lifespan and kinetics of human basophils and eosino-phils from their putative origin in bone marrow, through their release into the circulation and migration into tissues, are less well understood than those of the neutrophil; the relative infrequency of these cells, especially of the basophil, has made it difficult to isolate them and to perform kinetic studies in large numbers of subjects, including asymptomatic, normal individuals. Moreover, as will be stressed in this review, it is not at all clear that the only mechanism of tissue accumulation of basophils and eosinophils, or, for that matter, neutrophils, is the release of mature cells from bone marrow and their migration through the blood to tissues.

2

Mast cells

The bone marrow/peripheral blood/tissue compartmentalization model, as it has been applied to basophils and eosinophils, is not as readily applicable to the mast cell. Circulating mast cells are rare, and occur almost exclusively in neoplastic disorders such as severe systemic mastocytosis or mast cell leukaemia in man (which can also be accompanied by basophilia). Mast cells, originally defined, like basophils, by Ehrlich[5] as metachromatic granule-containing mononuclear cells were first seen in unstained preparations by von Recklinghausen[6]. They are clearly larger than basophils or eosinophils, containing morphologically distinct granules, and they populate tissues, primarily skin, the adventitia of blood vessels, serosal and mucosal surfaces[5,6]. In mice, the bone marrow origin of these 'sessile' metachromatic cells has now been formally demonstrated by Kitamura and his co-workers[7]; however, the kinetics of mast cell progenitor release and migration are unclear, and have only recently been measured, mainly in rodents during immune or inflammatory reactions (see later). It is also likely that some mast cells may originate from progenitors resident within tissues, such as the thymus gland, thoracic duct lymphocytes, or lymph nodes and even from mature mast cells themselves (e.g. at dermal sites); some mast cells may simply represent tissue forms of basophils. Morphology and cytochemistry, while providing important distinctions between mature forms of these two cell types in different species[8-11] are simply not sufficient to clarify these issues.

In the following, the complexity of basophil–mast cell–eosinophil ontogeny will be expanded upon, and an attempt will be made to provide new information on the basis of which the ontogenic inter-relationships of these lineages can be better understood.

Phylogenetic aspects of basophils, mast cells and eosinophils

The specialized granulocytes, basophils, mast cells and eosinophils (BME) contain many specific mediators of inflammation and immunity. Such cells are found in mammals and lower vertebrates, including fish, amphibians, birds and reptiles[6]. There is an inverse species variation with regard to the presence of subtypes of metachromatic cells: apparently 'basophil-rich' species with few recognizable mast cells (e.g. guinea pig, rabbit) and, conversely, 'mast cell-rich' ones (e.g. rat, mouse)[6,11]. The basis for this is not known, but it is assumed that one metachromatic cell type may functionally 'substitute' for the other phylogenetically[6]. In the human, both latter cell types occur in abundance, and, as will be discussed, the lineage relationships between basophils and mast cells or, among BME, are just coming to light.

Selye[6] documented that, at least in animals, mature mast cells appear to undergo mitosis during reactions which elicit their *in vivo* accumulation, anticipating more contemporary observations. The embryonic development of mast cells in the rat is accompanied by sequential changes in proteoglycan content, as evidenced by histochemical staining; the relationship of this to the phylogeny of BME is unknown, but peculiar, hybrid metachromatic

3

granule containing eosinophils are commonly found in some species (e.g. rabbit), suggesting their common evolution[6].

In any case, the presence of BME in reactions to parasitic infestation, in conjunction with IgE or other cytophilic ('homocytotrophic') antibodies[12, 13] (which are also found early in phylogeny), suggests that these cells form a primitive line of defence against particulate antigen primarily at mucosal surfaces. Therefore, from Ehrlich's description of metachromatic (i.e. colour change from blue to purple), granule-laden cells to the demonstrations of their content of histamine, serotonin and other mediators[14], it has become clear that the potential roles for BME in inflammation and immunity are numerous.

BASOPHILS, MAST CELLS AND EOSINOPHILS IN INFLAMMATION AND IMMUNITY

Cutaneous basophil hypersensitivity

BME are found in a wide range of allergic and inflammatory-immune reactions in both animals and man[1, 2, 9–14] (Table 1.1). These cells, which secrete many mediators of inflammation, are found not only during IgE-mediated immunity but also in the course of other immune reactions, including delayed-type hypersensitivity and cytotoxicity[9, 12, 15]. Experimental BME increases are seen in tissue reactions to parasites, especially to nematodes and ectoparasites, including a specific delayed-in-time hypersensitivity reaction in the skin of guinea pigs known as cutaneous basophil hypersensitivity (CBH), which is dependent upon T-cells, homocytotropic antibodies and vasoactive amines[9, 12]. Possible human counterparts to CBH or parasite-induced basophilia/mast cell hyperplasia include contact dermatitis, or IgE-dependent conditions such as atopic dermatitis, allergic respiratory

Table 1.1 Immune mechanisms involving basophils, mast cells and eosinophils

Type of reaction	Elements involved
Immediate hypersensitivity	basophils, mast cells, eosinophils homocytotropic antibodies chemotactic factors vasoactive and other inflammatory mediators
Cytotoxicity	mast cells, eosinophils IgG or homocytotropic antibodies vasoactive amines peroxides
Immune complex	basophils complement (C3a, C5a) vasoactive and other inflammatory mediators
Delayed hypersensitivity	mast cells, basophils T-lymphocytes vasoactive amines

4

Table 1.2 Tissue sites and models of basophil, mast cell and eosinophil accumulaton

Tissue	Mechanism	Examples
Skin	immediate hypersensitivity and/or immune complex	urticaria and angioɛdema
	cutaneous basophil hypersensitivity	atopic eczema Jones–Mote reacticns
	delayed hypersensitivity	contact allergy
Mucosal surfaces	immediate hypersensitivity	allergic rhinitis asthma
	immediate and/or delayed hypersensitivity	parasitic infection inflammatory bowel disease
Other	cytoxicity or delayed hypersensitivity	tumour or graft rejection

disease, late-phase skin reactions, skin allograft responses and some cases of urticaria or angioedema[9, 16] (Table 1.2). Various other inflammatory reactions in man involving lung or bowel, systemic vasculitidies and rheumatoid arthritis can involve BME mediator release or tissue accumulation as a component of inflammatory responses[16].

While it has been recognized that BME participate in many inflammatory and immune reactions, the mechanisms whereby these cells accumulate in tissues or gain access to sites of inflammation are poorly understood. A proper understanding of these mechanisms requires an overview of the appearance of BME in specific experimental and clinical situations, and of the ontogeny of these cells.

Basophils, mast cells and eosinophils in allergy

In human allergic and atopic disorders, BME have been found in tissues, and are postulated as representing the chief effector cells in allergic rhinitis, bronchial asthma and atopic dermatitis[16–21]. A functional role has been demonstrated for nasal mucosal basophils and mast cells in human allergic rhinitis, lending support to morphological observations of BME in secretions, epithelial scrapings and nasal mucosal biopsies from subjects with this condition. Similarly, an effector role for eosinophils and, more recently, basophils and mast cells and/or their granule constituents, has been inferred from their presence in sputum, bronchial brushings and bronchoalveolar lavage fluid in bronchial asthma. It has been postulated that intraepithelial migration of nasal mucosal mast cells occurs during the course of pollen allergy, but the source and mechanism of accumulation of these cells is still not clear. Likewise, it has been demonstrated that basophils accumulate at skin patch test (i.e. antigen-containing) sites in patients with atopic dermatitis, but the precise mechanism of this cellular reaction is unknown. Basophil counts in peripheral blood fluctuate before, during and after the pollen season along with IgE levels, but the relative contributions to this of either demargination or storage pool release (of mature cells) or of bone marrow basophil growth (of progenitors) have not been clarified.

5

MECHANISMS OF TISSUE ACCUMULATION OF BME IN ALLERGIC AND INFLAMMATORY STATES

Chemotaxis

It has been assumed that the tissue accumulation of mature, circulating, peripheral blood basophils or eosinophils is chiefly, if not exclusively, a result of chemotaxis, which may involve lymphokine-dependent or -independent stimuli. Included among such responses are antigen- and IgE-dependent reactions in which chemotactic stimuli for eosinophils are liberated from basophils or resident tissue mast cells[14]. In the CBH model, a variety of soluble factors, including antibodies of the IgG1 or IgE class and vasoactive amines, serve as important chemotactic stimuli for basophils, presumably contributing to their tissue accumulation. However, chemotaxis alone does not appear to explain basophil accumulation in guinea pig skin during CBH reactions[22], nor has there been any formal demonstration of the *in vivo* importance of chemotaxis on BME or other inflammatory cell recruitment to allergic or inflammatory reactions in man. The corollary of this is that the mechanisms of disappearance of BME from allergic inflammatory sites after treatment, such as with corticosteroids, are also unclear. Molecules which may functionally activate BME include haemopoietic growth and differentiation factors, such as purified neutrophil/macrophage colony-stimulating factor (GM-CSF)[23], which may thus play a role in BME-rich tissue responses.

An important marker of the allergic diathesis, total serum IgE, cannot itself account for the type or severity of symptoms in human seasonal allergic rhinitis[24]. Thus, it is reasonable to hypothesize that mechanisms other than chemotaxis may contribute to the accumulation of allergic effector cells in tissues, and that the number of cells may be an independent correlate of disease severity.

In situ haemopoiesis

The evidence for the contribution of the bone marrow to tissue accumulation of BME is indirect but considerable. First, mature, circulating basophils fluctuate *in vivo* during allergic, specifically IgE-dependent, reactions. These fluctuations appear to be dependent on antigen exposure and, although in part probably related to demargination and chemotaxis of mature cells, they may also result from BME progenitor proliferation/differentiation. The total number of basophilic cells accumulating in CBH reactions cannot be accounted for by chemotaxis even of the entire circulating pool of mature basophils at any one time, and in these reactions, serum basophil growth-stimulating factor fluctuates in accordance with basophilic responses in the bone marrow, peripheral blood and skin. Inhibitory as well as stimulatory activities can be demonstrated in serum in direct relation to the kinetics of *in vivo* basophil responses to antigen[10].

Vastly increased numbers of circulating BME progenitors are found in various human atopic states[10, 25], including significant and clinically relevant fluctuations of these progenitors in relation to seasonal exposure to the

6

allergen[10, 26], and an inverse relationship of the number of circulating progenitors to the number of (mature) progeny accumulating in tissue sites such as the nasal mucosa[10, 27]. These results suggest that progenitors traffic to tissue during allergic reactions; indeed, BME progenitors can be found within nasal mucosa and BME growth factors, which appear to be lineage- and phenotype-specific for BME, are elaborated by nasal epithelial scrapings and a variety of other tissues or cells[10]. These factors are produced in large amounts by nasal epithelium from severe atopics, as well as by epithelial scrapings or mononuclear cells present in nasal polyps[10]. Thus, the local environment can affect the expression of the allergic diathesis either by promotion of progenitor ingress from the blood, with growth and differentiation in the tissues, or by promotion of growth of those progenitor cells already present in tissues. It is likely that the epithelium can produce these factors in both the upper and lower respiratory tracts and possibly elsewhere; 'in situ haemopoiesis' is thus thought to play an important role in human BME accumulation in certain inflammatory states.

HUMAN BASOPHIL, MAST CELL AND EOSINOPHIL GROWTH AND DIFFERENTIATION

Parallelisms among BME

Until recently, there has been a relative lack of information on the growth and differentiation of human BME even though biochemical, functional and haematological studies have clearly demonstrated similarities among these specialized granulocytes in a variety of laboratory animals and man[13, 15, 28–32]. Although investigations in man may be crucial in understanding the ontogeny and lineage interrelationships of BME and their clinical importance, most of our understanding and analysis of these cells has come from studies in rodent models such as the mouse or rat[2, 10, 33, 34]. In the past few years, metachromatic cells fitting descriptions of either basophils or mast cells have been recognized in human haematopoietic cell cultures, paralleling experiments in nature such as chronic myeloid leukemia in which basophilia can be a prominent and important feature, or systemic mastocytosis, in which a neoplastic proliferation of mast cells occurs in various organs[35].

In vitro observations

Differentiation of metachromatic cells from progenitors in semi-solid and suspension cultures of bone marrow or peripheral blood from leukaemic patients was first observed only within the last decade[36–39], culminating in reports of human immature basophilic cell lines developed *in vitro*[36, 40]. Studies by a number of investigators have focused upon the regulation of normal human BME growth and differentiation; these have provided tools with which to examine the question of the contribution of BME growth and differentiation to the allergic tissue inflammatory response.

7

Table 1.3 Sources of human basophil, mast cell and eosinophil growth and differentiation factors

Source	Active component(s)
T-cells or T-cell lines	IL-3 GM-CSF basophil differentiation factor eosinophil differentiation factor (IL-5) nerve growth factor
Keratinocytes or keratinocyte cell lines	G-CSF
Bladder carcinoma cell line	G-CSF
Nasal polyp or epithelial scrapings	basophil differentiation factor G-CSF (?)
Placental trophoblast cells	GM-CSF G-CSF basophil differentiation factor eosinophil differentiation factor (IL-5?)
Osteogenic sarcoma cell line	G-CSF

Sources of BME growth and differentiation factors

Human BME growth and differentiation factors have been derived from specific antigen-stimulated lymphomononuclear cells of allergic patients, from mitogen-stimulated nasal polyp mononuclear cells, from human T-lymphoblasts (Mo leukaemic cell line), from human keratinocytes and from nasal polyp or allergic epithelial scrapings *in vitro*[10] (Table 1.3). Certain of these factors appear to be lineage-specific, promoting differentiation of basophils or mast cells or eosinophils, respectively[10]. *In vivo* models include the presence of circulating or resident mast cell progenitors in murine mast cell hyperplasia in response to antigen or other local stimuli[41-43], the specific production of a low molecular weight peptide with eosinophilopoietic activity following treatment of mice with anti-eosinophil serum[1], and the presence in serum of specific basophil growth stimulatory or inhibitory factors during guinea pig responses to heterologous antigens or ticks[10]. In addition, fluctuations in serum interleukin (IL)-3 (mast cell growth factor) are measurable during reactions to tumours and grafts[10,41,43]. Thus, there is evidence pointing to the pathophysiologic role of BME growth and differentiation responses in the local accumulation of these cells during specific hypersensitivity reactions. Until recently, however, there did not exist specific, quantitative assay systems for BME growth and differentiation, nor were the ontogenic inter-relationships of these cells fully appreciated. Moreover, the discovery of heterogeneity among mast cell populations has added complexity to our understanding of the ontogeny and phylogeny of BME.

MAST CELL HETEROGENEITY

Rat mast cells

Histochemical differences: rodents

While mast cells have long been recognized on the basis of their staining properties, the lineages to which they belong and the factors which control and regulate their growth and differentiation have only relatively recently been examined[10]. It was Enerback who first observed that mast cells in rat intestine stained differently from those found in connective tissue, depending on whether the tissue had been fixed in formaldehyde or other fixatives such as basic lead acetate. The rat intestinal mucosal mast cell loses its metachromatic staining after formaldehyde fixation (i.e. 'formaldehyde-sensitive'), while the rat peritoneal mast cell does not (i.e. 'formaldehyde-resistant'). This staining difference seems to be based on the relative capacity of aldehyde groups on the granular proteoglycans to be blocked by the fixative. Subsequently, it has become clear, at least in the rat and the mouse, that mast cells in the normal intestinal mucosal layer as well as those proliferating in the mucosa after *in vivo* infection with the nematode *Nippostrongylus brasiliensis* are different from the serosal or connective tissue mast cell, the latter best represented by cells derived from the peritoneal cavity.

Functional and biochemical differences: rodents

Differences between the above mast cell types include functional responses to a variety of secretagogues and anti-allergic compounds[10]. It is noteworthy that there are few morphological differences described among mast cells at different sites except that the intestinal mucosal mast cell is smaller, has less granules and less histamine than the peritoneal mast cell, and fewer high affinity IgE receptors. In addition, it has been observed that thymectomized or nude animals, or animals which have had their thoracic ducts drained do not mount an intestinal mast cell response to nematode infection. A soluble factor probably accounts for this and is likely to be T-cell-derived since the mastocytosis can be restored by thoracic duct lymphocytes or by immune serum.

Additional differences between intestinal and peritoneal mast cells have come to light, and include the synthesis and secretion of certain arachidonic acid metabolites, such as leukotriene C4 in preference to others (prostaglandin D2) upon stimulation of intestinal mast cells with antigen or calcium ionophores, whereas the reverse is true for peritoneal mast cells[10]. Furthermore, careful studies of mast cell proteoglycans have shown that in the rat, the cultured bone marrow mast cell, and the isolated intestinal mucosal mast cell both possess a uniquely sulphated proteoglycan, chondroitin sulphate di-B, not found in peritoneal mast cells but interestingly found in the rat basophilic leukaemia cell (RBL)[10,44]. In the mouse, both the bone marrow cultured cells and those derived from the intestine share another oversulphated proteoglycan, chondroitin sulphate E, not found in murine peritoneal

9

mast cells[45]. Finally, the serine proteases of the two types of mast cells differ[45]: the intestinal cell contains a unique protease, rat mast cell protease (RMCP) II, also found in the bone marrow-derived mast cell and in the RBL, but not in the peritoneal mast cells[46]. This interesting serine protease has homology with a serine protease cloned recently from cytotoxic T-cells, suggesting some 'family relationship' among T-cells and mast cells, an idea first proposed by Burnet. Thus, in rodents, there is evidence for mast cell heterogeneity which may well reflect ontogenic differences.

Morphological, functional and biochemical differences: humans and primates

In the human, evidence for mast cell heterogeneity such as is seen in the rat is available but not as extensive. Both formaldehyde-sensitive and formaldehyde-resistant mast cells have been described in human skin, nose, respiratory and gastrointestinal tracts[10, 47, 48]; basophils found in tissues and in peripheral blood are commonly formaldehyde-sensitive. Some variation in size of mast cells in the nose has also been observed[10, 17, 48]. On the basis of immunohistochemical staining for serine esterases in mast cells of human skin and respiratory tracts, there is also evidence for heterogeneity: chymotryptic proteinase and tryptase in skin mast cells, tryptase only in mucosa-associated mast cells[49]. Human colonic mucosa releases histamine and

Table 1.4 Evidence for *in vivo* human mast cell heterogeneity

Site	Method of demonstration
Nasal mucosa	morphological* histochemical†
Bronchus	histochemical biochemical‡
Alveolus	functional§ histochemical morphological biochemical
Gastrointestinal mucosa	histochemical biochemical
Skin	histochemical biochemical functional
Blood	morphological histochemical functional

*Differences in size, shape of nucleus, ultrastructure
†Formaldehyde blocking of metachromasia; basophils in peripheral blood are formaldehyde-sensitive
‡Proteases: chymotryptic and tryptic
§Response to secretagogues and anti-allergic compounds

chondroitin sulphate-E, indicating that a unique mast cell with this proteo-glycan may be present[50]. However, functional heterogeneity has been more difficult to demonstrate: elutriated, small mast cells derived from human lung parenchyma appear to have different functional characteristics from the majority of the rest[10, 51]. By analogy, monkey lung lavage mast cells, after recurrent Ascaris infection, differ both histochemically and functionally from those derived from lung tissue proper[10]. No unequivocal functional heterogeneity has been demonstrated for mast cells derived from human or monkey intestine or human lung. However, circumstantial evidence is accumulating to suggest that, at least at some sites, there may exist human mast cell heterogeneity similar to that found in the rodent[10] (Table 1.4).

These types of observations have led to the postulation of the existence of a specific mucosal mast cell in man. In this regard, of interest is that a new anti-allergic compound has been shown to be considerably more active against broncho-alveolar mast cells than against those obtained from lung fragments. It is also interesting that cortisone has been shown to eliminate mucosal but not other mast cells in the Nippostrongylus infected rat model of intestinal mast cell hyperplasia[52], a phenomenon similar to corticosteroid ablation of mast cells in human allergic rhinitis[10]. There may thus be important practical and clinical implications of mast cell heterogeneity, in whatever form it may be present in the human.

LINEAGE INTER-RELATIONSHIPS OF BASOPHILS, MAST CELLS AND EOSINOPHILS

Rodent basophils, mast cells and eosinophils

In most species, on light and electron microscopy it is easy to differentiate the polymorphonuclear appearance of a peripheral blood basophil from that of the mononuclear mast cell[8, 9]; however, whether a cell belongs to a specific lineage cannot be judged solely on the basis of morphology, even including painstaking cytochemical analysis[2], although the latter techniques are extremely useful in dealing with questions of ontogeny and phylogeny. In rodents, very low numbers of basophils, if any, are found in peripheral blood, but parallel increases in both basophils and eosinophils in tissues and in blood may be found after parasitic infection which also elicits tissue mastocytosis[13, 28].

In the rat, a basophilic leukaemia cell may be misnamed since it has biochemical characteristics similar to an intestinal mast cell[46]; this cell has been used for many years to study mediator release and IgE receptors. The rat blood basophil found during nematode infection may not contain RMCP II, making it less likely to be identical or directly related to the intestinal mast cell. Thus, caution must be taken in utilizing morphological criteria alone to determine lineage, especially since cells which appear similar or identical by the former method may be found to be dissimilar by the latter. This may often be the case with *in vitro* established cell lines.

11

Cultured rodent basophils

In mice, it is estimated that up to 0.3% of all nucleated bone marrow cells are basophil progenitors, increasing to 10% in the peripheral blood after immunization. However, in general, murine basophils are rare and even their morphological identification is difficult[8, 9]. A cloned, natural cytotoxic cell with basophil features has been reported to possess, like mast cells, high affinity IgE receptors, but no histamine; these cells take up and store serotonin[9, 10]. No other cytotoxic cell line has been shown to have similar properties, but the presence of RMCP II-like material in cytotoxic T-cells (above), suggests a lineage relationship among basophils, cytotoxic cells and intestinal mast cells.

In guinea pigs, the growth of basophils from bone marrow has been shown to be T-cell dependent and inducible by specific antigen[53]. The factor responsible appears to be a relatively large, heat stable glycoprotein separable from other lymphokines and haemopoietic growth factors, including IL-3[10]. Basophil and eosinophil growth stimulatory factors are present in serum during *in vivo* tick infection, paralleling *in vivo* basophilia and eosinophilia in these situations; the stimulatory factors are succeeded by inhibitory factors in serum as the tissue responses reach their maximum[10]. The inhibitors have not yet been characterized.

Human basophils and eosinophils

In the human, basophil precursors have been found in cord blood, fetal liver, peripheral blood and bone marrow; these are non-adherent, non-B non-T cells[10, 38]. Human leukaemic cells which can differentiate to basophils[36, 40] or other lineages have been described, but their relationship to mature basophils or to tissue mast cells is unclear. Cultured human cord blood basophils possess high affinity IgE receptors, contain low level of histamine, synthesize chondroitin-4-sulphate, and surprisingly take up and release arachidonic acid without incorporation into metabolites (unlike fetal liver derived basophilic cells *in vitro*, which do), suggesting that a differentiation factor is likely to be missing from the conditioned media in which they are grown[10].

Human tissue mast cells

Human mast cells are found in most tissues, with increases found in a variety of inflammatory states including allergic rhinitis, eczema and asthma. Increased mast cell numbers are also found in association with neurofibromata and other tumours, and in tissue repair processes such as scar or callus formation (particularly keloids) and in pulmonary fibrosis[54]. In urticaria pigmentosa or systemic mastocytosis, large numbers of (presumably) neoplastic mast cells are found in skin, bone, gastrointestinal tract and bone marrow[35]. The increases in basophils found in association with myeloproliferative disorders as well as in allergic conditions are almost exclusively in the circulating compartment, and not necessarily accompanied by tissue mast cell increases, although basophils and mast cells may share some morphological features in these conditions (see below).

Common human and rodent basophil–eosinophil progenitor

The observation of: parallel increases, decreases, or absence of basophils and eosinophils in tissue or in circulation[13, 15, 28]; their shared granular contents and anomalies[29–32]; specific chromosomal aberrations associated with atypical basophils or eosinophils[55]; and specific antigen/T-cell regulated basophil/eosinophil growth and differentiation *in vivo* and *in vitro*[10, 53], point circumstantially to a shared basophil/eosinophil haemopoietic lineage. Indeed, several investigators have now observed the presence of a common, clonally-derived human basophil/eosinophil colony-forming cell (CFU-c)[56], which responds to separable, specific differentiation factors in human T-cell leukaemic conditioned media, allowing it to express either basophil or eosinophil phenotype during terminal differentiation[10, 57]. Similar observations have been made concerning guinea pig basophil and eosinophil progenitors in reponse to splenic T-cell products[10, 52].

Basophils and mucosal mast cells

Mast cell heterogeneity, present in rodents prototypically in the rat and, to a lesser extent, in man, is evidenced by the aforementioned distinctions between mucosal and non-mucosal mast cells, which include T-cell dependence of growth and differentiation. There is an inverse relationship, in general, between the frequency of mast cells and that of basophils as the predominant metachromatic cell type in various species. The precise lineage relationships between basophils and mast cells have only recently begun to be explored. In many respects basophils resemble mucosal mast cells rather than connective tissue mast cells. In the rat, the basophil leukaemic cell (RBL) contains the same oversulphated proteoglycan (chondroitin sulphate di-B)[46] found in the intestinal and bone marrow cultured cell, but not in the peritoneal mast cell. Similarly, the serine protease RMCP II is associated with RBL, intestinal and not peritoneal mast cells. Recent observations have suggested that a serine esterase analogous to RMCP II is not found in the circulating peripheral blood basophil in the rat. It is most likely, therefore, that the RBL cell may better resemble a mucosal type of mast cell rather than a basophil, in lineage.

The histochemical staining properties of basophils do however resemble intestinal mast cells in that they are formaldehyde-sensitive. The only other significant difference so far found between intestinal mast cells and basophils in rodents is the segmented nucleus. Recent experiments on human nasal metachromatic cells in allergic rhinitis suggest that basophils are related to mucosal mast cells histochemically and in lineage. For example, peripheral blood basophils and metachromatic cells in haemopoietic colonies from allergic individuals both stain after fixation in Mota's basic lead acetate but not after formaldehyde. The predominant intra-epithelial nasal metachromatic cell (NMC) which also correlates best with symptoms and signs in allergic rhinitis and responds to corticosteroids likewise is a formaldehyde-sensitive cell, the morphology of which resembles mast cells[10, 48]. Thus, the

13

metachromatic cells found in colonies grown from circulating progenitors in allergic patients may correspond to NMC.

Up to recently, the assignment of a cell to the basophil, as opposed to the mast cell, lineage has been on a morphological basis alone. Using these criteria it may be that the T-cell derived factors which stimulate the growth of mucosal mast cells are different and separable from those responsible for basophil growth[10, 58]; these may ultimately prove to underly terminal differentiation steps of cells having a common origin. Mucosal mast cell growth factor in the mouse corresponds to interleukin (IL)-3, counterparts to which may exist in the human. Moreover, a human IL-3-like activity, probably identical with granulocyte colony-stimulating factor (G-CSF), is separable from a basophil growth-stimulating factor[10, 39, 58], implying separate lineages for human basophils and mast cells.

Human basophils and eosinophils in relation to human mast cells

Indirect evidence for the separation of human basophil/eosinophil from mast cell lineage has come from studies of patients with urticaria pigmentosa and systemic mastocytosis, in whom mast cells or their progenitors appear to lack granular proteins found in both basophils and eosinophils[10, 37, 56, 59]. Thus, human basophils, eosinophils and possibly mucosal-type mast cells may be derived from one progenitor, and connective tissue-type mast cells from another, each regulated by (a) distinct growth factor(s).

It has been reported that some leukaemic basophils are, ultrastructurally, hybrid basophil–mast cells[8]; in fact, many blast cells in chronic myeloid leukaemic peripheral blood are seen by electron microscopy to contain 'primitive' or immature basophil and mast cell granules. Whether one can infer from these observations of leukaemic cells that human basophils and mast cells share a common progenitor is totally unclear. In any case, *in vitro*, it is difficult to tell morphologically whether a metachromatic cell is definitely a basophil or a mast cell, since polymorphonuclearity is often incomplete, and granule structure not fully developed. Nonetheless, it is possible to observe rare mast cells as well as basophils in cultures of human cord blood, and immature mast cell or basophil granulation in colony metachromatic cells grown in semi-solid media. There is no known morphological uniqueness to a human mucosal mast cell which can reliably distinguish it from a connective tissue mast cell*. Thus, unless human cells can be grown in large enough amounts to fully study function, biochemistry and morphology simultaneously and to manipulate differentiation patterns to one lineage (e.g. mast cell) or another (e.g. basophil), the inter-relationships among human basophil and mast cell lineages will simply not be known with any precision, as they appear to be in the rodent (especially the rat).

---

*Very recent observations using immunological localization of proteases by electron microscopy may allow such distinctions to be made.

MAST CELL GROWTH AND DIFFERENTIATION

Murine Interleukin 3

Long-term murine bone marrow cultures have provided evidence for the growth of a specific subtype of murine mast cell[10, 33, 43, 60]. The survival and proliferation of this mast cell is dependent on a factor isolated from myelomonocytic leukaemic cells (see above), or from mitogen- or antigen-stimulated T-cells, and has been termed IL-3[61] Murine IL-3 is a large (30 000 dalton) protein which induces lymphocyte differentiation, as quantitated by surface marker expression or specific enzymes. IL-3 is identical with a number of haemopoietic factors orginally termed murine mast cell growth factor, erythroid burst-promoting activity and multi-CSF, and it has been sequenced, its gene isolated and cloned[62]. A related human IL-3 has also recently been cloned[63], but the relationship of this molecule to basophil or eosinophil colony stimulating (haemopoietic) activities is unclear; it is *not* GM-CSF. The convergence of several haemopoietic growth factor activities in one, distinct IL-3-like molecule has not yet been found in man as it has in the mouse, even though the IL-3 gene appears to have been conserved in evolution[63].

Other possible haemopoietic factors for mast cells

Murine IL-3 is distinct from more lineage restricted CSFs for macrophages and neutrophils/eosinophils, respectively[23, 60-64]. In man, G-CSF promotes bone marrow mast cell growth and is biochemically distinct from GM-CSF and, apparently, from basophil/eosinophil CSF or differentiation activities[10, 58, 60-64]. G-CSF is secreted by human urinary bladder carcinoma cells, and has also been called 'multi-CSF' because of its wide range of activities involving most haemopoietic lineages[65]. Other sources of G-CSF include human placental cells, keratinocytes and nasal epithelial cells, but not T-cells (including T-leukaemic cells, Mo) (Table 1.3)[10]. Murine or human T-cell derived lymphokines with mast cell, eosinophil and B-cell growth factor activity have recently been proposed to be distinct from IL-3 and other CSFs, although controversy has arisen regarding the distinctiveness of some molecules related to this 'IL-4'[66]. The field of lymphokines is rapidly expanding; many different biological functions have been found to be the consequence of single, cloned protein molecules (e.g. recently an 'IL-5' has also been isolated with B-cell differentiating activity).

From the work suggesting a T-cell origin for a factor involved in murine mucosal mast cell growth, has come a significant body of literature concerning IL-3. However, the most significant source of IL-3 has been the (non-T) murine myelomonocytic leukaemic cell line, WEHI-3B; similar activity has been derived from murine epidermal or related cells, suggesting a physiological role for this material. In large amounts, this and possibly other factors do permit or stimulate the growth of human mast cells *in vitro*. Non-mucosal (e.g. peritoneal) mast cells in the rodent may require a factor distinct from IL-3 for orderly growth and differentiation, IL-4.

15

Mast cell phenotypes and specific differentiation factors

In this regard, recent investigations have now shown conclusively that other tissue-specific factors, distinct from IL-3, are important in determining mast cell growth and differentiation[67, 68]. For example, cloned mast cells adopt different staining and other phenotypic characteristics (such as heparin content) depending on the tissue environment. Thus, clonally derived peritoneal cells bearing 'beige' granular defects, adoptively transferred into mast cell-deficient recipients, develop the staining characteristics typical of intestinal mucosal cells when placed in the stomach, but that of connective tissue-type of mast cells when put into the skin. The progenitor for subtypes of mast cells is thus common to both[67].

In addition, mouse fibroblasts have been shown to provide factors which may selectively promote the growth of connective tissue type mast cells[10, 11]; this may be the mechanism underlying the known association between mast cell increases and fibrosis or tissue repair[10, 54]. The fibroblast-dependent factor as well as other tissue-specific mast cell differentiation factors appear to be distinct from IL-3; some may act via cell-to-cell contact, while others may be required only at terminal stages of differentiation for the orderly maturation of mast cells, by regulating expression of cell surface receptors. Indeed, one such mast cell growth factor has been identified which acts in concert with IL-3, but does not by itself promote mast cell growth[68]. This factor may in fact be the same as IL-4 (see above).

Mast cell (or basophil) differentiation factors may thus be as heterogenous and as numerous as the cell lineages which they can stimulate, and may be proteins with wide-ranging biological functions; local haemopoietic processes for different cell types may involve such factors, thus providing a biologically plausible mechanism for rapid accumulation of specific effector cells in tisues where they are required. Indeed, stromal cells derived from bone marrow in long-term cultures have now been recognized as having important growth and differentiation regulatory functions; i.e. a bone marrow haemopoietic microenvironment exists and is probably duplicated in many tissues.

Inhibitory factors

Many inhibitory factors also exist which regulate haemopoiesis, including T-cell products, antibodies, T-suppressor cells, prostaglandins and isoferritins. Factors derived from mesenteric lymphocytes of Lewis rats infected with nematodes drastically inhibit the growth of mast cells *in vitro*, depending on the nature of stimulant used to derive the conditioned medium and the time after initial infection at which lymphocytes are taken[34]. Thus, it is likely that factors capable of the physiologic inhibition of basophil, eosinophil or mast cell growth will be found and may in fact be identical with some stimulatory factors[69]. Such factors may prove to be therapeutically useful in regulating BME proliferation in allergic or leukaemic conditions.

16

Relationship of multipotential haemopoietic factors to BME growth

The capacity of purified haemopoietic growth factors to promote basophil or mast cell growth is not fully known at present, although several studies point to the effects of G-CSF, GM-CSF, as well as other more specific basophil or eosinophil differentiation factor(s)[57, 58]. Human T-cells, whether normal or leukaemic, keratinocyte cell lines, placental trophoblast conditioned medium, urinary bladder carcinoma cell lines and an osteogenic sarcoma cell line, all have been shown to secrete GM-CSF or G-CSF, or other differentiation factors which can at least represent co-factors in BME growth and differentiation. Interestingly, GM-CSF itself can activate mature neutrophils and eosinophils[23], and nerve growth factor can induce *in vivo* and *in vitro* myelopoiesis, including apparently preferential effects on basophils, mast cells and eosinophils[70]. This implies the presence of receptors for haemopoietic or other growth factors on the progeny, as well as the progenitors for BME, and provides at least one explanation for the existence of abnormally activated basophils or eosinophils in allergic disease (see later). A summary of the known or postulated haemopoietic growth factors in relation to BME growth and differentiation is given in Table 1.3.

BASOPHILS, MAST CELLS AND EOSINOPHILS IN NEOPLASIA

BME proliferation in bone marrow disorders

BME are known to proliferate abnormally or be present in increased numbers in the bone marrow or peripheral blood in various bone marrow disorders, including: chronic myeloid leukaemia (CML), myeloproliferative disorders, preleukaemia, certain types of acute myeloid leukaemia (AML) and MCPD[10, 36]. Reports have indicated that basophilia or eosinophilia may be associated with a poor prognosis in CML, and that atomic bomb survivors exhibit basophilia as the earliest sign of clinical CML, even before the Philadelphia (Ph[1]) chromosomal abnormality is detected. Blast cells with primitive ultrastructural features of both basophils and mast cells have been reported in CML peripheral blood, and these can express abnormal growth and differentiation patterns *in vitro*[8, 10, 36]. Short-lived basophil or mast cell lines derived from CML blood, bone marrow or fetal liver progenitors have also been described, as have Philadelphia chromosome-positive CML in blast crisis and acute leukaemia with abnormal granulocytic granules in which BME phenotypes are preferentially expressed[40, 55]. Moreover, an increase in the numbers of circulating BME progenitors in CML and MCPD has prognostic significance, since it is associated, respectively, with earlier blastic transformation or death from the time of diagnosis, or with evolution of the localized dermal MCPD, urticaria pigmentosa, to its systemic counterpart, systemic mastocytosis[10, 36].

17

BME and retroviruses

Neoplastic transformation of mast cells

Murine leukaemia virus infection of IL-3 dependent murine myeloid cells causes their neoplastic transformation to tumorigenic, IL-3 independent myeloid/mast cell lines[10]. Such observations suggest that retroviruses could play a role in self-renewal mechanisms of myeloid cells in response to growth factors such as IL-3 or to other human and murine cloned haemopoietic growth factors[63]. In this regard, CML patients can be shown to have circulating immune complexes which contain retroviral proteins, suggesting that retroviral infection and immunity may be occurring in these patients; however, the relationship of retroviral infection to the onset of CML or to phenotypic expression of CML blasts as basophil/mast cells is unknown. Recently, a human T-cell lymphotropic virus, HTLV-I, which is associated with endemic T-cell leukaemia/lymphoma, has been used to transform normal human T-cells into haemopoietic growth factor-producing cell lines (including an eosinophil differentiation factor). This may present a mechanism whereby retroviruses lead to aberrant haemopoiesis *in vivo*. The aforementioned T-cell leukaemic (Mo) line which produces BME and other haemopoietic growth factors is infected with the unique HTLV-II, but the relationship of retroviral gene insertion to the production of these activities is not yet known.

Leukaemogenesis and mast cell phenotype

The mast cell phenotype expressed in long-term murine cultures may be due in part to a selection artefact or to retroviral infection; however, if the latter is true, there is no explanation for the apparent selection of mast cells or mast cell progenitors as targets for these retroviruses. It is not unreasonable to hypothesize that retroviral infection and/or leukaemic transformation may stimulate BME differentiation programmes in murine or human haemopoietic pluripotent progenitors. Alternatively, a molecular association between a leukaemogenic event (e.g. chromosomal translocation) and a basophil/mast cell differentiation event (e.g. IL-3 receptor expression) may occur in certain human and murine haemopoietic stem cells. In man, the clinicopathologic associations between abnormal BME lineage expression and CML, preleukaemia or acute myeloid leukaemia may represent the experiments in nature analogous to retrovirus-infected, IL-3 independent, tumorigenic murine mast cell lines.

Human oncogenes, chromosomal aberrations and leukaemia

The abnormal activation of human cellular oncogenes (c-onc) as a result of chromosomal translocation is presumed to be a proximal cause of a number of haematologic malignancies, including Burkitt's lymphoma, CML, AML and possibly other human leukaemias[71], as a result of direct or indirect stimulation of growth regulatory proteins. Several growth factor associated c-onc encode proteins such as macrophage colony-stimulating factor receptor and platelet-derived growth factor[72, 73]. Little is known regarding the precise relationship between c-onc activation and leukaemic phenotype. For example, increased expression of the GM-CSF receptor does not adequately explain the pathogenesis of acute myeloid leukaemia.

Chromosomal abnormalities and BME growth

There are some associations between chromosomal abnormalities and BME phenotype in leukaemic cells which could prove instructive. For example, the inversion or translocation of chromosome 16 (inv16;p13q22 or t16;16) in a subtype (M4) of human acute myelomonocytic leukaemia is associated with the presence of abnormal eosinophils with basophilic granulation and with a relatively good prognosis[55]. A specific translocation (t6;9) in another type of acute non-lymphocytic leukaemia is accompanied by increased bone marrow basophils[74]. The human promyelocytic leukaemia cell line, HL-60, when cultured at alkaline pH can preferentially express eosinophil[75] and basophil/mast cell[76] lineages. HL-60 cells themselves can be shown to have abnormalities on the long arm of chromosome 16, similar to those seen *in vivo* in the M4 leukaemia with dysplastic eosinophils[55, 75].

These observations suggest that, as in CML, chromosomal abnormalities may be specifically associated with a preferential phenotypic pattern of haemopoietic differentiation, conceivably arising as a result of translocations in an area of the genome encoding important differentiation-specific proteins (in this case, for BME lineages). The inv16 abnormality involves a split in the metallothionine gene cluster which may account in part for the dysplastic eosinophil–basophil phenotype. HL-60 cells, which produce an autostimulatory glycoprotein closely related to macrophage-CSF, could conceivably produce BME growth and differentiation factors, especially those HL-60 lines differentiating to BME. Since CML blast cells can also be shown to produce transforming growth factors, the preferential expression of BME lineage *in vivo* and *in vitro* in CML and related bone marrow disorders may also represent autostimulation. This makes it even more important to identify BME differentiation-specific factors, since one can foresee their clinical application to the diagnosis and treatment of specific leukaemias. The knowledge gained from aberrant leukaemic cells could then be used in clinical studies in a variety of inflammatory disorders.

BASOPHILS, EOSINOPHILS AND MAST CELLS IN HUMAN RESPIRATORY DISEASE

Introduction

In lower animals and in man, especially in underdeveloped countries, parasitic infestations are common, eliciting IgE responses together with BME accumulation. In many of these situations, BME act as primary effector cells against parasites. In developed countries, much less parasitism and, instead, a very high prevalence of allergic diseases are observed. It has been speculated that the persistence of such IgE- and BME-mediated responses even in non-parasitized areas of the world is a result of the persistence of a parasite-directed immune mechanism in phylogeny. Given that BME accumulate in a wide variety of inflammatory disorders, not only those that are IgE-mediated, it is possible that a number of non-allergic disorders also represent persistence of part, if not all, of the phylogenetic apparatus involved in response to parasites. It is in this light that the problem of BME involvement in inflammatory respiratory disease may be seen.

Nasal challenge studies

Allergic rhinitis is the most common clinical manifestation of IgE-dependent sensitization. The observation that there is a correlation between serum IgE and the occurrence of respiratory allergy, i.e. IgE levels predict positive skin tests in patients with these conditions[77], has focused attention on mast cells and basophils in its pathogenesis[17,21,48]. The involvement of mast cells and basophils in allergen-induced reactions has been best demonstrated by nasal challenge studies. Nasal mucosal biopsies processed by both light and electron microscopy after intranasal administration of allergens have demonstrated progressive degranulation of such cells in the mucosa over a period of time[10,78]. In addition, the appearance in nasal secretions of inflammatory mediators corresponds in time to early and late nasal airway obstruction[18]. As a result of these observations it is a reasonable conclusion that preformed and newly formed basophil and mast cell products have a major involvement in the early events after allergen challenge.

IgE levels not sufficient to explain symptoms

While total IgE antibody levels are directly statistically related to the propensity to become sensitized to environmental allergens and to develop respiratory disease[77], the level of specific serum IgE antibody to ragweed pollen does not correlate with severity of symptoms in the seasonal form of ragweed-allergic rhinitis[24]. The likely basis for this discrepancy presumably lies with the effector cell population, including accumulation of neutrophils and eosinophils at tissue sites, but more importantly, with quantitative aspects of nasal mucosal mast cell infiltration. A dynamic state for basophils (and, by implication, mast cells) has been suggested in the past by the observation that the peripheral blood basophil count rises in the ragweed pollen season in ragweed allergic individuals, but not in non-allergic controls[79]. The precise enumeration of mast cells in mucosal tissues has until recently been hindered by the inability to recognize histochemical heterogeneity, including special requirements for fixation techniques. It has now become possible, however, to quantitate the continuing contribution of mucosal mast cell accumulation in allergic respiratory disease. In fact, it has become clear that increased numbers of progenitors for basophils and mucosal mast cells represent a marker of the allergic state[10,25-27,48] and possibly of non-allergic states such as chronic rhinitis with nasal polyposis.

20

Heterogeneity of metachromatic cells in human nose

Histochemically distinct metachromatic cells (NMC) can be identified in the nasal mucosa and secretions of patients with allergic rhinitis, most of whom have perennial rather than seasonal disease[48]. An abundance of eosinophils as well as mast cells has been observed in nasal polyps, usually a non-allergic condition. In nasal secretions the predominant metachromatic cell is a basophil, with a diameter of 5–6 μm, containing few granules but larger than other granulated cells; this cell is formaldehyde-sensitive, and is rarely seen in nasal biopsies or nasal scrapings performed with a curette. In the latter, more than 80% of the metachromatic cells are 5–12 μm diameter, formaldehyde-sensitive, and possess smaller, more numerous granules. It has been established that the reproducibility and reliability of methods to obtain nasal epithelial scrapings, upon which one can base clinical conclusions, are very high; indeed, there is a significant correlation of severity of symptomatology (e.g. nasal swelling and pallor) with numbers of formaldehyde-sensitive NMC. Thus, a correlate of the occurrence and severity of rhinitis in general would be predicted as being the number of mucosal mast cells derived from progenitors by amplification mechanisms. Antigenic challenge may provide a stimulus for this type of amplification in BME growth and differentiation.

Bronchial asthma

Just as it has been shown that basophils predominate in nasal secretions of allergic individuals, and that mast cells occur in nasal scrapings, both basophils and mast cells can be identified in the sputum, or bronchoalveolar lavage or bronchial brushings of patients with bronchial asthma, with or without allergy and/or nasal polyposis. Mast cells in sputum and bronchial secretions or tissue may represent a biological correlate of severe atopic asthma or of steroid-resistant asthma, or both, and may accumulate in the lower airway by mechanisms similar to those operative in the upper airway[80]. Moreover, positive correlations can be shown to hold between numbers of basophils, basophiloid cells, mast cells or eosinophils and bronchial hyper-reactivity in asthma[10, 18–20]. BME products in secretions or BME release of mediators likewise can be positively associated with asthmatic airway hyper-responsiveness[78]. All this implies that the numbers of BME are as important, potentially, as their function in determining the pathogenesis of bronchial asthma.

One is tempted to speculate that genes encoding a propensity for BME growth and differentiation persist in being activated in patients with allergic and some non-allergic types of inflammatory disorders of the respiratory tract, best represented by bronchial asthma of the so-called intrinsic type. The availability of genetic probes for BME growth and differentiation may revolutionize our understanding of the pathophysiology of asthma and provide more precise diagnostic modalities than simple analysis of airway hyper-responsiveness or enumeration of cells and mediators.

Functional activation of basophils and growth factors

A high turnover stage of basophils in asthma is circumstantially supported by the observation of increased 'releasability' of mediators from such cells in the peripheral blood of these patients[10, 18]. Sera from patients with nasal allergies can also confer this releasability upon basophils from non-allergics; perhaps this phenomenon reflects immaturity of cells, or cells in a high turnover state or activation of cells by haemopoietic factors present in the circulation as a concomitant of cell proliferation/differentiation.

Nasal epithelial scrapings from atopic individuals, or from patients with chronic rhinitis and polyposis, or polyp-derived mononuclear cells secrete putative growth factors for BME, as measured in haemopoietic cultures. Using the methylcellulose colony assay system, non-atopic subject scrapings can be shown to produce almost no CSF for BME, while increasing amounts are produced, respectively, by scrapings from mild and severe atopic patients. Similarly, the epithelium from polyps (polyp scrapings) secretes what appears to be a specific basophil/mast cell colony stimulating factor. In addition, mitogen-stimulated polyp mononuclear cells and confluent nasal epithelial cell monolayer cultures secrete BME colony-stimulating factors, while tonsillar tissue does not secrete factors with similar activity[10].

Corticosteroids and human allergy involving BME responses

It is known that steroids are associated with amelioration of symptoms of both early and late-phase allergic, as well as non-allergic, inflammatory responses in the respiratory tract and skin. The precise mechanisms of action of topical or systemic corticosteroids in treating allergic or non-allergic inflammatory diseases of the airways are not known but involve inhibition of mediator release mechanisms. Tissue or secretion examinations also reveal marked decreases in BME after such therapy. Since corticosteroids can cause a diminution in eosinophil or basophil growth *in vitro*, they may act in part by interfering with *in situ* haemopoietic mechanisms leading to tissue accumulation of BME.

Clinical implications

The discovery of mast cell heterogeneity and the development of sophisticated biochemical and tissue culture techniques has opened new doors in our approach to allergy. For example, the functional differences among mast cell subpopulations are now being exploited in the design of new drugs. The mechanism(s) of action of topical corticosteroids in selectively decreasing, for example, nasal mucosal mast cell numbers[80] can now be examined, with the hope of developing more potent and specific derivatives. Moreover, characterization and purification of haemopoietic factors which stimulate or inhibit BME development may lead to the use of physiological regulatory agents capable of reversing several allergic and non-allergic inflammatory disorders. Finally, a more precise understanding of the cell biology of BME may have wide applications in a variety of neoplastic and inflammatory processes.

22

ACKNOWLEDGEMENTS

I wish to thank my colleagues Drs J. Bienenstock, J. Dolovich, D. Harnish, D. Sauder and D. Befus for their constant stimulation and knowledge; postdoctoral fellows, Drs H. Otsuka, M. Ohnisi, H. Matsuda, Y. Tanno, J. Ruhno and S. Mattolli, for their important contributions; graduate student, S. Hutt-Taylor, for his patience, and research assistants S. Telizyn, J. Switzer and M. Davison for their loyalty and untiring efforts. Special gratitude goes to Drs B. Stadler, G. Roupe, S. Ahlstedt, G. Gleich, P. Askenase, S. Brown, S. Ackerman and H. Messner for their important collaborations, and to Drs T. Ishizaka and L. Enerback for their intellectual candour and collegiality.

Work by the author referred to in this chapter is supported by grants from the Medical Research Council and National Cancer Institute of Canada.

References

1. Beeson, P. B. and Bass, D. A. (1977). *The Eosinophil. Vol. XIV, Major Problems in Internal Medicine.* pp. 3–13. (Philadelphia, London, Toronto: W. B. Saunders)
2. Parwaresh, M. R. (1976). *The Human Blood Basophil. Morphology, Origin, Kinetics, Function and Pathology.* pp. 77–99. (Berlin, Heidelberg, New York: Springer-Verlag)
3. Suda, T., Suda, J. and Ogawa, M. (1983). Single-cell origin of mouse hemopoietic colonies expressing multiple lineages in variable combinations. *Proc. Natl. Acad. Sci. (USA)*, **80**, 6689–93
4. Leary, A. G., Ogawa, M., Strauss, L. C. and Civin, C. I. (1984). Single cell origin of multilineage colonies in culture: evidence that differentiation of multipotent progenitors and restriction of proliferative potential of monopotent progenitors are stochastic processes. *J. Clin. Invest.*, **74**, 2193–7
5. Ehrlich, P. (1897). Uber die spezifischen granulationen des blutes. *Arch. Anat. Physiol. Phys. Abt.*, **3**, 571–9
6. Selye, H. (1965). *The Mast Cells.* (Washington: Butterworths & Co.)
7. Kitamura, Y., Yokoyama, M., Matsuda, H., Ohno, T. and Mori, K. J. (1981) Spleen colony-forming cell as common precursor for tissue mast cells and granulocytes. *Nature*, **291**, 159–60
8. Zucker-Franklin, D. (1981). Eosinophils and basophils. In Zucker-Franklin, D., Greaves, M. F., Grossi, C. E. and Marmont, A. M. (eds.) *Atlas of Blood Cells (Function and Pathology).* pp. 257–317. (Milan: Edi. Ermes, Philadelphia: Lea & Febiger)
9. Dvorak, H. F. and Dvorak, A. M. (1975). Basophilic leukocytes: structure, function and role in disease. *Clin. Hematol.*, **4**, 651–83
10. Befus, A. D., Bienenstock, J. and Denburg, J. A. (eds.) (1986). *Mast Cell Differentiation and Heterogeneity.* (New York: Raven Press)
11. Padawer, J. (ed.) (1963). Mast cells and basophils. *Ann. NY Acad. Sci.*, **103**, 1–492
12. Askenase, P. W. (1977). Role of basophils, mast cells and vasoamines in hypersensitivity reactions with a delayed time course. *Prog. Allergy*, **23**, 199–327
13. Rothwell, T. L. W. (1975). Studies of the responses of basophil and eosinophil leucocytes and mast cells to the nematode *Trichostrongylus colubrimformis.* I. Observations during the expulsion of first and second infections by guinea-pig. *J. Pathol.*, **116**, 51–60
14. Lagunoff, D., *et al.* (1980). In Weissman, G. (ed.) *The Cell Biology of Inflammation. Vol. 2, Handbook of Inflammation.* pp. 217–65. (Amsterdam: Elsevier-North Holland)
15. Capron, M., Rousseaux, J., Mazingue, C., Bazin, H. and Capron, A. (1978). Rat mast cell–eosinophil interaction in antibody-dependent eosinophil cytotoxicity to *Schistosoma mansoni* schistosomula. *J. Immunol.*, **121**, 2518–25
16. Pepys, J. and Edwards, A. M. (eds.) (1979). *The Mast Cell: Its Role in Health and Disease.* (Kent, UK: Pitman Medical)

17. Okuda, M. (1977). Mechanisms in nasal allergy. *O.R.L. Digest*, **39**, 22–34
18. Schleimer, R. P., Fox, C. C., Naclerio, R. M., Plaut, M., Creticos, P. S., Togias, A. G., Warner, J. A., Kagey-Sobotka, A. and Lichtenstein, L. M. (1985). Role of human basophils and mast cells in the pathogenesis of allergic diseases. *J. Allergy Clin. Immunol.*, **76**, 369–74
19. Durham, S. R. and Kay, A. B. (1985). Eosinophils, bronchial hyperreactivity and late-phase asthmatic reactions. *Clin. Allergy*, **40**, 411–18
20. Frigas, E. and Gleich, G. J. (1986). The eosinophil and the pathophysiology of asthma. *J. Allergy Clin. Immunol.*, **77**, 527–37
21. Hastie, R., Heroy, J. H. and Levy, D. A. (1979). Basophil leucocytes and mast cells in human nasal secretions and scrapings studied by light microscopy. *Lab. Invest.*, **49**, 554–61
22. Leonard, E. J., Lett-Brown, M. A. and Askenase, P. W. (1979). Simultaneous generation of tuberculin-type and cutaneous basophilic hypersensitivity at separate sites in the guinea pig. *Int. Arch. Allergy Appl. Immunol.*, **58**, 460–9
23. Gasson, J. C., Weisbart, R. H., Kaufman, S. E., Clark, S. C., Hewick, R. M., Wong, G. G. and Gold, D. W. (1984). Purified human granulocyte-macrophage colony-stimulating factor: direct action on neutrophils. *Science*, **226**, 1339–42
24. Nickelsen, J. A., Georgitis, J. W. and Reisman, R. E. (1986). Lack of correlation between titers of serum allergen-specific IgE and symptoms in untreated patients with seasonal allergic rhinitis. *J. Allergy Clin. Immunol.*, **77**, 43–8
25. Denburg, J. A., Telizyn, S., Belda, A., Dolovich, J. and Bienenstock, J. (1985). Increased numbers of circulating basophil/mast cell progenitors in atopic patients. *J. Allergy Clin. Immunol.*, **76**, 466–72
26. Otsuka, H., Dolovich, J., Bienenstock, J. and Denburg, J. A. (1986). Basophilic cell progenitors, nasal metachromatic cells and peripheral blood basophils in ragweed allergic patients. *J. Allergy Clin. Immunol.*, **78**, 365–71
27. Otsuka, H., Dolovich, J., Befus, A. D., Bienenstock, J. and Denburg, J. (1986). Basophilic cell progenitors, peripheral blood basophils and nasal metachromatic cells in patients with allergic rhinitis. *Am. Rev. Resp. Dis.*, **133**, 757–61
28. Ogilvie, B. M., Askenase, P. W. and Rose, M. E. (1980). Basophils and eosinophils in three strains of rats and in athymic (nude) rats following infection with the nematodes *Nippostrongylus brasiliensis* or *Trichinella spiralis*. *Immunology*, **39**, 385–9
29. Juhlin, L. and Michaelsson, G. (1977). A new syndrome characterized by absence of eosinophils and basophils. *Lancet*, **1**, 1233–5
30. Tracey, R. and Smith, H. (1978). An inherited anomaly of human eosinophils and basophils. *Blood Cells*, **4**, 291–8
31. Ackerman, S. J., Weil, G. J. and Gleich, G. J. (1982). Formation of Charcot–Leyden crystals by human basophils. *J. Exp. Med.*, **155**, 1597–609
32. Ackerman, S. J., Kephart, G. M., Habermann, T. M., Greipp, P. R. and Gleich, G. J. (1983). Localization of eosinophil granule major basic protein in human basophils. *J. Exp. Med.*, **158**, 946–61
33. Nagao, K., Yokoro, K. and Aaronson, S. A. (1981). Continuous lines of basophil/mast cells derived from normal mouse bone marrow. *Science*, **212**, 333–5
34. Denburg, J. A., Befus, A. D. and Bienenstock, J. (1980). Growth and differentiation *in vitro* of mast cells from mesenteric lymph nodes of *Nippostrongylus brasiliensis*-infected rats. *Immunology*, **41**, 195–202
35. Lennert, K. and Parwaresch, M. R. (1979). Mast cells and mast cell neoplasia: a review. *Histopathology*, **3**, 349–65
36. Denburg, J. A., Wilson, W. E. C. and Bienenstock, J. (1982). Basophil production in myeloproliferative disorders: Increases during acute blastic transformation of chronic myeloid leukemia. *Blood*, **60**, 113–20.
37. Denburg, J. A., Richardson, M., Telizyn, S. and Bienenstock, J. (1983). Basophil/mast cell precursors in human peripheral blood. *Blood*, **61**, 775–80
38. Ogawa, M., Nakahata, T., Leary, A. G., Sterk, A. R., Ishizaka, K. and Ishizaka, T. (1983). Suspension culture of human mast cells/basophils from umbilical cord blood mononuclear cells. *Proc. Natl. Acad. Sci. (USA)*, **80**, 4494–8
39. Tadokoro, K., Stadler, B. M. and deWeck, A. L. (1983). Factor-dependent *in vitro* growth of human normal bone marrow-derived basophil-like cells. *J. Exp. Med.*, **158**, 857–71

24

40. Kishi, K. (1985). A new leukemia cell line with Philadelphia chromosome characterized as basophil precursors. *Leuk. Res.*, **7**, 381–90
41. Guy-Grand, D., Dy, M., Luffau, L. and Vassali, P. (1984). Gut mucosal mast cells: origin, traffic and differentiation. *J. Exp. Med.*, **160**, 12–28
42. Mayrhofer, G. and Bazin, H. (1981). Nature of the thymus dependency of mucosal mast cells. III. Mucosal mast cells in nude mice and nud. rats, in B rats and in a child with the Di George Syndrome. *Int. Arch. Allergy Appl. Immunol.*, **64**, 320–31
43. Crapper, R. M. and Schrader, J. W. (1983). Frequency of mast cell precursors in normal tissues determined by an *in vitro* assay: antigen induces parallel increases in the frequency of P-cell precursors and mast cells. *J. Immunol*, **131**, 923–8
44. Stevens, R. L., Lee, T. G., Seldin, D. C., Austen, K. F., Befus, A. D. and Bienenstock, J. (1986). Intestinal mucosal mast cells from rats infected with *Nippostrongylus brasiliensis* contain protease-resistant chondroitin sulfate di-B proteoglycans. *J. Immunol.*, **137**, 291–4
45. Woodbury, R. G., Everitt, M., Sanada, Y., Katunuma, N., Lagunoff, D. and Neurath, H. (1978). A major serine protease in rat skeletal muscle: Evidence for its mast cell origin. *Proc. Natl. Acad. Sci. USA*, **75**, 5311–13
46. Seldin, D. C., Adelman, S., Austen, K. F., Stevens, R. L., Hein, A., Caulfield, J. P. and Woodbury, R. G. (1985). Homology of the rat basophilic leukemia cell and the rat mucosal mast cell. *Proc. Natl. Acad. Sci. USA*, **82**, 3871–5
47. Befus, D., Goodacre, R., Dyck, N. and Bienenstock, J. (1985). Mast cell heterogeneity in man: I. Histologic studies of the intestine. *Int. Arch. Allergy Appl. Immunol.*, **76**, 232–6
48. Otsuka, H., Denburg, J. A., Dolovich, J., Hitch, D., Lapp, P., Rajan, R. S., Bienenstock, J. and Befus, A. D. (1985). Heterogeneity of metachromatic cells in human nose: significance of mucosal mast cells. *J. Allergy Clin. Immunol.*, **76**, 695–702
49. Irani, A. A., Schechter, N. M., Craig, S., DeBlois, M. D. and Schwartz, L. B. (1986). Two types of human mast cells that have distinct neutral protease compositions. *Proc. Natl. Acad. Sci. USA*, **83**, 4464–8
50. Eliakim, R., Gilead, L., Ligumsky, M., Okon, E., Rachmilewitz, D. and Razin, E. (1986). Histamine and chondroitin sulfate E proteoglycan released by cultured human colonic mucosa: indication for possible presence of E mast cells. *Proc. Natl. Acad. Sci. USA*, **83**, 461–4
51. Schulman, E. S., Kagey-Sobotka, A., MacGlashan, D. W., Adkinson Jr., N. F., Peters, S. P., Schleimer, R. P. and Lichtenstein, L. M. (1983). Heterogeneity of human mast cells. *J. Immunol.*, **131**, 1936–41
52. King, S. J., Miller, H. R. P., Newlands, G. J. F. and Woodbury, R. G. (1985). Depletion of mucosal mast cell protease by corticosteroids: effect on intestinal anaphylaxis in the rat. *Proc. Natl. Acad. Sci. USA*, **82**, 1214–18
53. Denburg, J. A., Davison, M. and Bienenstock, J. (1980). Basophil production: stimulation by factors derived from guinea pig splenic T-lymphocytes. *J. Clin. Invest.*, **65**, 390–9
54. Bienenstock, J., Tomioka, M., Stead, R., Ernst, P., Jordana, M., Gauldie, J., Dolovich, J. and Denburg, J. (1987). Mast cell involvement in various inflammatory processes. *Am. Rev. Resp. Dis.* (In press)
55. LeBeau, M. M., Larson, R. A., Bitter, M. A., Vardiman, J. W., Golomb, H. M. and Rowley, J. D. (1983). Association of an inversion of chromosome 16 with abnormal marrow eosinophils in acute myelomonocytic leukemia: a unique cytogenetic–clinicopathological association. *N. Engl. J. Med.*, **309**, 630–6
56. Denburg, J. A., Telizyn, S., Messner, H., Lim, B., Jamal, N., Ackerman, S. J., Gleich, G. J. and Bienenstock, J. (1985). Heterogeneity of human peripheral blood eosinophil-type colonies: evidence for a common basophil–eosinophil progenitor. *Blood*, **66**, 312–18
57. Tanno, Y., Bienenstock, J., Richardson, M., Lee, T. G., Befus, A. D. and Denburg, J. (1987). Reciprocal regulation of human basophil and eosinophil growth by separate factors in cord blood cultures. *Exp. Hematol.*, **15**, 24–33
58. Stadler, B. M., Hirai, K., Tadokoro, K. and deWeck, A. L. (1985). Distinction of human basophil promoting activity from human interleukin-3. *Int. Arch. Allergy Appl. Immunol.*, **77**, 151–4
59. Denburg, J. A., Messner, H., Lim, B., Jamal, N., Telizyn, S. and Bienenstock, J. (1985). Clonal origin of human basophil/mast cells from circulating multipotent hemopoietic progenitors. *Exp. Hematol.*, **13**, 185–8.

60. Razin, E., Cordon-Cardo, C. and Good, R. A. (1981). Growth of pure populations of mouse mast cells *in vitro* with conditioned medium derived from concanavalin A-stimulated splenocytes. *Proc. Natl. Acad. Sci. USA*, **78**, 2559–61

61. Ihle, J. N., Keller, J., Oroszlan, S., Henderson, L. E., Copeland, T. D., Fitch, F., Prystowsky, M. B., Goldwasser, E., Schrader, J. W., Palaszynski, M. D. and Lebel, B. (1983). Biological properties of homogeneous interleukin 3. I. Demonstration of WEHI-3 growth factor activity, P cell-stimulating factor activity, colony-stimulating factor activity, and histamine-producing cell-stimulating factor activity. *J. Immunol.*, **131**, 282–7

62. Fung, M. C. *et al.* (1984). Molecular cloning of cDNA for murine interleukin-3. *Nature*, **307**, 233–6

63. Yang, Y.-C., Ciarletta, B. B., Temple, P. A., Chung, M. P., Kovacic, S., Witek-Giannotti, J. S., Leary, A. C., Kriz, R., Donahue, R. E., Wong, G. G. and Clark, S. C. (1986). Human IL-3 (multi-CSF): identification by expression of cloning of novel hematopoietic growth factor related to murine IL-3. *Cell*, **47**, 3–10

64. Gough, N. M. *et al.* (1984). Molecular cloning of cDNA encoding a murine hematopoietic growth regulator, granulocyte–macrophage colony stimulating factor. *Nature*, **309**, 763–7

65. Watson, J. D., Crosier, P. S., March, C. J., Conlon, P. J., Mochizuki, D. Y., Gillis, S. and Urdal, D. L. (1986). Purification of homogeneity of a human hematopoietic growth factor that stimulates the growth of a murine interleukin-3-dependent cell line. *J. Immunol.*, **137**, 854–7

66. Sanderson, C. J., O'Garra, A., Warren, D. J. and Klaus, G. G. B. (1986). Eosinophil differentiation factor also has B-cell growth factor activity: proposed name interleukin-4. *Proc. Natl. Acad. Sci. USA*, **83**, 437–40

67. Kobayashi, T., Nakano, T., Nakahata, T., Asai, H., Yagi, Y., Tsuji, K., Komiyama, A., Akabane, T., Kojima, S. and Kitamura, Y. (1986). Formation of mast cell colonies in methylcellulose by mouse peritoneal cells and differentiation of these cloned cells in both the skin and the gastric mucosa of W/W^v mice: evidence that a common precursor can give rise to both "connective tissue-type" and "mucosal" mast cells. *J. Immunol.*, **136**, 1378–84

68. Smith, C. A. and Rennick, D. M. (1986). Characterization of a murine lymphokine distinct from interleukin 2 and interleukin 3 (IL-3) possessing a T-cell growth factor activity and a mast cell growth factor activity that synergizes with IL-3. *Proc. Natl. Acad. Sci. USA*, **83**, 1857–61

69. Gullberg, U., Nilsson, E., Sarngadharan, M. G. and Olsson, I. (1986). T-lymphocyte-derived differentiation-inducing factor inhibits proliferation of leukemic and normal hemopoietic cells. *Blood*, **68**, 1333–8

70. Stanisz, A., Scicchitano, R., Stead, R., Matsuda, H., Tomioka, M., Denburg, J. and Bienenstock, J. (1987). Neuropeptides and immunity. *Am. Rev. Resp. Dis.* (In press)

71. Rowley, J. D. (1983). Human oncogene locations and chromosome aberrations. *Nature*, **301**, 290–1

72. Sherr, C. J., Rettenmier, C. W., Sacca, R., Roussel, M. F., Look, A. T. and Stanley, E. R. (1985). The *c-fms* proto-oncogene product is related to the receptor for the mononuclear phagocyte growth factor, CSF-1. *Cell*, **41**, 665–76

73. Niman, H. L. (1984). Antisera to a synthetic peptide of the *sis* viral oncogene product recognize human platelet-derived growth factor. *Nature*, **307**, 180–3

74. Pearson, M. G., Vardiman, J. W., LeBeau, M. M., Rowley, J. D., Schwartz, S., Kerman, S. L., Cohen, M. M., Fleischman, E. W. and Prigogina, E. L. (1985). Increased numbers of marrow basophils may be associated with a t(6;9) in ANLL. *Am. J. Hematol.*, **183**, 83–403

75. Fischkoff, S. A., Pollak, A., Gleich, G. J., Testa, J. R., Misawa, S. and Reber, T. J. (1984). Eosinophilic differentiation of the human promyelocytic leukemia cell line, HL-60. *J. Exp. Med.*, **160**, 179–96

76. Taylor, S. R., Harnish, D. and Denburg, J. A. (1986). Basophilic differentiation of the promyelocytic leukemia cell line HL-60. *Blood*, **68**(S), 193a

77. Burrows, B. and Barbee, R. A. (1976). Respiratory disorders and allergy skin-test reactions. *Ann. Intern. Med.*, **84**, 134–9

78. Holgate, S. T., Hardy, C., Robinson, C., Agius, R. M. and Howarth, P. H. (1986). The mast cell as a primary effector cell in the pathogenesis of asthma. *J. Allergy Clin. Immunol.*, **77**, 274–82

79. Hirsch, S. R. and Kalbfleisch, J. H. (1976) Circulating basophils in normal subjects and in subjects with hay fever. *J. Allergy Clin. Immunol.*, **58**, 676–82
80. Otsuka, H., Denburg, J. A., Befus, A. D., Hitch, D., Lapp, P., Rajan, R., Bienenstock, J. and Dolovich, J. (1987). Effect of beclomethasone diproprionate on nasal metachromatic cell populations. *Clin. Allergy* (In press)

2
The Fine Structure of
Human Basophils and Mast Cells

A. M. DVORAK

INTRODUCTION

Paul Ehrlich first described human mast cells[1] and basophils[2] in the 1870s with the light microscope based on their metachromatic staining properties. In 1986, using ultrastructural analyses, we can confirm the existence of two different cell types in man; we know that both cells undergo release reactions which are rapid or slow and can define the effect on the morphological expression of each cell of these functional events; and we can describe morphological events associated with maturation of both cell types. We here review the fine structural properties of human basophils and mast cells at rest, during slow, piecemeal degranulation, during rapid, anaphylactic degranulation, and during differentiation and maturation stimulated either by growth factor(s) or by an antecedent degranulation event. We also discuss the potential relevance of cytoplasmic lipid bodies in arachidonic acid metabolism in mast cells.

HUMAN BASOPHILS

Fine structure of mature, resting human basophils

Human basophils[3-19] are small cells with polylobed nuclei (Figure 2.1). The nuclear chromatin is condensed and nucleoli are absent. The Golgi area is inapparent and rough endoplasmic reticulum and free ribosomes are scarce. The cell surface displays irregularly placed blunt processes. The cytoplasm contains mitochondria, vesicles, glycogen and granules. Mature granules are generally filled with dense particles (Figure 2.2A). Some granules contain multiple membrane arrays which compartmentalize the granule (Figure 2.2B). A second minor and smaller granule type contains homogeneous content and is located near the nucleus (Figure 2.3). Rarely, Charcot–Leyden

29

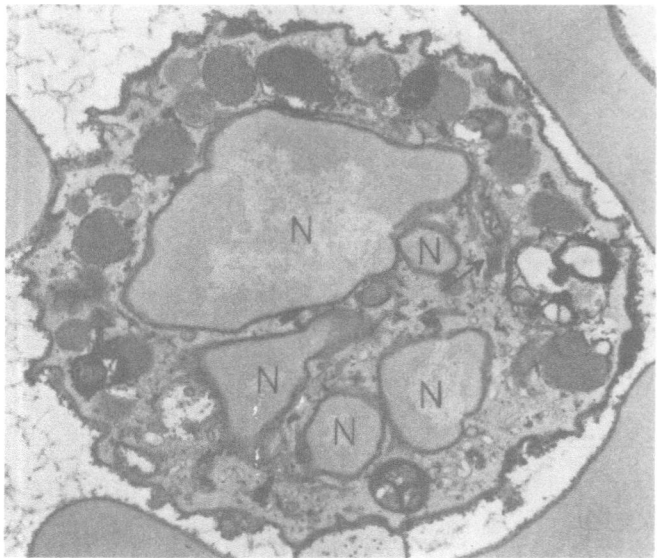

Figure 2.1 Peripheral blood basophil shows polylobed nuclei (N), short irregular blunt surface processes and numerous granules filled with particles. Cationized ferritin stains the cell surface. The Golgi area is small (arrow). Monoparticulate glycogen and vesicles are present in the cytoplasm. OPF, CF, ×13 700

crystals are present in basophils, either within particle-containing granules or free in the cytoplasm (Figure 2.4)[8]. While most basophils are rounded cells, prominent elongated, narrow uropods, or tails have been described in human (Figure 2.5)[4, 6, 12] and guinea pig basophils[20].

Fine structure of degranulating human basophils

Morphologic expressions of human basophil release reactions can be classified in two general categories. These are (1) slow release reactions which occur over days; we have called these piecemeal degranulation[16]; (2) rapid release reactions which are complete in minutes; these are called anaphylactic degranulation, so named for their initial description as immunoglobulin E (IgE)-mediated events. We have studied the ultrastructural morphology of rapid release reactions from human basophils stimulated by a wide variety of triggering events. Since the morphologic expression is similar in all

All methods for the preparation of cells for electron microscopy are described in detail in references 4, 14, 23, 25, 27, 30, 31, 33, and referred to in individual legends by the following abbreviations: OCUB, osmium collidine, uranyl en bloc; OPF, osmium potassium ferrocyanide; CF, cationized ferritin; [³H]AA, tritium-labelled arachidonic acid autoradiography; ³⁵S, ³⁵sulphur-labelled sulphate autoradiography; DAB, diaminobenzidine substrate for peroxidase demonstration. All pictures are of human cells.

30

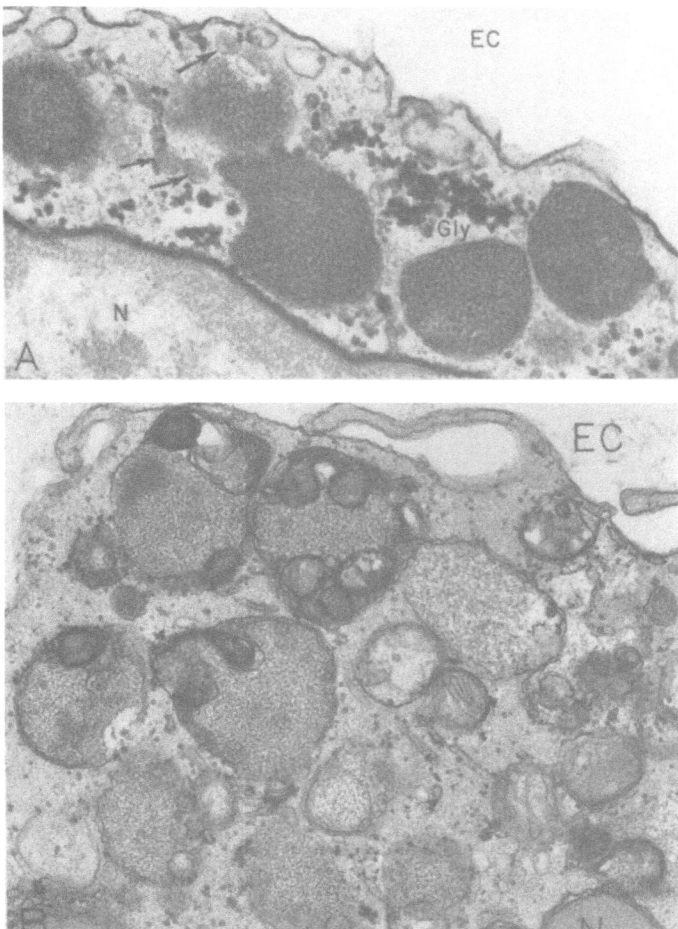

Figure 2.2   High magnification micrographs of peripheral blood basophils show particle-filled granules in (**A**) and vesicles (arrows in **A**) and granules which contain numerous membrane arrays in (**B**). N = nucleus; Gly = glycogen; EC = extracellular space. OPF, (**A**) ×31 500; (**B**) ×26 250

instances, we routinely refer to these rapid release events as anaphylactic degranulation to distinguish them from the morphologically distinctive piecemeal degranulation of human basophils.

Piecemeal degranulation

We studied experimentally-produced contact allergy reactions in human skin and found basophils to be a major component of the inflammatory infiltrate in them[3, 15]. Skin reactions were biopsied sequentially over days after their

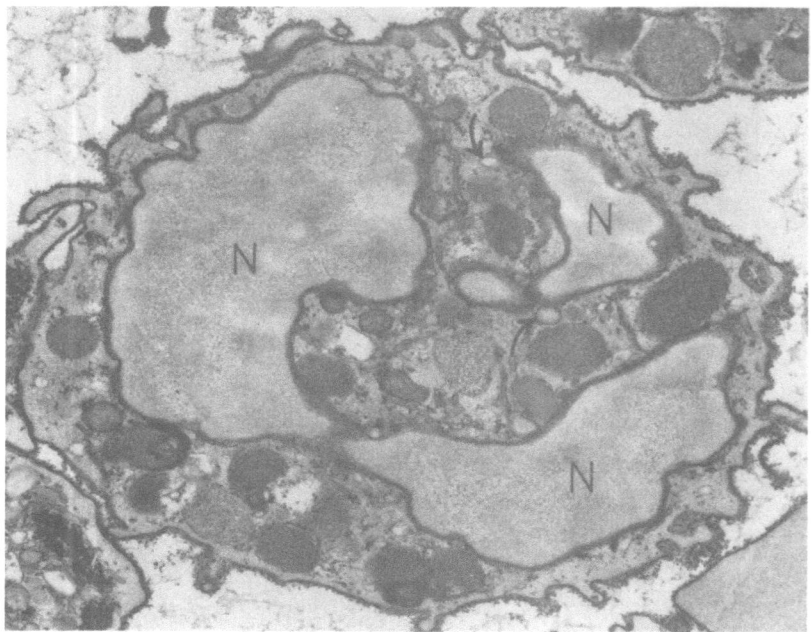

Figure 2.3 Peripheral blood basophil with polylobed nucleus (N) shows a mixture of large, particle-filled granules and a second minor granule type. The latter granules are small, homogeneous granules located in the nuclear area (arrows). OPF, CF, ×17 200

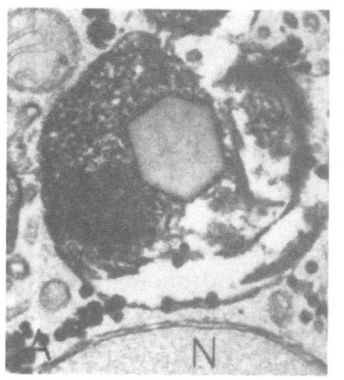
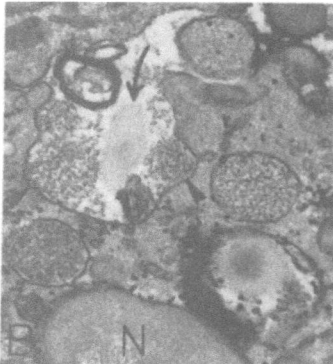

Figure 2.4 Charcot–Leyden crystal in peripheral blood human basophil granule is a hexagonal structure when seen in cross-section (**A**). Particulate granule contents (arrowheads) and a Charcot–Leyden crystal (arrow) are extruded to the basophil's exterior after stimulation with C5 peptide(s) in (**B**). N = nucleus. OPF, (**A**) ×46 400; (**B**) ×28 000

32

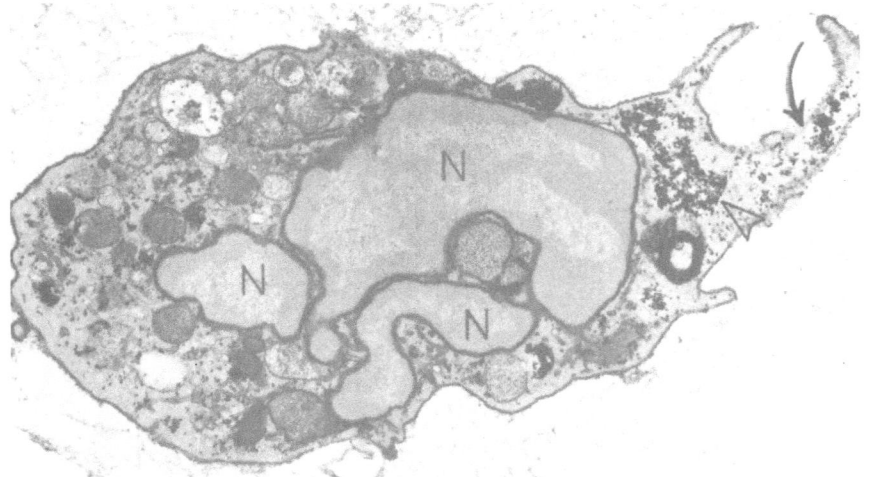

Figure 2.5 Peripheral blood basophil shows elongated tail-like uropod (arrow). N = nucleus; arrowhead = glycogen (with permission, ref. 6), OPF, ×12 000

induction. We found that basophils in these lesions remained viable, but progressively lost their dense particulate granule content over this time. Completely degranulated basophils retained their empty granule chambers (Figure 2.6). This process occurred by vesicular transport of small packages of granule particles which budded from granule membranes (Figure 2.7), traversed the cytoplasm (Figure 2.8), and fused with the plasma membrane.

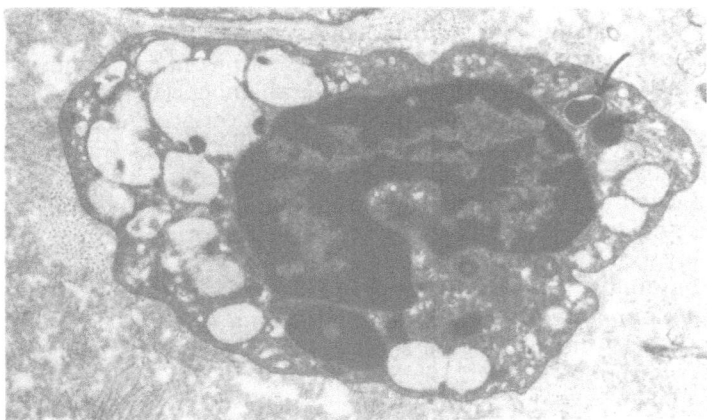

Figure 2.6 Basophil *in vivo* from the ileum of a patient with Crohn's disease shows piecemeal degranulation characterized by empty granule chambers. One granule retains its contents (arrow). OCUB, ×8800

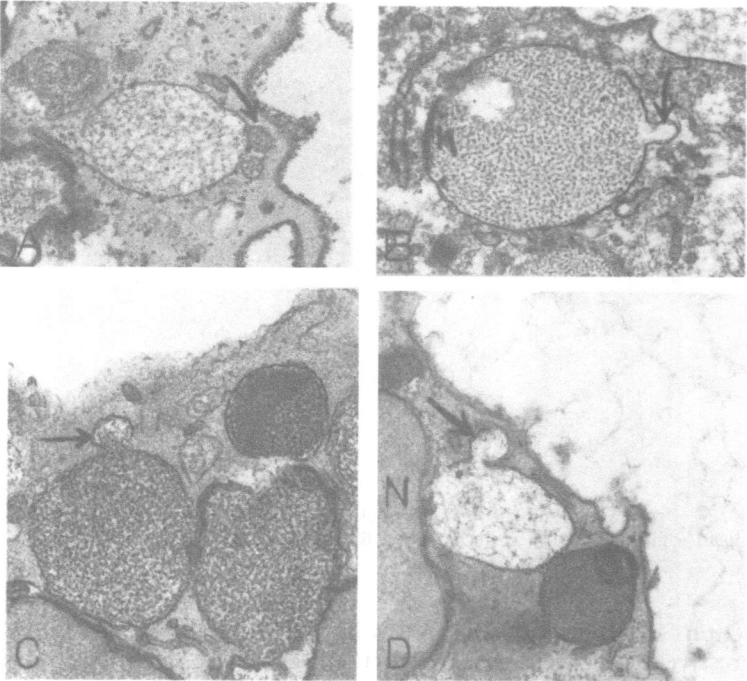

Figure 2.7 High magnification micrographs of peripheral blood basophils show vesicles (arrows) budding from granules (**A–D**). Some of these vesicles contain particles (**A, C**) and some appear empty (**B, D**). N = nucleus. (**A**) OPF, CF, ×28 800; (**B**) OCUB, ×24 400; (**C**) OPF, ×34 400; (**D**) OPF, ×24 400

Granule membranes did not fuse with each other to form intracytoplasmic degranulation channels nor did individual granules fuse with the plasma membranes. The morphologic endpoint of these piecemeal granule losses was a viable basophil filled with empty granule chambers (Figure 2.6). Over the six-day study period, basophils displayed all variations of a progressive event. For example, we could find cells with full granules (Figure 2.9), cells with partially depleted granules (Figure 2.10) and cells with nearly all empty granules (Figure 2.11). The co-existence in the same cell of completely filled granules and granules in the process of depletion or completely empty was commonly seen (Figure 2.10). Since the completion of these studies, we have found basophils in the inflammatory infiltrate undergoing piecemeal degranulation *in vivo* in biopsy material from a variety of diseases. These include Crohn's disease (Figure 2.12)[5], bullous pemphigoid (Figure 2.13)[21] and graft rejection (Figure 2.8)[22].

Since human basophils have the capacity to transport granule materials to the cells' exterior in vesicles, we postulated that the reverse event could also occur. To prove this we showed that guinea pig basophils (Figure 2.14) could endocytose the electron-dense tracer, horseradish peroxidase, and transport

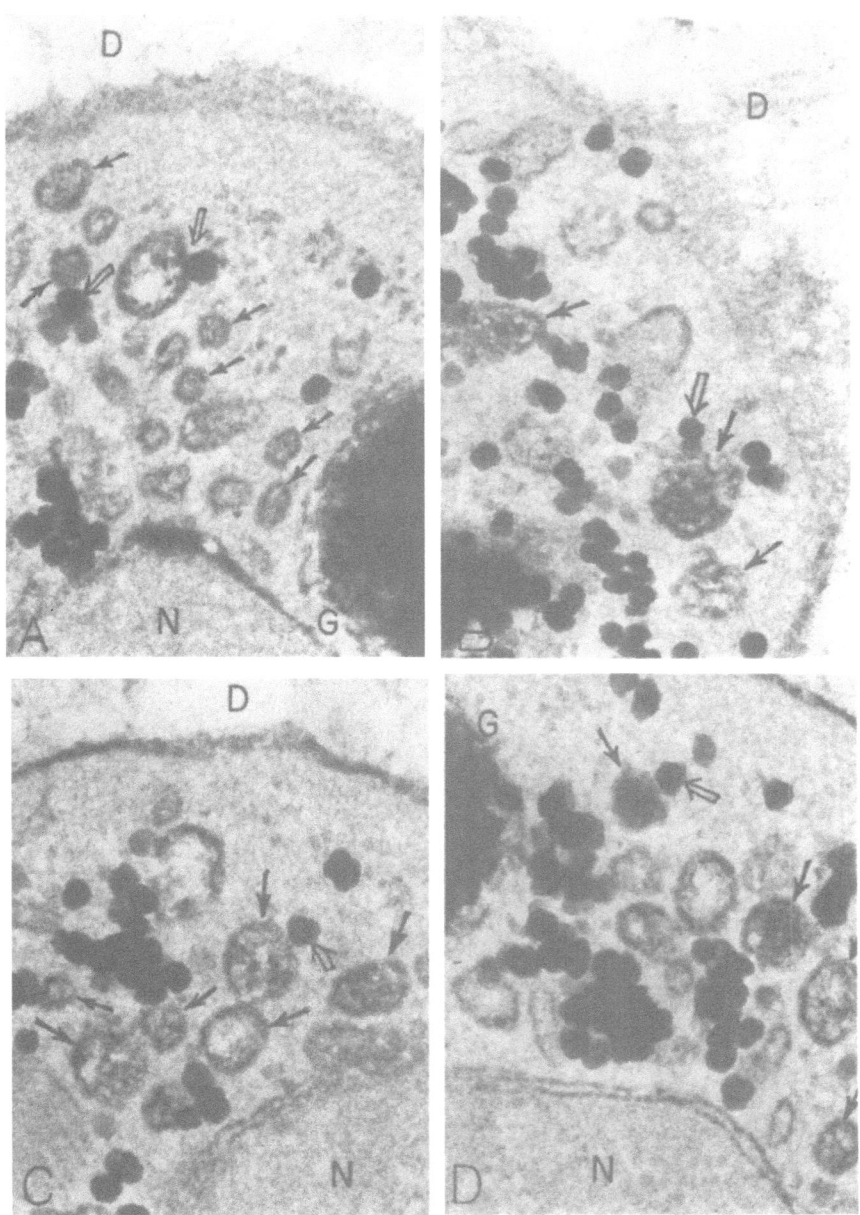

Figure 2.8 High magnification micrographs of basophils *in vivo* in skin graft rejection. Peripheral cytoplasmic vesicles with dense particulate contents are present (arrows). Glycogen particles are closely associated with these vesicles (open arrows). N = nucleus; D = dermis; G = granule. OPF, **(A–D)** ×98 000

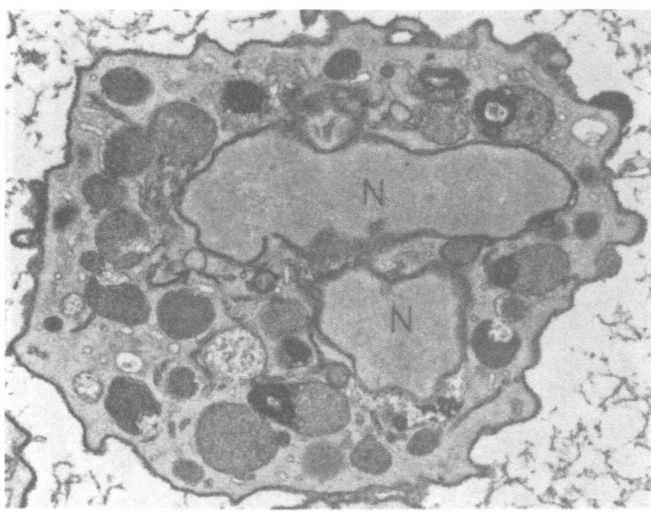

Figure 2.9 Basophil with nearly all cytoplasmic granules filled with particles. Some granules also have dense membranes. Arrow = small granule; N = nucleus. OPF, CF, ×15 100

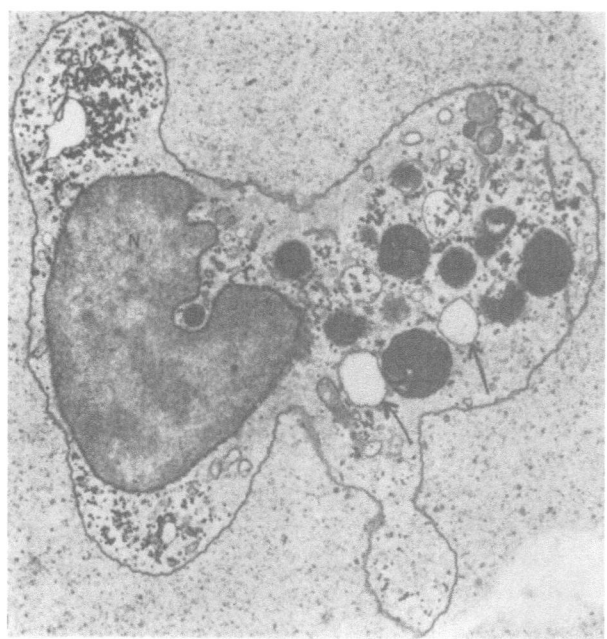

Figure 2.10 Basophil in the skin in contact allergy shows partial depletion of granules secondary to piecemeal degranulation. Note adjacent empty granule chambers (arrows) and full granules in the cytoplasm. Gly = glycogen; N = nucleus (with permission, ref. 16). OPF, ×8100

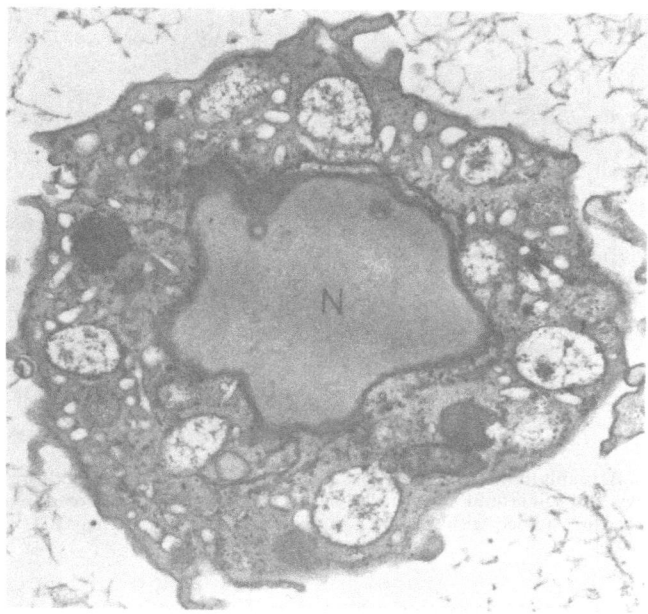

Figure 2.11 Basophil with nearly all empty cytoplasmic granules. Three nearly full granules remain. The cytoplasm is filled with large numbers of small empty vesicles. N = nucleus. OPF, ×17 500

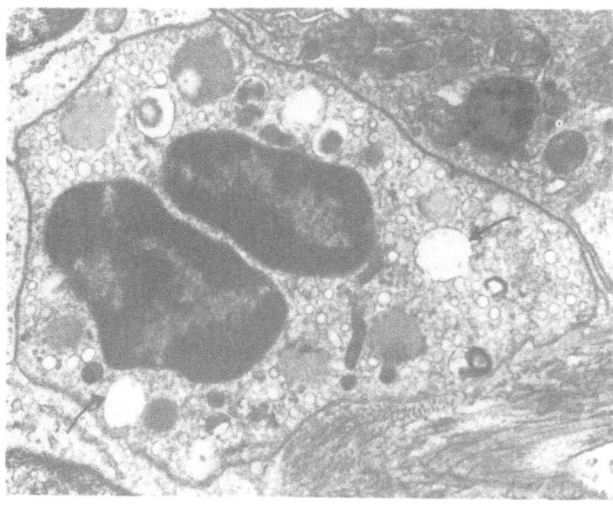

Figure 2.12 Basophil in the ileum in Crohn's disease shows piecemeal degranulation. Empty granules (arrows), full granules and numerous cytoplasmic vesicles are seen (with permission, ref. 11). OCUB, ×8400

37

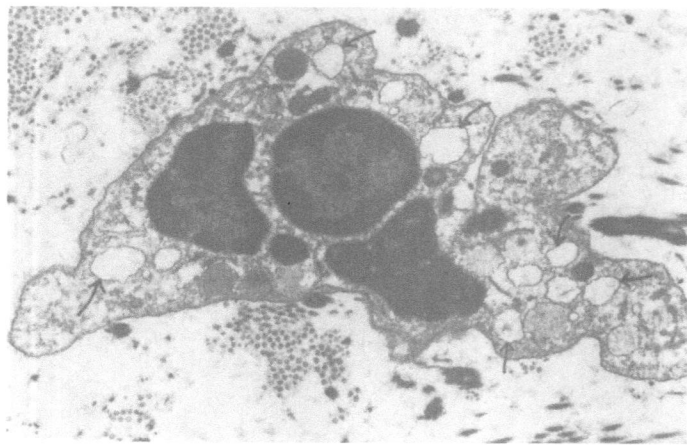

Figure 2.13 Basophil in the skin in bullous pemphigoid shows piecemeal degranulation with empty (arrows) and full granules in the cytoplasm. Cytoplasmic lucent areas are glycogen-rich areas which are not stained with this method (with permission, ref. 21). OCUB, ×8100

it in small cytoplasmic vesicles which then fused with cytoplasmic granules where peroxidase was bound and stored[23, 24]. Wash-out experiments showed the transport of this granule-bound peroxidase in vesicles from granules to the cells' exterior[24]. More recently we have shown that guinea pig baso-phils[25], mouse mast cells[25] and human basophils (Figures 2.15–17)[14] can use a similar mechanism to transport exogenous eosinophil peroxidase into their interiors and bind it to cytoplasmic storage granules. This mechanism may also, then, represent an important function for basophils, e.g. the sequestration of potentially toxic materials released by eosinophils in inflammatory exudates. Whether re-release of this material by vesicular transport is also possible is not yet known.

Anaphylactic degranulation

We have studied the morphologic expression of these rapid release reactions induced in isolated, partially purified human blood basophils (Figure 2.18)[4, 6, 7, 12, 13] or in cultured human basophils (Figure 2.19)[13] stimulated by a variety of triggers. We examined multiple time points in the basophils of four separate allergic donors that were stimulated to degranulate by exposure to antigen E (Figure 2.20)[4]. We found that human basophils rapidly extruded intact membrane-free granules to the cells' exterior through multiple openings in their cell circumference (Figure 2.21). Rarely, we found granule-to-granule fusions which produced chains of granules being extruded through a single pore in the cell membrane (Figure 2.22). The earliest event we were able to identify was narrow openings between cell surface and individual granules (Figure 2.23). These widened (Figure 2.24) to allow extrusion of

38

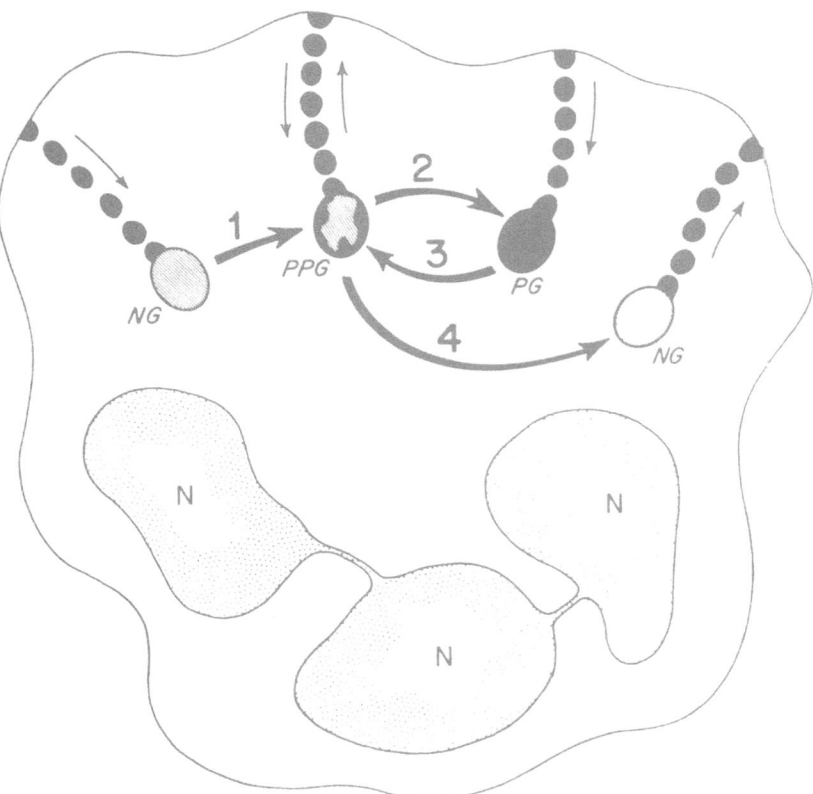

Figure 2.14 This schematic diagram illustrates the vesicular transport of horseradish peroxidase (HRP) by guinea pig basophils. Negative granules (NG), partially-positive granules (PPG), and positive granules (PG) are depicted in relationship to flow of HRP in vesicles (dark circular structures). Uptake of HRP from the extracellular space proceeds via pinocytotic vesicles which flow through the cytosol and attach to granules. **Arrow 1** depicts the consequent development of granules with focal areas of HRP (PPG). Further uptake may result in additional numbers of PPG and of PG **(arrow 2)**. During washout, as depicted by **arrow 3**, PG may revert to PPG and ultimately, with continuing release of HRP-positive vesicles from PPG **(arrow 4)**, to NG. HRP-positive cytoplasmic vesicles in the presence of negative granules may occur either in the earliest stages of uptake (before granules become positive) or in the final stages of washout (after granules have released their HRP content). N = nucleus (with permission, ref. 24)

granule material which often remained attached to the cells' surface (Figure 2.25) for the duration of the kinetic experiments (30 minutes) (Figure 2.24). This process was accompanied by an extraordinary elongation of and development of complexity to the cell surface processes (Figure 2.22). The minor paranuclear granule type did not participate in this release reaction, and often served to help to identify a completely degranulated basophil with a markedly activated cell surface (Figures 2.26, 27).

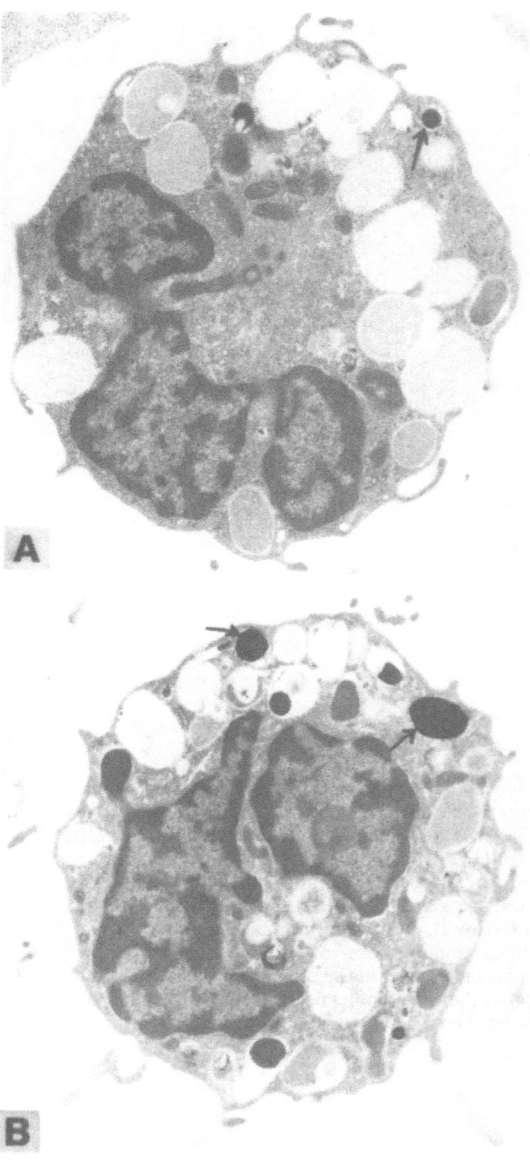

Figure 2.15 Cultured human basophils which developed in growth factor-supplemented media contain several peroxidase-positive granules (arrows), but most are negative (with permission, ref. 14). DAB, (A) ×10 400; (B) ×8800

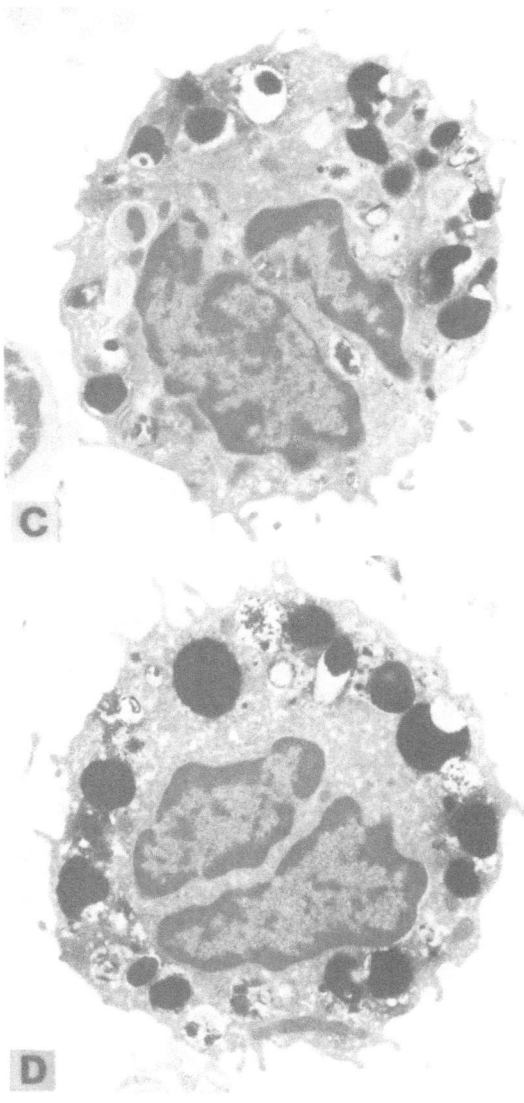

Figure 2.16 Cultured basophils prepared as in Figure 2.15 contain nearly all peroxidase-positive granules (with permission, ref. 14). DAB, **(C)** ×9200; **(D)** ×8800

41

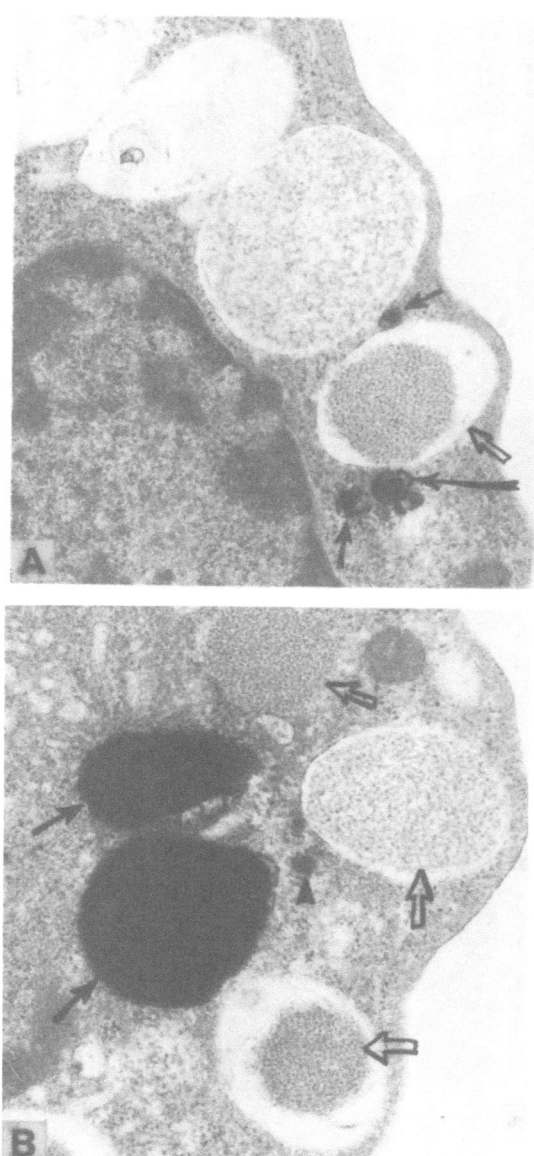

Figure 2.17 Higher magnification micrographs of cultured basophils prepared as in Figure 2.15 show peroxidase-positive vesicles (**A**, arrow; **B**, arrowhead) close to basophil granules. The granules are peroxidase-negative (**A, B**, open arrows) and strongly peroxidase-positive (**B**, arrows) (with permission, ref. 14). DAB, (**A**) ×28 000; (**B**) ×29 600

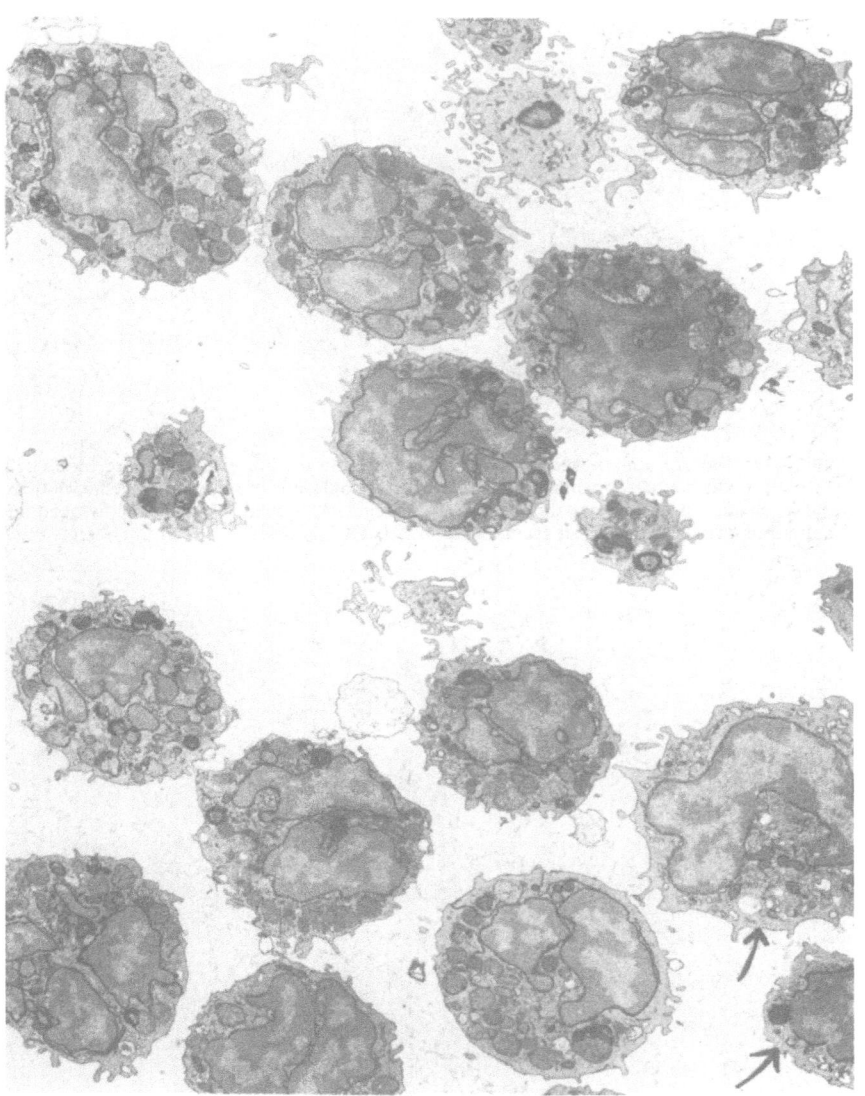

Figure 2.18 Purified peripheral blood basophils. The principal contaminating cells are lymphocytes and monocytes (arrows) (with permission, MacGlashan, D. W., Jr., Lichtenstein, L. M., Galli, S. J., Dvorak, A. M. and Dvorak, H. F. (1982). Purification of basophilic leukocytes from guinea pig and human blood and from guinea pig bone marrow. In Pretlow II, T. G. and Pretlow, T. P. (eds.) *Cell Separation: Methods and Selected Applications.* Vol. 1, pp. 301–20. (New York: Academic Press)). OPF, ×4950

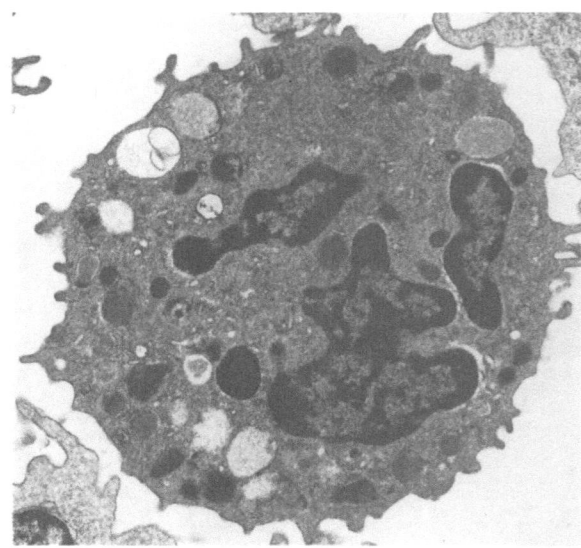

Figure 2.19 Mature human basophil which developed in a culture of fetal cord blood cells grown in growth factor-supplemented media. Most cytoplasmic granules are filled with dense particles. Surface processes are short, blunt and irregularly spaced. Nucleus is polylobed and chromatin is condensed as in all granulocyte nuclei. OCUB ×9300

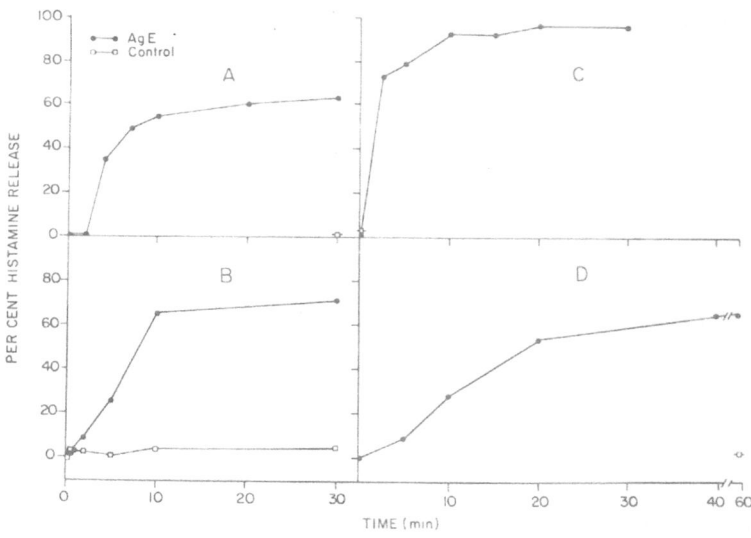

Figure 2.20 Histamine release kinetics of four ragweed-sensitive patients (**A–D**). □ , Control points; ●, antigen-induced histamine release points. Concentration of antigen E: $1 \times 10^{-2}\,\mu g/ml$, experiments **A** and **B**; $1 \times 10^{-3}\,\mu g/ml$, experiments **C** and **D** (with permission, ref. 4)

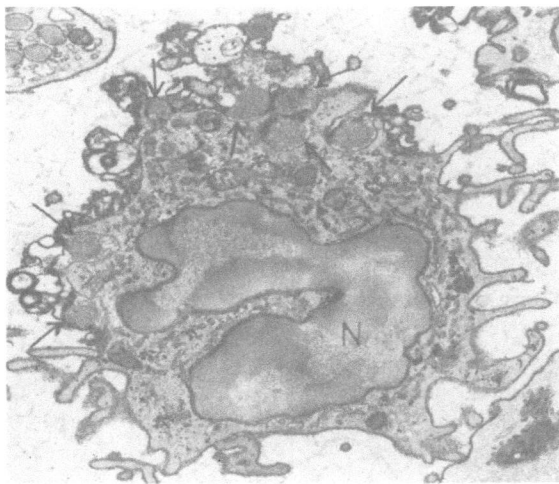

Figure 2.21 Sensitized peripheral blood basophil from an allergic donor fixed 2 min after exposure to antigen-E shows anaphylactic degranulation. All granules have been extruded from the cell at different points (arrows). They are attached to the cell, and their surfaces are stained with cationized ferritin. Surface processes are elongated. N = nucleus (with permission, ref. 4). OPF, CF, ×9750

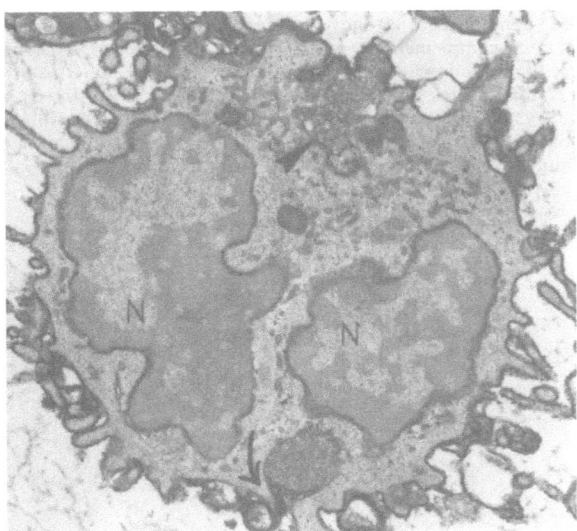

Figure 2.22 Sensitized peripheral blood basophil from an allergic donor fixed 30 minutes after exposure to antigen-E shows anaphylactic degranulation characterized by extrusion of an interconnected chain of granules through a single opening in the plasma membrane (arrowhead). All granules have been released. One granule is within a cationized ferritin-stained narrow cul-de-sac (arrow). Surface processes are increased in number, complexity and length. N = nucleus (with permission, ref. 4) OPF, CF, ×13 200

45

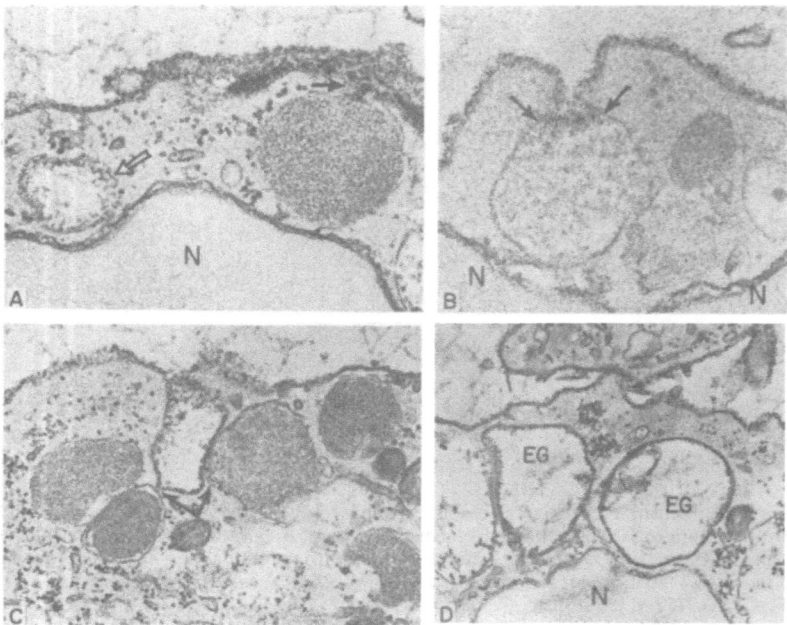

Figure 2.23 These higher magnification micrographs of basophils exposed to C5 peptide(s) for 15 seconds (**A, B**) or 2 minutes (**C, D**) show the entry of cationized ferritin into these cells as the result of exposure to complement. In (**A**), ferritin is seen entering a narrow pore opening into a granule (arrow) and lining an empty granule (open arrow). In (**B**), ferritin has entered a larger pore that communicates with an underlying granule (arrows). In (**C**), a large ferritin-positive surface invagination contacts two granules but does not yet fill them with tracer (arrows). In (**D**), two large empty granule spaces (EG) are stained with cationized ferritin and thus are in continuity with exterior. N = nucleus (with permission, ref. 6). OPF, CF, (**A**) ×28 200; (**B**) ×51 000; (**C**) ×21 000 (**D**) ×17 400

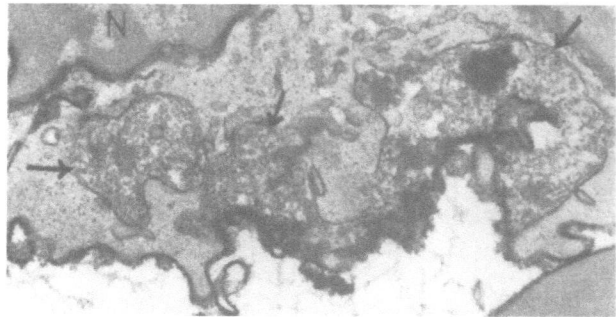

Figure 2.24 Peripheral blood basophil from a sensitized donor fixed 30 minutes after exposure to antigen E shows widened opening (arrows) to the cells' exterior filled with extruded granule particulate contents. These extruded granules bind cationized ferritin on their outermost aspects. OPF, CF, ×21 700

46

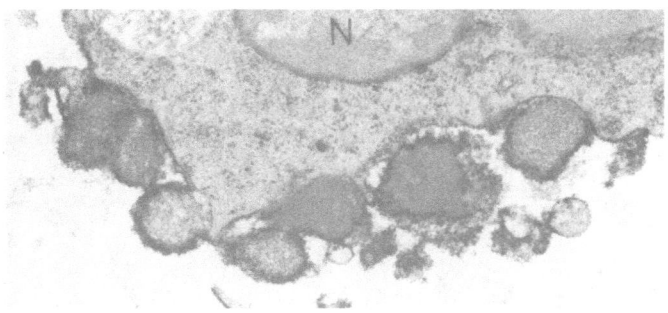

Figure 2.25 Passively sensitized, cultured human basophil which developed in growth factor-supplemented media, 15 minutes after exposure to anti-IgE shows seven membrane-free, particle-filled extruded granules attached to the cells' surface. Extruded granule surfaces and plasma membrane bind cationized ferritin. N = nucleus. OPF, CF, ×24 500

We also examined non-allergic human basophils which were induced to develop in cultures of human cord blood cells grown in basophil growth factor (BGF)-containing conditioned media (Figure 2.19)[13]. These cells were passively sensitized, and subsequent exposure to antigen produced images identical to those described above (Figure 2.25)[13]. Three other degranulation stimuli were examined with similar results. These included an hyperosmolar agent, mannitol[7], a complement factor (C5A) (Figure 2.28)[6], and a lymphocyte-derived product, histamine-releasing agent (HRA) (Figure 2.29)[12]. We have proposed a general model for degranulation of basophils which encompasses both slow and rapid release reactions (Figure 2.30). This general scheme could also apply to slow and rapid release reactions from mast cells.

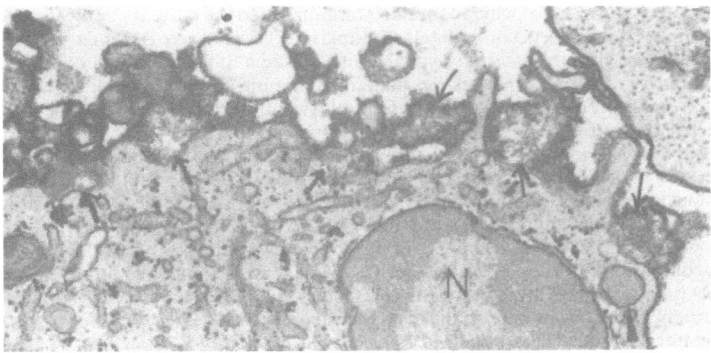

Figure 2.26 Peripheral blood basophil from an allergic donor fixed seven minutes after exposure to antigen E has numerous cationized ferritin-covered, extruded granules attached to the cell's surface at multiple points (arrows). Second granule type (arrowhead) is not extruded. N = nucleus (with permission, ref. 4). OPF, CF, ×27 000

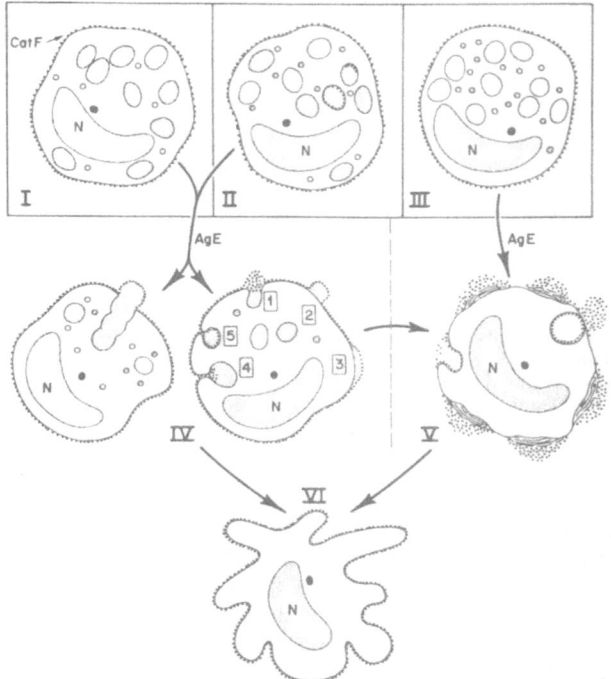

Figure 2.27 Schematic diagram of antigen E-induced human basophil degranulation. Cationized ferritin was employed after cell fixation as an ultrastructural tracer for demonstrating communications between granules and the cell surface. Prior to antigen exposure, Hypaque-Ficoll-isolated basophils from specifically allergic patients could be classified into types I–III. A uniform layer of cationized ferritin was bound to the negatively charged cell surface membrane of each cell type. Type I basophils had a full complement of full granules (stippled), one or two smaller granules of a different type in the nuclear area (small, black) and numerous cytoplasmic vesicles, most of which were empty. Type II cells had a mixture of full (stippled) and empty granules, only a few of which contained cationized ferritin particles, indicating continuity with the cell surface at other cellular levels. Cytoplasmic vesicles were either empty or contained particles similar to granule material. Type III cells showed a full complement of empty granules and the majority of cytoplasmic vesicles contained granule-like particles. Following exposure to antigen, extrusion of full granules or of empty granules led to the appearance of types IV and V cells, respectively. Type IV cells (left) rarely exhibited extrusion of interconnected granules. More commonly, granule extrusion involved openings at multiple points of the cell with extrusion of individual granules. In either event, cationized ferritin particles (black dots) were bound to extruded granules. Aggregated ferritin deposits were generally present over granule-sized openings (1); uniformly distributed over completely extruded, plasma membrane-attached granules (2,3); deep within narrow necks opening to full granules (4); and surrounding granules contained within open cul-de-sacs (5). Type V cells showed multiple, focal piled-up areas of extra membranes attached to the cell surface. Increased binding of cationized ferritin was invariably present over these extruded membranes. Occasional residual empty granules contained the tracer, indicating cell surface continuity at other planes of section. These cells were devoid of vesicles. By the time histamine release was complete, as measured biochemically, completely degranulated basophils (type VI) showed marked surface folding with a uniform layer of bound cationized ferritin, no full or empty granules or vesicles, but the minor population of small perinuclear granules remained unchanged. At this time occasional type I cells remained, but type III cells were no longer present (with permission, ref. 4)

48

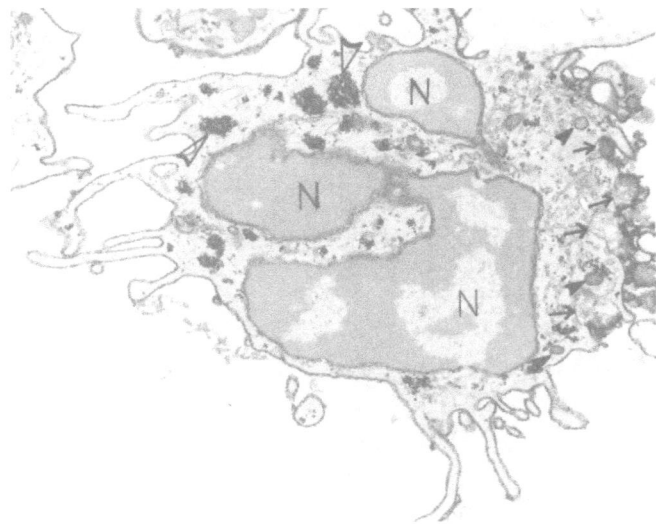

Figure 2.28 Peripheral blood basophil fixed 3 minutes after stimulation with C5 peptide(s) shows anaphylactic degranulation. Small granules are not extruded (closed arrowhead). Arrows = extruded granules; N = nucleus; open arrowhead = glycogen. OPF, CF, ×7000

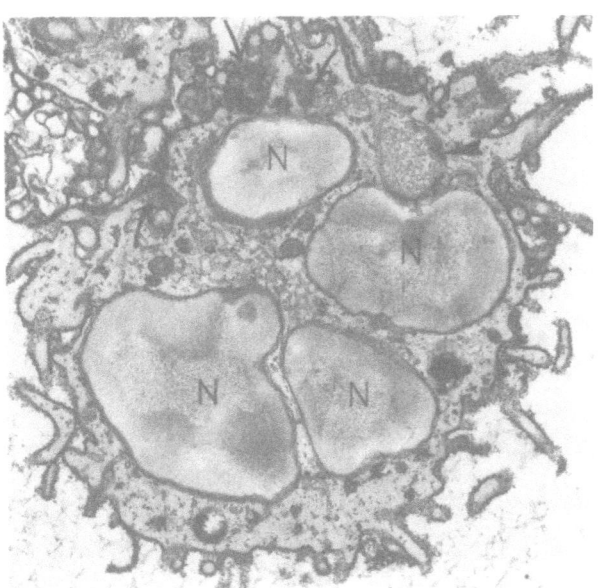

Figure 2.29 Peripheral blood basophil fixed 3 minutes after exposure to HRA shows extrusion of all granules (arrows). One granule contains cationized ferritin (arrowhead) indicating an opening to the cell surface at a level out of this plane of section. N = nucleus. OPF, CF ×13000

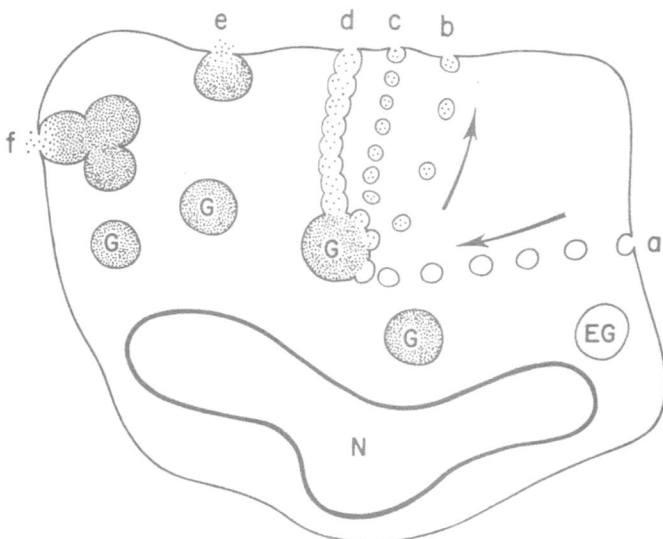

Figure 2.30 Model of basophil degranulation involving transport of endocytotic (a) and exocytotic (b, c) vesicles. At sufficiently rapid rates of discharge, vesicles may fuse to form channels (d). Direct fusion of granules (G) with cell membrane (e) or other granules (f) may also occur. EG = empty granule; N = nucleus. Arrows indicate direction of vesicle movement (with permission, ref. 16)

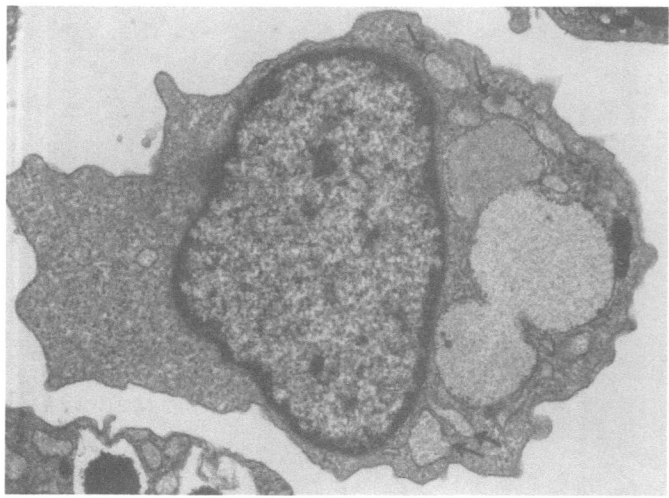

Figure 2.31 Young basophilic myelocyte which developed from fetal cord blood cells grown in growth factor-supplemented media has a single large nucleus with dispersed chromatin, dilated rough endoplasmic reticulum cisternae (arrows) and several large immature granules (with permission, ref. 14). OCUB, ×9500

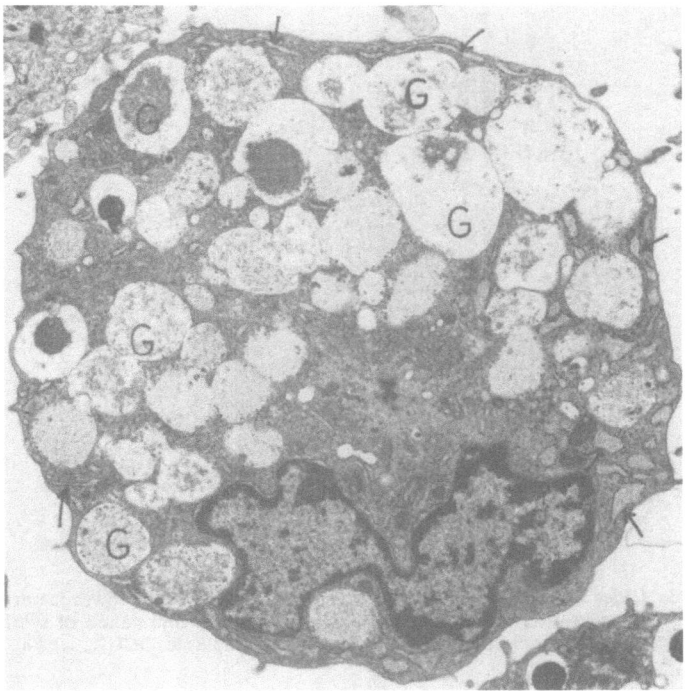

Figure 2.32 Cultured, middle-aged basophilic myelocyte which developed in growth factor-containing media. Note non-segmented, lobular nucleus, large immature granules (G) with lightly dense content and cisterns of rough endoplasmic reticulum (arrows) (with permission, ref. 38). OCUB, ×7400

Fine structure of human basophil maturation

Until recently, and because of the rarity of basophils, human basophil maturation has not been described. Malignant mature and immature basophils from patients with basophil leukaemia and chronic myelogenous leukaemia have been used for this purpose, but nuclear, cytoplasmic and granule developmental asynchrony in this malignant population of cells make it difficult to infer normal maturational events from their study[26, 27]. We found that appropriate growth factor-containing conditioned media of human or mouse origin stimulated, sustained or drove to completion the differentiation and maturation of human basophils derived from stem cells present in human cord blood cells[13, 14]. Our ultrastructural and cytochemical analysis of these events allow us now to demonstrate that human basophil development follows the morphologic rules for granulocyte development in general and specifically for basophil development, as we have described for other species, e.g. guinea pig[28] and mouse[29]. Since eosinophils also developed and matured in this system, we were able to compare and contrast their development with that of basophils.

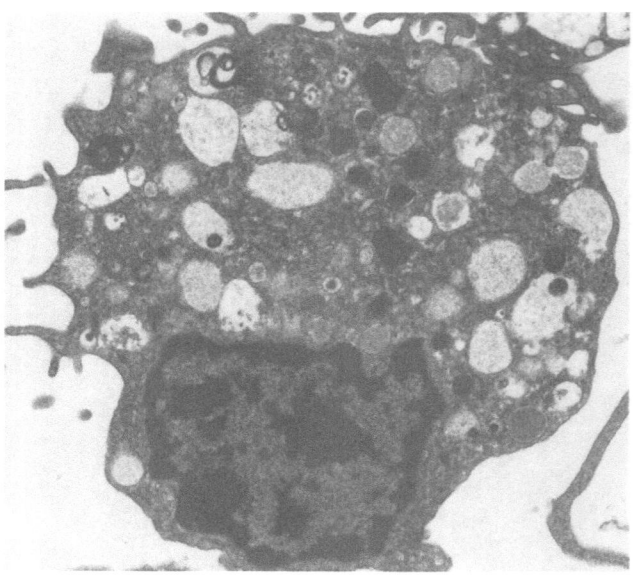

Figure 2.33 Older cultured basophilic myelocyte which developed in growth factor-containing media shows condensation of chromatin and nearly complete elimination of synthetic structures, such as rough endoplasmic reticulum, from the cytoplasm. OCUB, ×9800

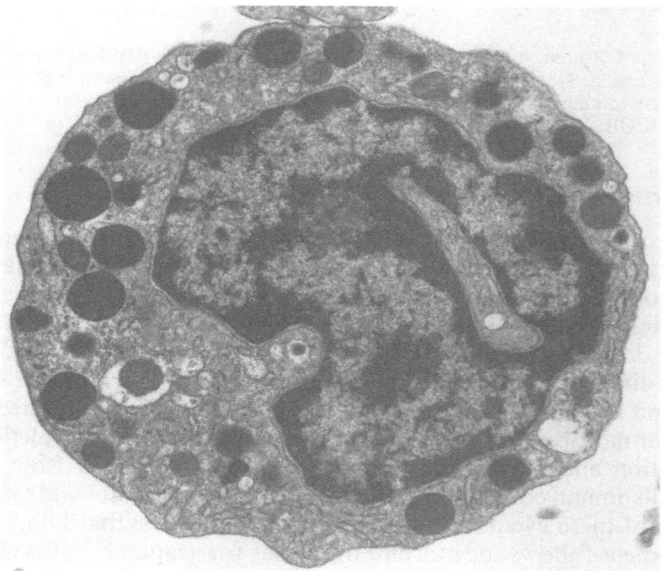

Figure 2.34 Cultured eosinophilic myelocyte from growth factor-supplemented media shows numerous round, homogeneously dense immature granules and dilated cisterns of rough endoplasmic reticulum. OCUB, ×11 200

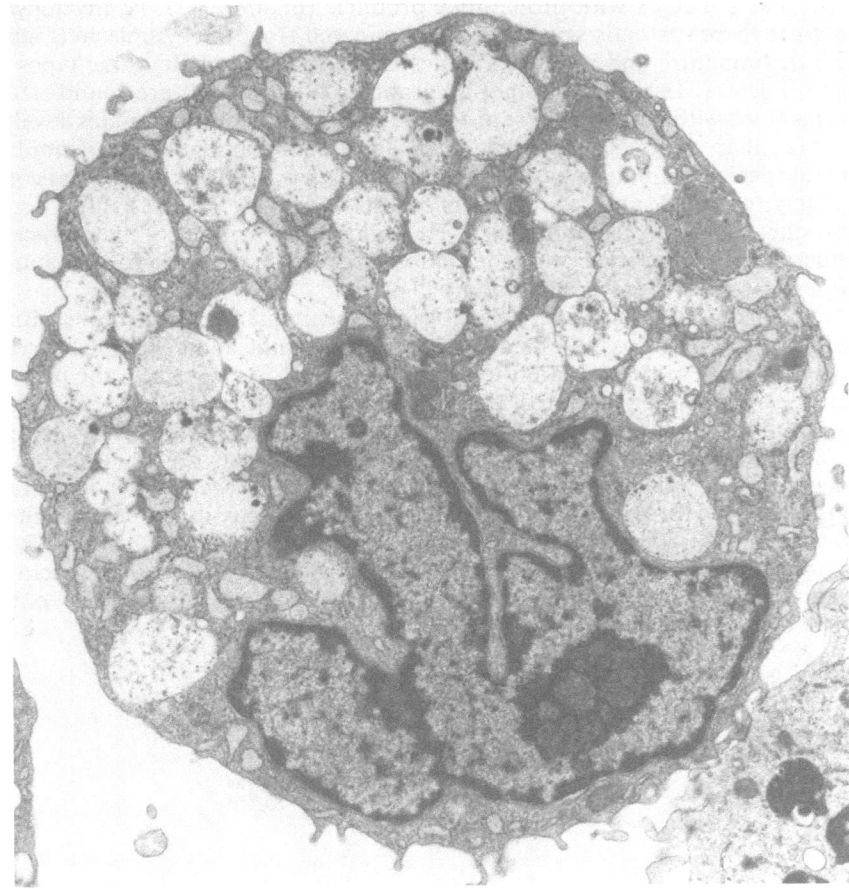

Figure 2.35 Cultured basophilic myelocyte from growth factor-supplemented media shows lobular nucleus with dispersed chromatin and large nucleolus. The cytoplasm is filed with immature granules and cisterns of rough endoplasmic reticulum (with permission, ref. 14). OCUB, ×8800

Myelocytes are first specifically named when the appearance of specific immature or mature granules allows one to do so. These large cells display morphologic evidence of immaturity. These include nuclear, synthetic and granular features. For example, nuclei are large, contain nucleoli, display a dispersed chromatin pattern and are often eccentrically located in the cell. They are non-segmented in young myelocytes (Figure 2.31). As maturation proceeds, these immature nuclei undergo size reduction, segmentation, loss of nucleoli, and chromatin condensation to produce the typical segmented nucleus common to all granulocytes. Young myelocytes have an expanded cytoplasm which contains a large Golgi area actively producing immature granules and parallel arrays of rough endoplasmic reticulum whose dilated

53

cisternae are filled with protein-like products (Figure 2.32). As myelocytes mature these synthetic structures are eliminated from the cytoplasm (Figure 2.33). Immature and mature granules differ for each of the three types of granulocytes. Immature eosinophil granules (Figure 2.34) are round structures filled with uniform dense products; mature eosinophil granules develop the familiar spherical shape and central dense core that identifies eosinophils in all species. Immature basophil granules (Figure 2.35) are larger, less completely rounded and contain flocculent and particulate, lightly dense products as well as small vesicles. These immature structures undergo considerable size reduction as condensation occurs to produce mature granules filled with particles and membranous arrays[14].

We also used Graham and Karnovsky's technique for the demonstration of endogenous peroxidase to distinguish eosinophilic and basophilic myelocytes during their maturation to mature cells[14, 23]. As expected, the perinuclear cisterna, the cisternae of the rough endoplasmic reticulum, some Golgi structures, immature granules and mature granules (except their central cores) were all strongly positive in eosinophilic myelocytes (Figure 2.36)[14]. By contrast, none of these synthetic structures, none of the immature granules, and rare mature granules (see the above discussion under piecemeal degranulation) were positive in basophilic myelocytes (Figure 2.37)[14]. Thus, cytochemistry of endogenous peroxidase, as well as routine ultrastructural morphology, serve to aid in the identification of human basophilic myelocytes[14].

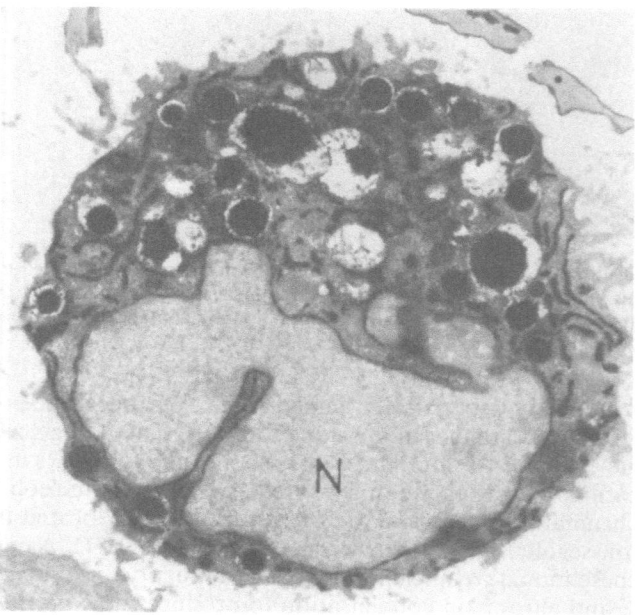

Figure 2.36 Cultured eosinophilic myelocyte shows peroxidase in the perinuclear cistern, the cisterns of rough endoplasmic reticulum and in immature, round, crystal-free granules (with permission, ref. 14). N = nucleus. DAB, ×7200

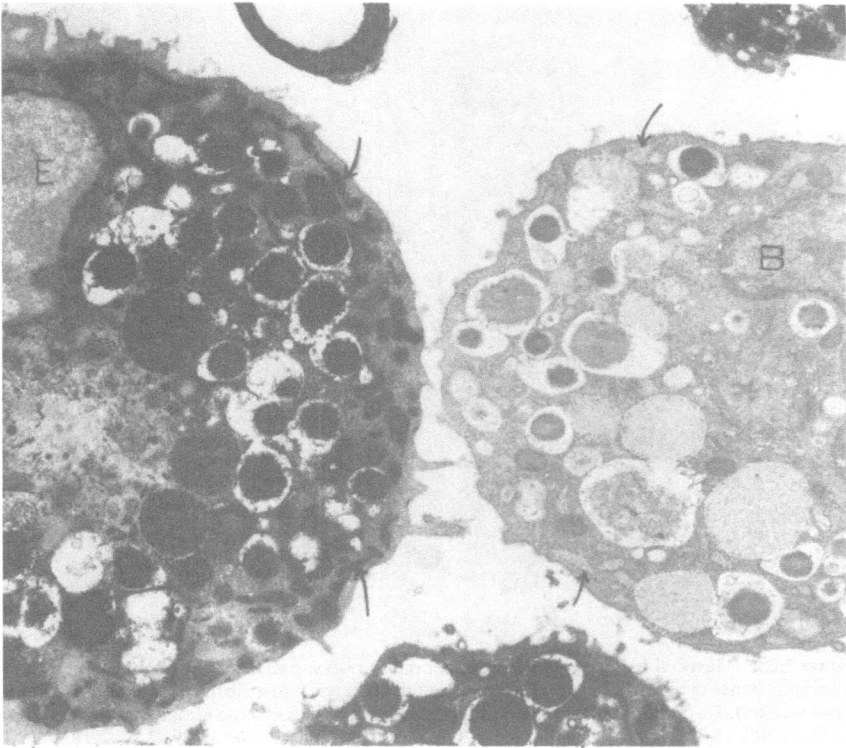

Figure 2.37 Eosinophilic myelocyte (**E**) and basophilic myelocyte (**B**) in growth-factor supplemented media are peroxidase-positive (**E**) and -negative (**B**). Immature granules and synthetic cisterns (arrows) in the myelocytes are strongly positive (**E**) or negative (**B**) (with permission, ref. 38). DAB, ×7800

HUMAN MAST CELLS

Fine structure of mature, resting human mast cells[5, 9-11, 21, 30-38]

Human mast cells are large mononuclear cells with numerous cytoplasmic granules (Figure 2.38). These granules are smaller, more variable in size, and more numerous than are the cytoplasmic granules of human basophils. Cell surfaces are adorned with regularly spaced, short, narrow folds. The nuclear chromatin pattern is partially dispersed, nucleoli are absent, Golgi structures are small and membrane-bound ribosomes are extremely rare. Glycogen is generally absent from the cytoplasm. Mitochondria, lipid bodies, free ribosomes, intermediate filaments and small vesicles complete the cytoplasmic substructural organelles. Some mast cells display canalicular structures which reflect internalized surface folds within plasma membrane-lined intracellular cavities (Figure 2.39). These structures may or may not be in continuity with the cells' surface at the time of fixation for study by electron microscopy.

55

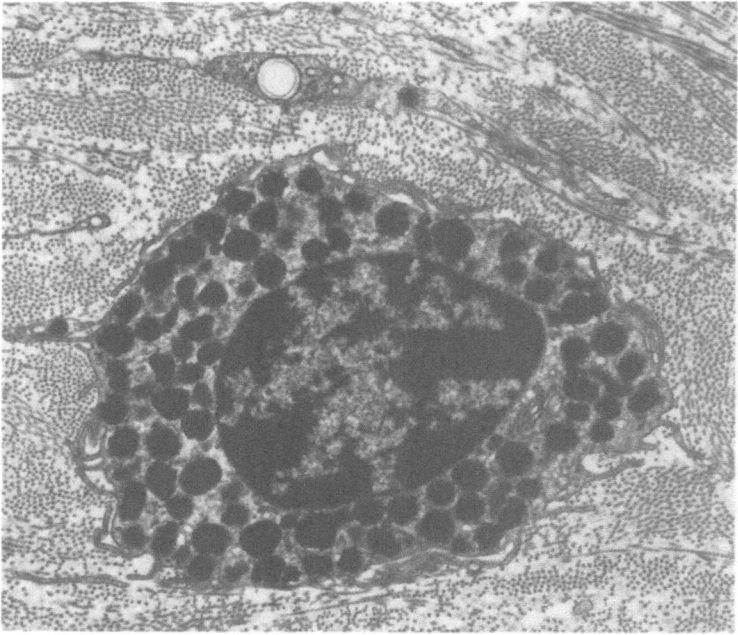

Figure 2.38 Mast cell from a breast fibroadenoma *in vivo* shows a large mononuclear cell with numerous dense cytoplasmic granules enmeshed in collagen (most fibrils of collagen are cut in cross-section). Note that nuclear chromatin is partially condensed, the Golgi area is small, and surface folds are narrow and elongated. OCUB, ×9500

Human mast cell granules have extremely complex substructural patterns[31, 37]. These have been described in detail by numerous reports (reviewed in Reference 37). We refer to the major types of patterns seen simply as:

(1)   Scroll granules (Figures 2.40, 41),
(2)   Crystal granules (Figure 2.42),
(3)   Particle granules (Figure 2.43),
(4)   Mixed granules.

In addition to these major patterns, some granules with entirely homogeneous, very dense contents (Figure 2.44) occur as well as patterns variously described as 'reticular', 'beaded threads', etc. (Figure 2.45). The latter are rare and seem to reflect a single type of granule pattern with variable expressions. Scroll granules display extremely regular lamellar arrays of multiple membranes. These may be straight or curved and oriented in multiple directions. Some lamellar structures are extremely dense, others are much less dense. Some have dense material in their centres (Figure 2.41), others do not. A horizontal periodicity can be seen to traverse some lamellae in appropriate sections (Figure 2.41). Crystal granules (Figure 2.42) contain extremely regular periodic parallel arrays which display two periodicities, 60 Å and

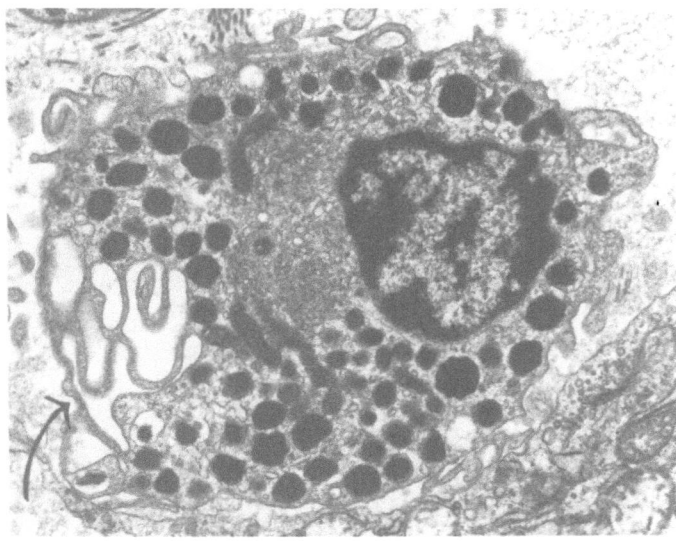

Figure 2.39 Ileal mast cell *in vivo* shows canaliculi (arrow) (with permission, Dvorak, A. M. and Dickersin, G. R. (1979). Crohn's disease, electron microscopic studies. In Sommers, S. C. and Rosen, P. P. (eds.) *Pathology Annual Part II*, Vol. 14, pp. 259–306. (New York, Appleton-Century-Crofts)). OCUB, ×8400

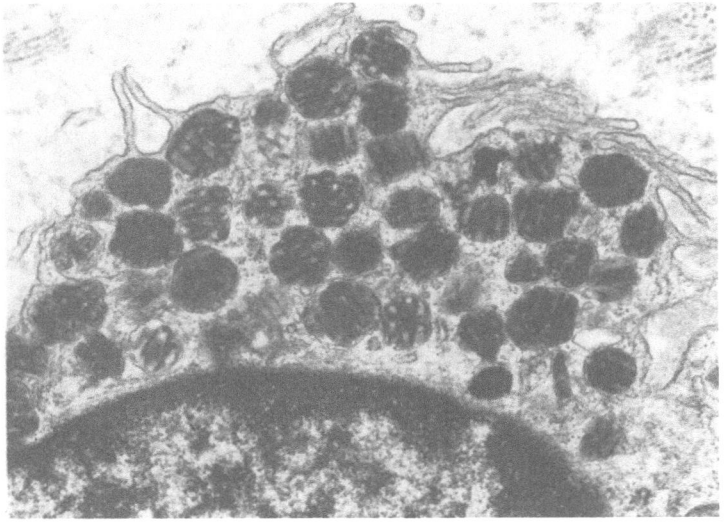

Figure 2.40 Heart mast cell *in vivo* contains scroll granules. OCUB, ×14 700

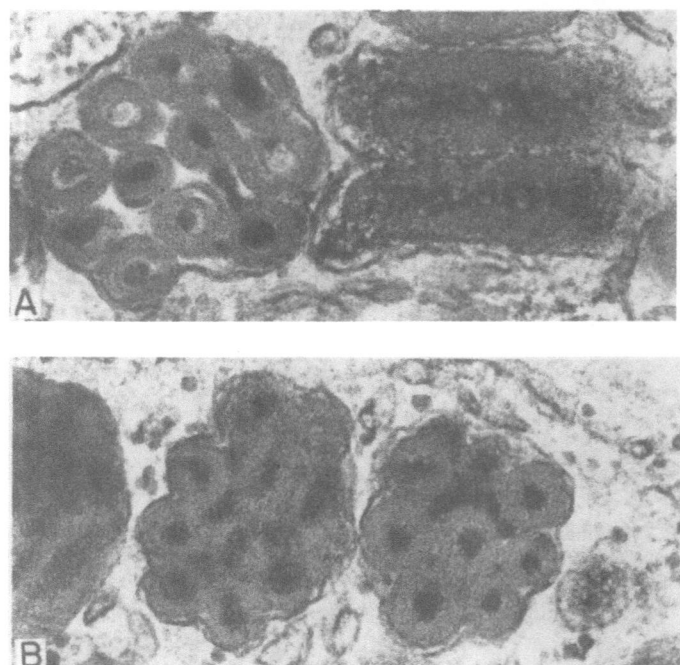

Figure 2.41 Isolated human lung mast cell scroll granules seen in cross- **(A, B)** and longitudinal **(A)** -section show central dense material within lamellae which display cross-striations. OPF, ×56 100

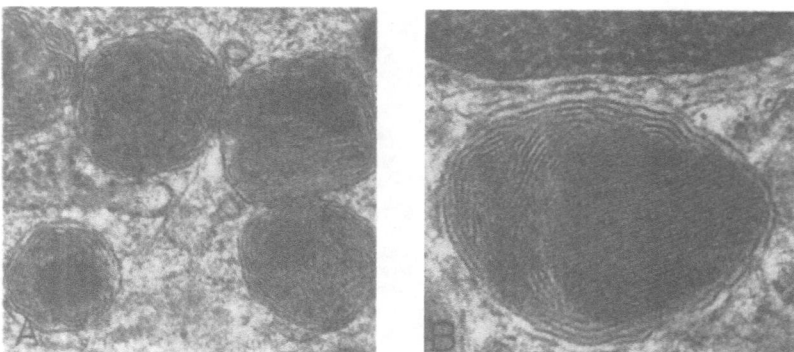

Figure 2.42 Skin mast cell crystal granules *in vivo* seen at high magnifications show two periodicities, 8 nm **(A)** and 12 nm **(B)**, that are oriented in multiple directions. OCUB, **(A)** ×43 400 **(B)** ×60 200

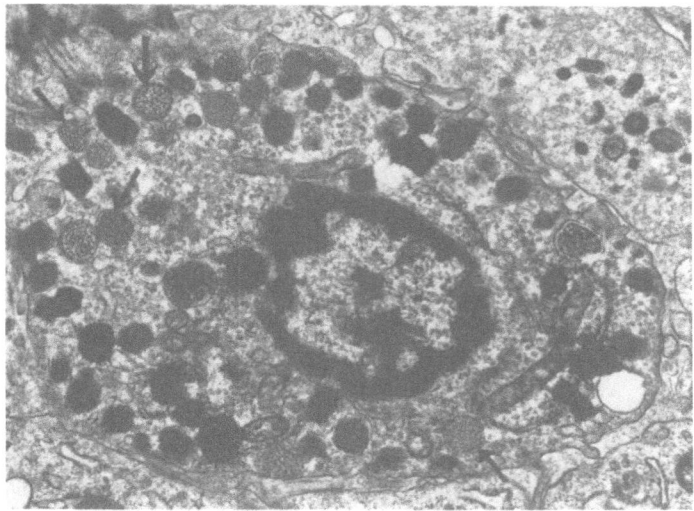

Figure 2.43 Ileal mast cell *in vivo* contains particle granules (arrows). OCUB, ×11 600

120 Å[39] and can also be oriented in multiple directions. Particle granules (Figure 2.43) are filled with electron-dense particles enmeshed within a less dense background material with no substructural distinctions. Mixed granules contain variable mixtures of scrolls, crystals and particles, or any combination of two of these patterns.

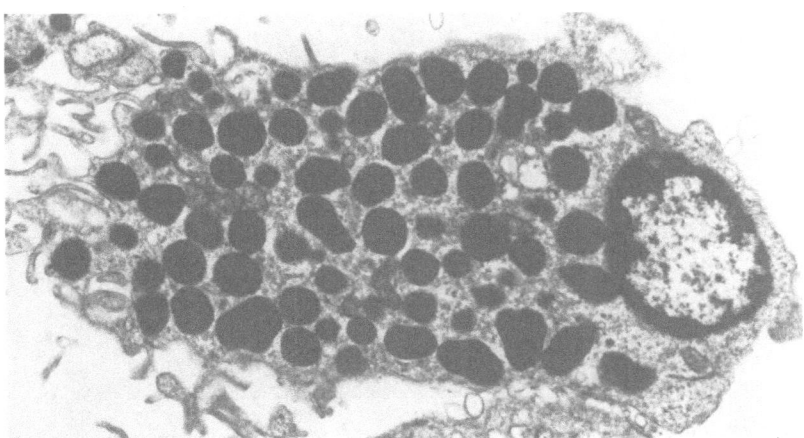

Figure 2.44. Isolated human lung mast cell is filled with homogeneous membrane-bound dense granules which lack substructural patterns. OCUB, ×8400

59

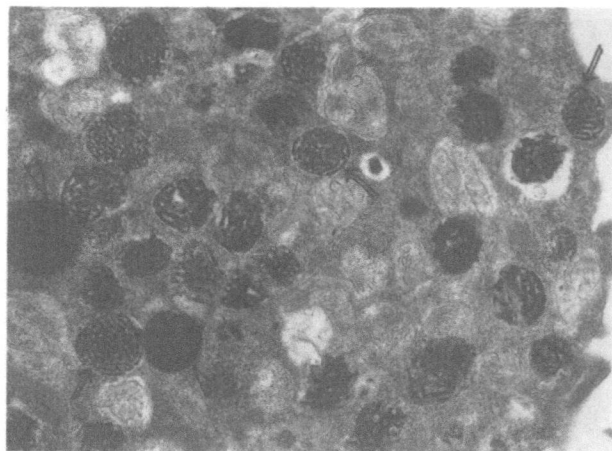

Figure 2.45 Isolated human lung mast cell contains 'reticular', 'beaded thread' granule contents (arrows). Two lipid bodies (arrowheads) and scroll granules are also present. OCUB, ×16 950

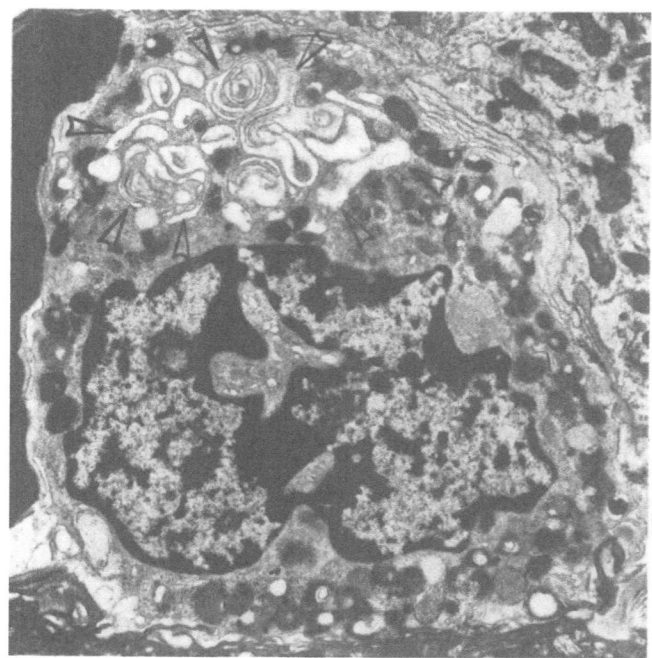

Figure 2.46 Lung mast cell *in vivo* from a patient with adenocarcinoma of the lung is filled with particle granules and a few reticular granules. A large canalicular structure is present (arrowheads) and the irregular, immature nucleus has dispersed chromatin and a large nucleolus. Narrow surface folds are present. OCUB, ×8400

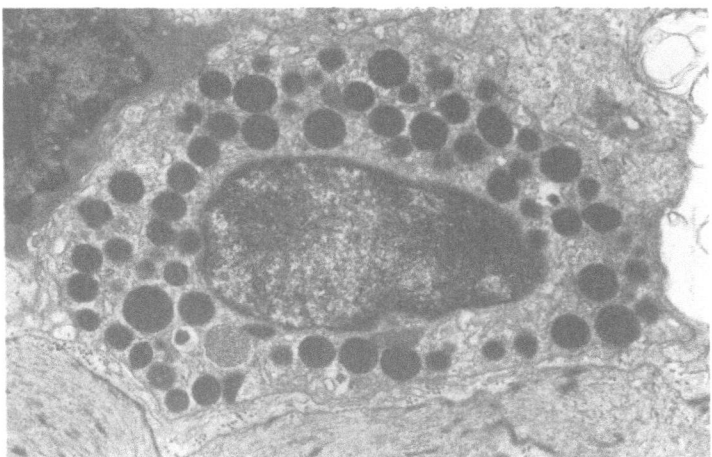

Figure 2.47 Ileal mast cell *in vivo* contains homogeneously dense granules OCUB, ×8100

The meaning of these various granule patterns in human mast cells is obscure. It is important to realize that human mast cells can have particle granules, as do human basophils, as well as to realize that human basophils can display lamellar arrays in some granules, as do human mast cells. Given all ultrastructural criteria for identification, however, it is generally possible to properly classify normal mast cells and basophils. The marked heterogeneity of mast cell granule patterns serves to distinguish them from the more homogeneous expression of human basophil granule patterns.

We have examined human mast cells *in vivo* in large studies of lung (Figure 2.46), gut (Figure 2.47) and skin (Figure 2.48) specimens as well as in biopsy

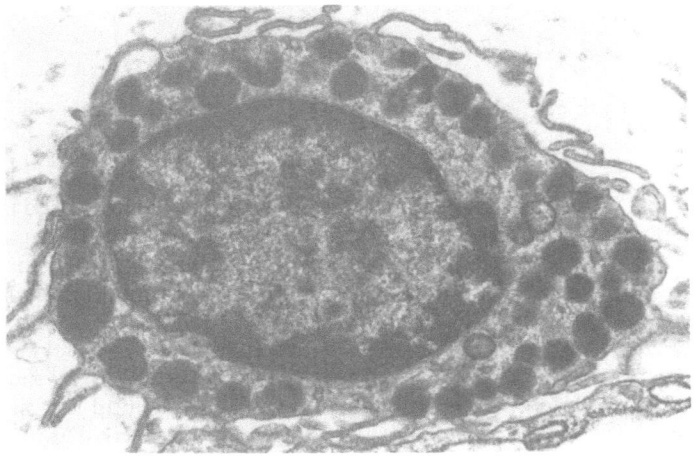

Figure 2.48 Skin mast cell *in vivo* contains crystal granules. OCUB, ×14 300

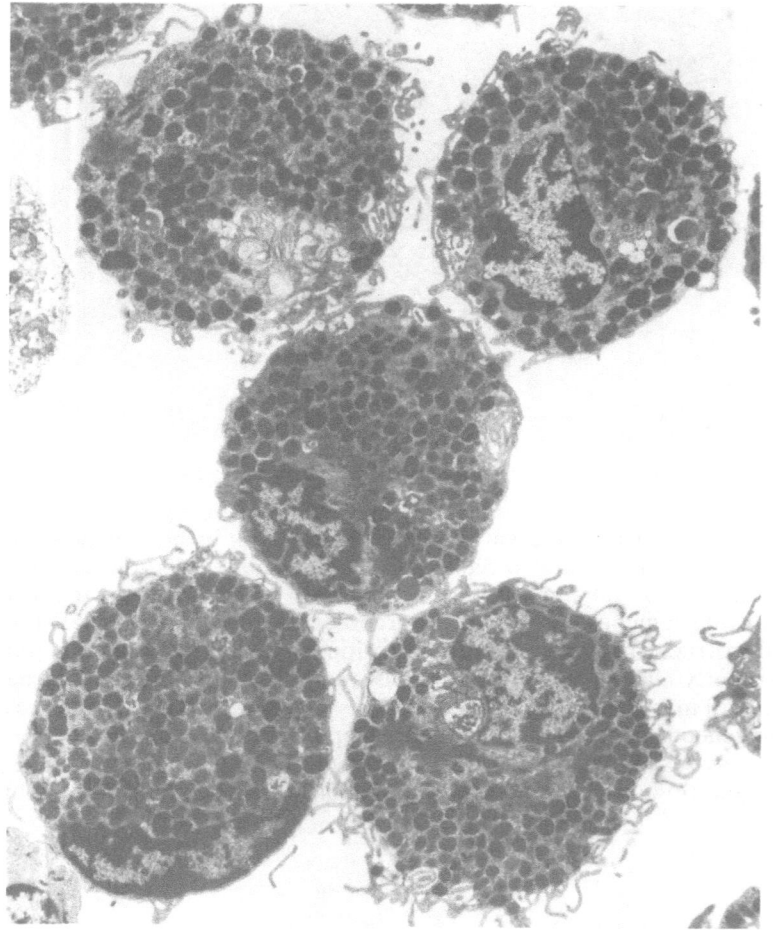

Figure 2.49 Isolated, purified human lung mast cell preparation (with permission, ref. 33). OCUB, ×5900

material from all accessible sites in humans. We have also examined isolated, partially purified preparations of human mast cells from lung (Figure 2.49)[9–11, 31–33, 36–38], colon (Figure 2.50)[34], synovium[38a] and skin (A. M. Dvorak, unpublished). In all instances it is possible to find human mast cells with predominant granule patterns reflecting one of the four above-listed major categories. It is essential to document this type of background of cellular heterogeneity in order to interpret ultrastructural changes induced by a variety of experimental stimuli. In general, we have found that skin mast cells more often express crystal granules; lung mast cells, scroll granules; and gut mast cells, particle granules. All granules types, however, can be found in mast cells from all tissue locations.

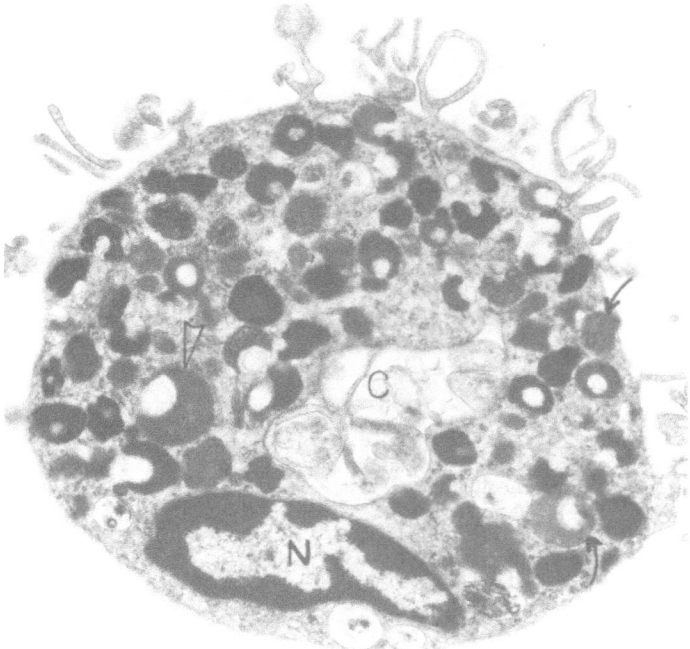

Figure 2.50 Isolated human gut mast cell shows irregularly shaped granules which vary in size. Many granules are particle granules (arrows). A lipid body (arrowhead) and canalicular structure (C) are present. N = nucleus. OCUB, ×9800

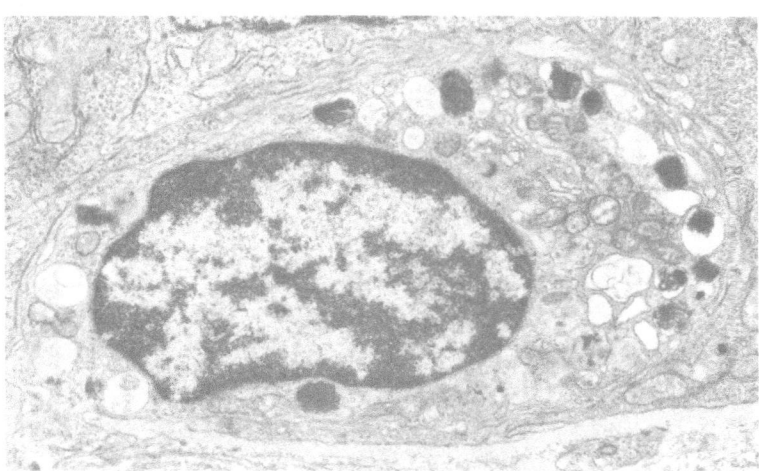

Figure 2.51 Ileal mast cell *in vivo* from a patient with Crohn's disease shows piecemeal degranulation. Some scroll granules remain, but many granules have lost nearly all of their contents. OCUB, ×9800

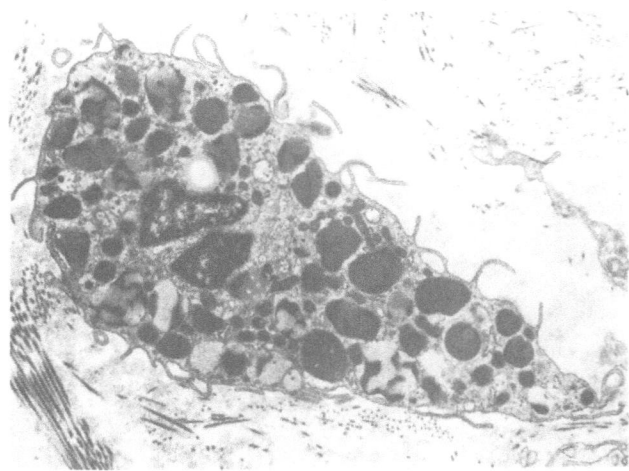

Figure 2.52 Skin mast cell *in vivo* in bullous pemphigoid shows irregular, geographic piecemeal degranulation losses of nearly all granules (with permission, ref. 21). OCUB, ×5600

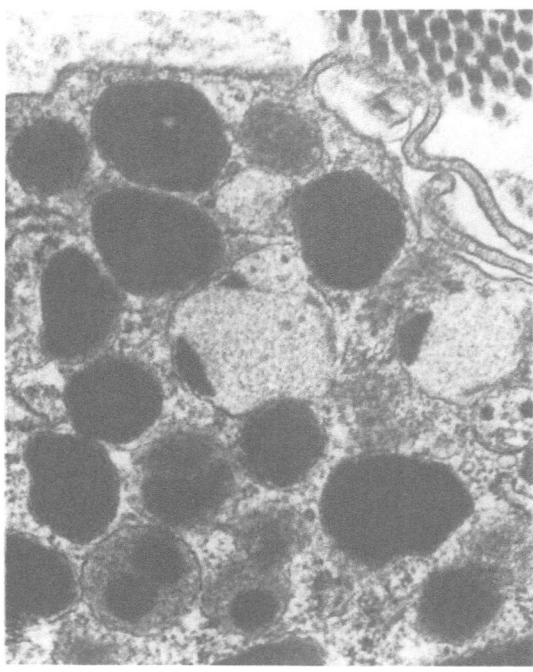

Figure 2.53 Focal piecemeal losses of individual granule contents in a skin mast cell from a patient with bullous pemphigoid. OCUB, ×28 400

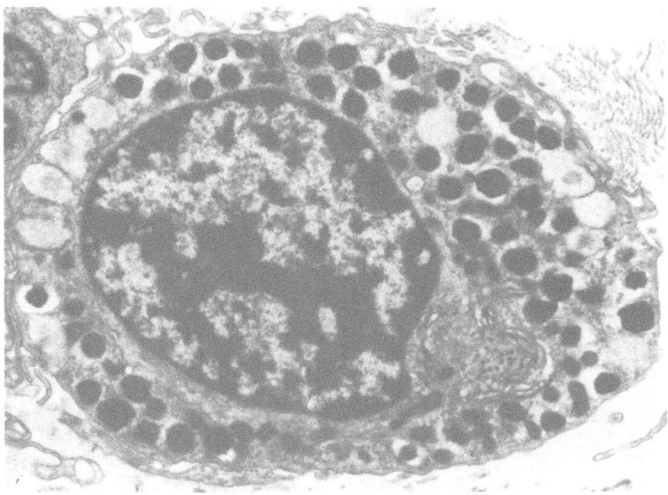

Figure 2.54 Complete loss of individual granule contents in an ileal mast cell from a patient with Crohn's disease. Most granules are unaltered. OCUB, ×7700

Fine structure of degranulating human mast cells

Like human basophils, human mast cells may also undergo two general morphologic categories of release reactions. These are (1) piecemeal degranulation and (2) anaphylactic degranulation. The kinetics of the latter are rapid. There is no available experimental data that can document the kinetics of the former in human mast cells. By morphologic analogy to human basophils, however, we also propose that piecemeal granule content losses from human mast cells occurs in days, not minutes, as in anaphylactic degranulation.

Piecemeal degranulation

We have described piecemeal losses from mast cell granule contents in systematic studies of two diseases, (1) Crohn's disease (Figure 2.51)[5] and (2) bullous pemphigoid (Figure 2.52)[21]. We have also seen similar losses of granule contents in mast cells found in a wide variety of biopsies of inflammatory and neoplastic disorders. As in human basophils, the ultrastructural diagnostic hallmark for this process is a mast cell filled with empty granule chambers whose membranes are not fused with each other or with the plasma membrane. All possible variations of these slow release processes from human mast cells are evident. Thus, we can find cells with focal, irregular losses from individual granules (Figure 2.53), from nearly all granules (Figure 2.52), to complete losses from single granules (Figure 2.54) to complete losses from all granules (Figure 2.55). Many individual mast cells contain completely full, unaltered granules side-by-side with granules displaying piecemeal losses (Figure 2.54). As in basophils, we feel piecemeal

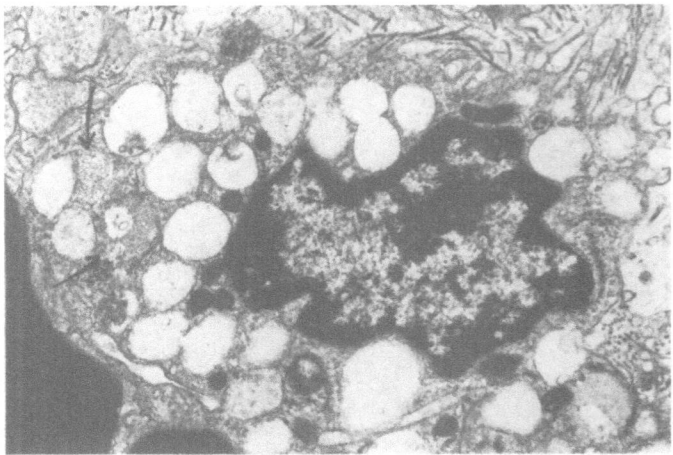

Figure 2.55 Piecemeal degranulation *in vivo* of a gut mast cell in Crohn's disease shows empty granule chambers. Some granules with particles remain (arrows). OCUB, ×11 200

granule loss from human mast cells is mediated by the budding of small vesicles from granules (Figure 2.56) and vesicular transport of quanta of granule materials through the cytoplasm to be released at the plasma membrane.

Anaphylactic degranulation

We have studied the kinetics of IgE-mediated degranulation and recovery using isolated, purified human lung mast cells (Figures 2.49, 57)[31-33, 36, 37, 40,41]. These studies include multiple times in the early release period (Figure 2.58)

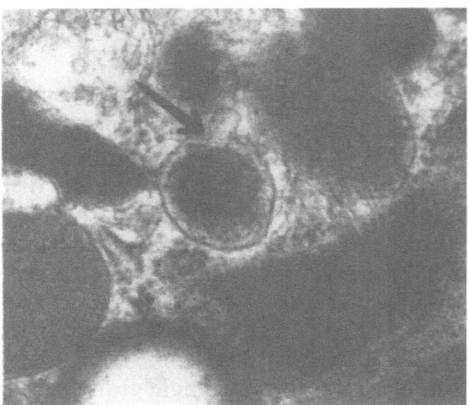

Figure 2.56 Higher magnification micrograph of a mast cell *in vivo* in a leiomyoma of the oesophagus shows budding of a vesicle from a granule (arrow). OCUB, ×33 500

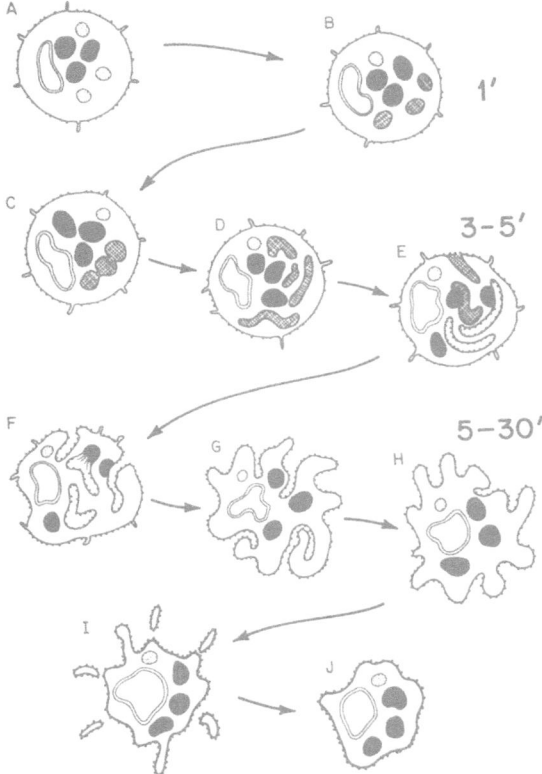

Figure 2.57 Schematic diagram of the ultrastructural changes exhibited by human lung mast cells stimulated to undergo degranulation by exposure to anti-IgE *in vitro*. Unstimulated cell (**A**) has a surface with short ridges and folds (shown labelled with cationized ferritin) and contains both granules (stippled) and larger, homogeneously electron-dense lipid bodies. By 1 minute of stimulation (**B**), many of the granules appear swollen and show dissolution of their matrix material (indicated by cross-hatching). Note that at this interval the altered granules exclude the electron-dense tracer cationized ferritin. By 3–5 minutes after stimulation (**C–E**), the membranes limiting swollen granules clearly appear fused (**C**) and the tortuous channels formed by granule–granule fusion (**D**) open to the exterior at multiple locations in the plasma membrane (**E**). At this interval, the contents of some degranulation channels impede access of cationized ferritin to membranes lining the deeper regions of the channels (see upper channel in **E**). Other channels, electron-lucent because of the loss of granule contents, are lined by membranes uniformly labelled with cationized ferritin (**E**). The number of unaltered granules (stippled) is markedly reduced compared to baseline values. By contrast, lipid bodies are unchanged in aggregate volume[31], but many of them appear in close proximity to the degranulation channels (**E**). At later intervals after stimulation (5–30 minutes, **F–J**), the exteriorization of degranulation channel membranes results in a more complex surface architecture with numerous narrow processes (**F–H**). Many of these surface processes and membranes ultimately appear discontinuous with the cell surface and are labelled with cationized ferritin (**I**). At the latest intervals studied (20–30 minutes, **J**), the mast cell surface assumes a more regular and smooth configuration. In this period we also observed rare lipid bodies that appeared to discharge their contents into electron-lucent degranulation channels (**F**), but the aggregate volume of the cytoplasmic lipid bodies remained unchanged from baseline levels[31] (with permission, ref. 33)

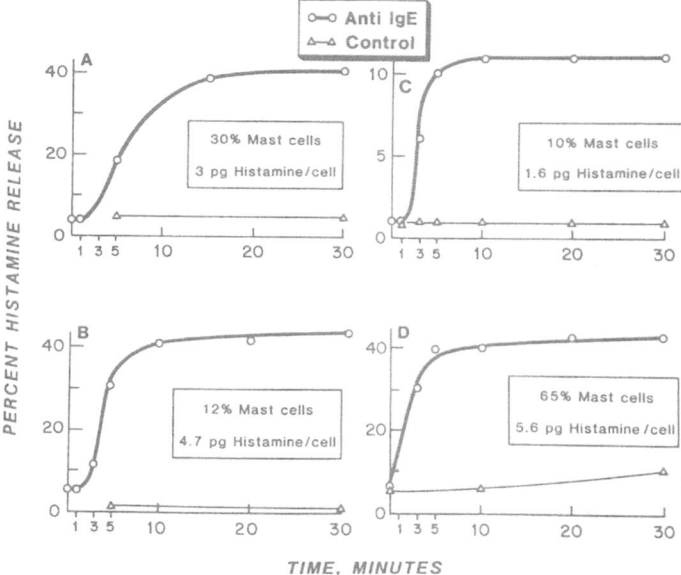

Figure 2.58 Mast cell purity, histamine content, and histamine release kinetics of isolated, partially purified human lung mast cells. △ — △ , control points; ○—○, anti-IgE-induced histamine release points. Concentration of anti-IgE: 3 μg/ml, experiments **A, C, D**; 2 μg/ml, experiment **B** (with permission, ref. 33)

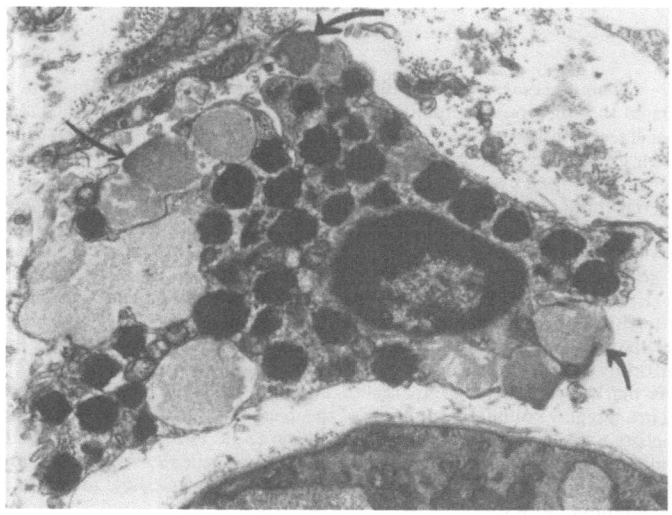

Figure 2.59 Heart mast cell *in vivo* shows anaphylactic degranulation characterized by formation of degranulation channels filled with swollen, altered granules and extrusion through plasma membrane pores of membrane-free swollen altered granules (arrows) (with permission, ref. 42). OCUB, ×9800

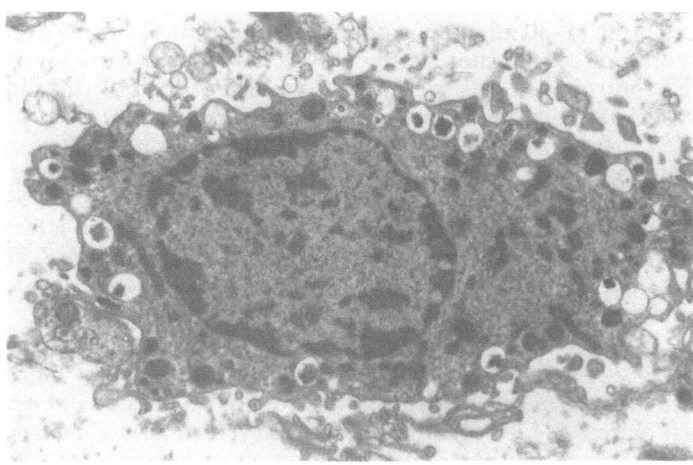

Figure 2.60 Mast cell *in vivo* from a kidney adenoma shows shedding of surface processes (with permission, ref. 35). OCUB, × 5900

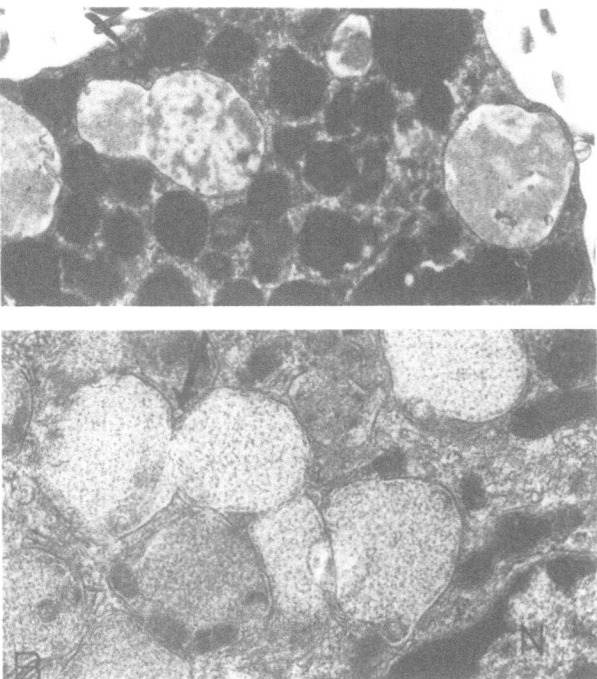

Figure 2.61 Isolated human lung mast cells fixed 1 minute after stimulation with anti-IgE show swelling and fusion of granules (arrows). In (**A**), the swollen, fused granules show focal ring patterns of lost contents in the altered granule matrix and numerous dense unaltered granules remain. N = nucleus. OCUB, (**A**) ×15 200; (**B**) ×23 100

after stimulation (1–30 minutes), and multiple early and later recovery intervals thereafter of cells in short-term cultures (30 minutes to 72 hours). Non-stimulated control mast cells were also examined at each of these intervals. The ultrastructural expression of certain aspects of these events *in vitro* (Figure 2.57) has allowed us to identify some of their counterparts in *in vivo* biopsy material. For example, degranulation channel formation and granule extrusion was present in interstitial cardiac mast cells in biopsies from two patients with unexplained cardiomyopathies of acute onset in a large series of 70 cardiac biopsies examined by electron microscopy (Figure 2.59)[42], and shedding of mast cell surface folds was evident from mast cells associated with a renal adenoma (Figure 2.60)[35].

Early degranulation period (1–30 minutes)[31, 33]: The earliest morphologic change which we were able to identify was swelling and fusion of cytoplasmic granules (Figure 2.61). Swollen granules displayed an altered matrix characterized by the spreading apart and dissolution of scrolls, particles and crystals (Figures 2.62, 63). Eventually, as tortuous chains of granules (Figure 2.64) widened and elongated to form cytoplasmic degranulation channels, the altered matrix pattern often no longer reflected recognizable granule substructural elements. Non-participating granules and lipid bodies did not show changes in their identifying substructural characteristics.

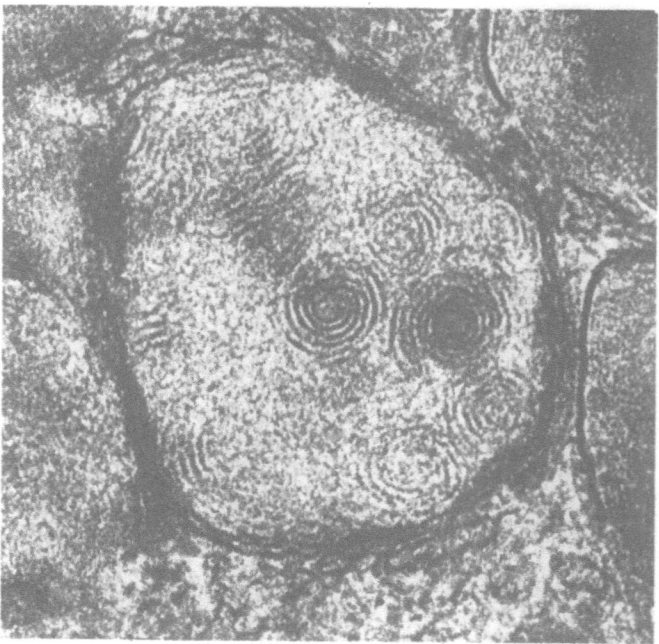

Figure 2.62 High magnification micrograph of isolated human lung mast cell granule fixed 3 minutes after stimulation with anti-IgE shows swelling and partial solubilization of scrolls (with permission, ref. 35). OCUB, ×105 000

70

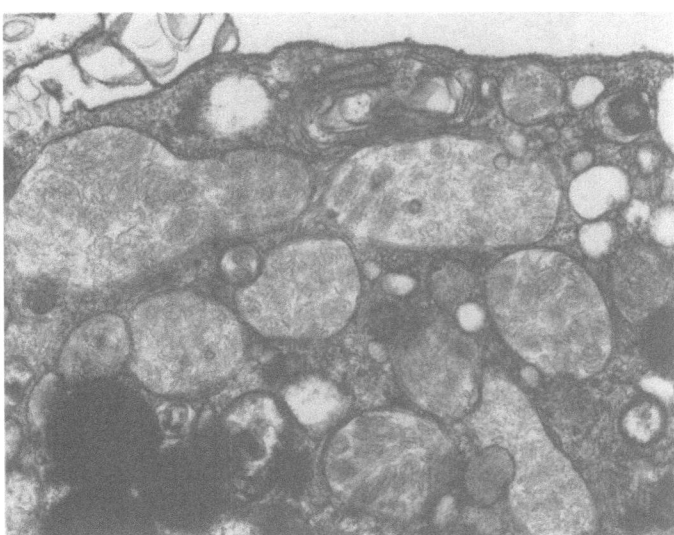

Figure 2.63 Isolated human lung mast cell fixed 15 minutes after stimulation with anti-IgE shows swelling of scroll granule contents characterized by spreading apart, stretching and dissolution of scroll structures. Several unaltered osmiophilic lipid bodies remain. OCUB, ×19 800

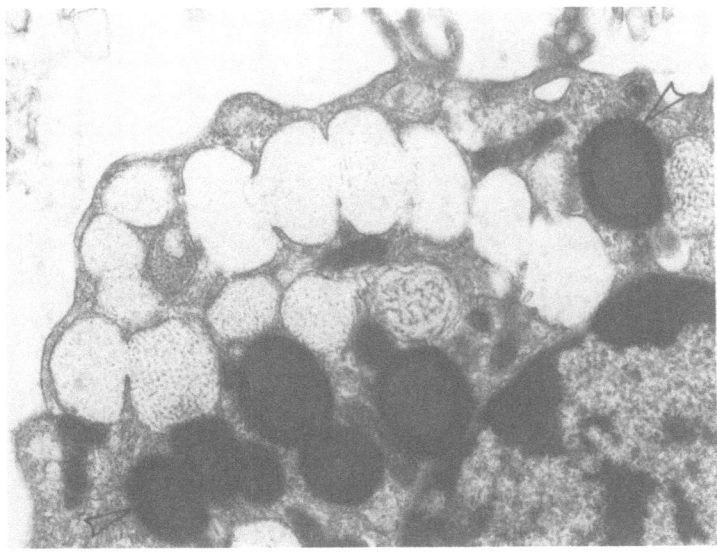

Figure 2.64 Isolated human lung mast cell fixed 3 minutes after stimulation with anti-IgE shows the formation of chains of interconnected, fused granules with altered contents. Lipid bodies (arrowheads). OCUB, ×17 500

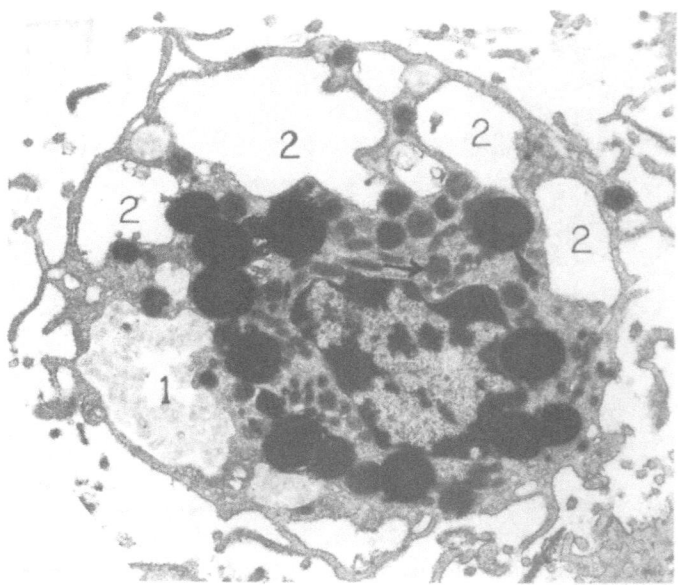

Figure 2.65 Isolated human lung mast cell fixed 10 minutes after stimulation with anti-IgE shows a mixture of closed (1) and open (2) degranulation channels. Closed channels (1) contain altered granule material and their membranes do not bind cationized ferritin; open channels (2) are devoid of granule materials and, like the plasma membrane, their membranes bind cationized ferritin. Numerous unaltered lipid bodies abound (arrowhead). A few unaltered granules remain (arrow) (with permission, ref. 11). OCUB, CF, ×8400

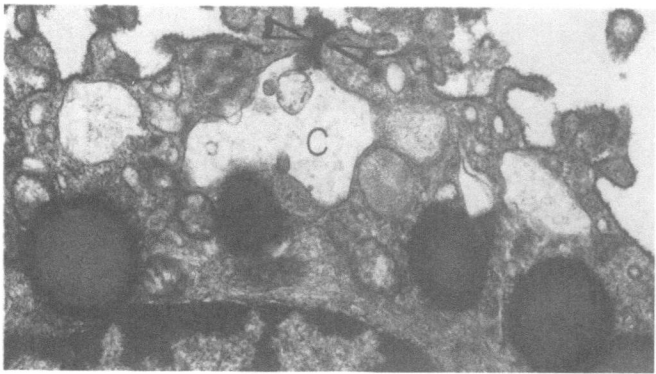

Figure 2.66 Isolated human lung mast cell fixed 20 minutes after exposure to anti-IgE shows a narrow opening of a degranulation channel (C) to the cell's exterior. This pore is filled with cationized ferritin (arrowheads). OCUB, CF, ×18 700

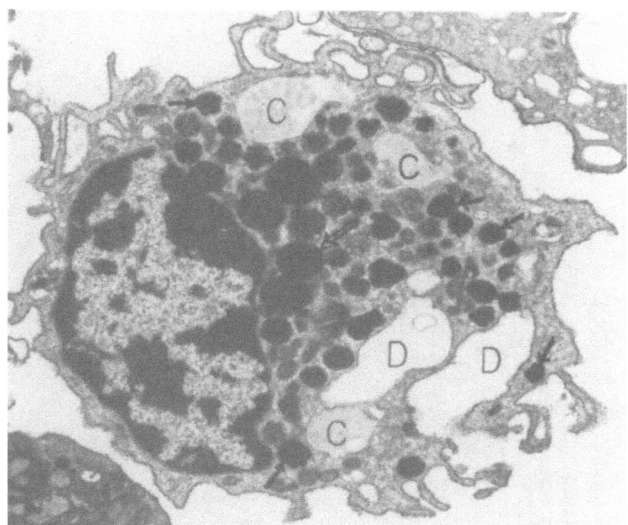

Figure 2.67 Isolated human lung mast cell fixed 5 minutes after exposure to anti-IgE shows a mixture of open, empty, cationized ferritin-stained degranulation channels (D), closed channels filled with altered granule matrix materials (C), unaltered scroll granules (arrows) and lipid bodies (open arrow) (with permission, ref. 33). OCUB, CF, ×8450

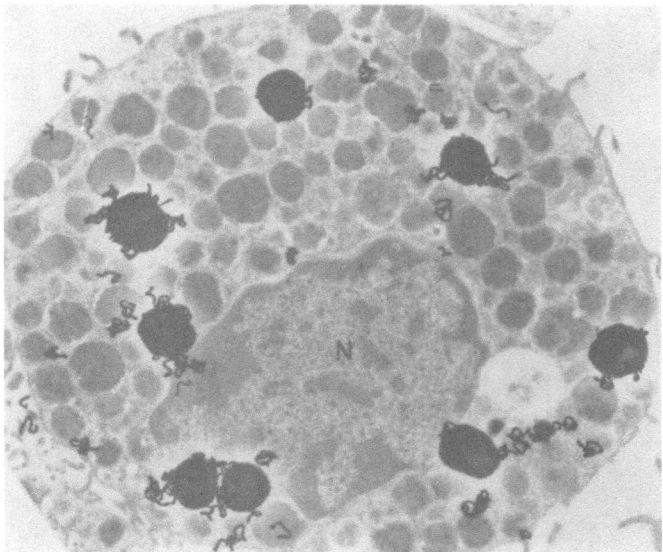

Figure 2.68 Isolated lung mast cell exposed to [³H]arachidonic acid before fixation shows numerous silver grains incorporated into lipid bodies. N = nucleus (with permission, ref. 30). OCUB, [³H]AA, ×6500

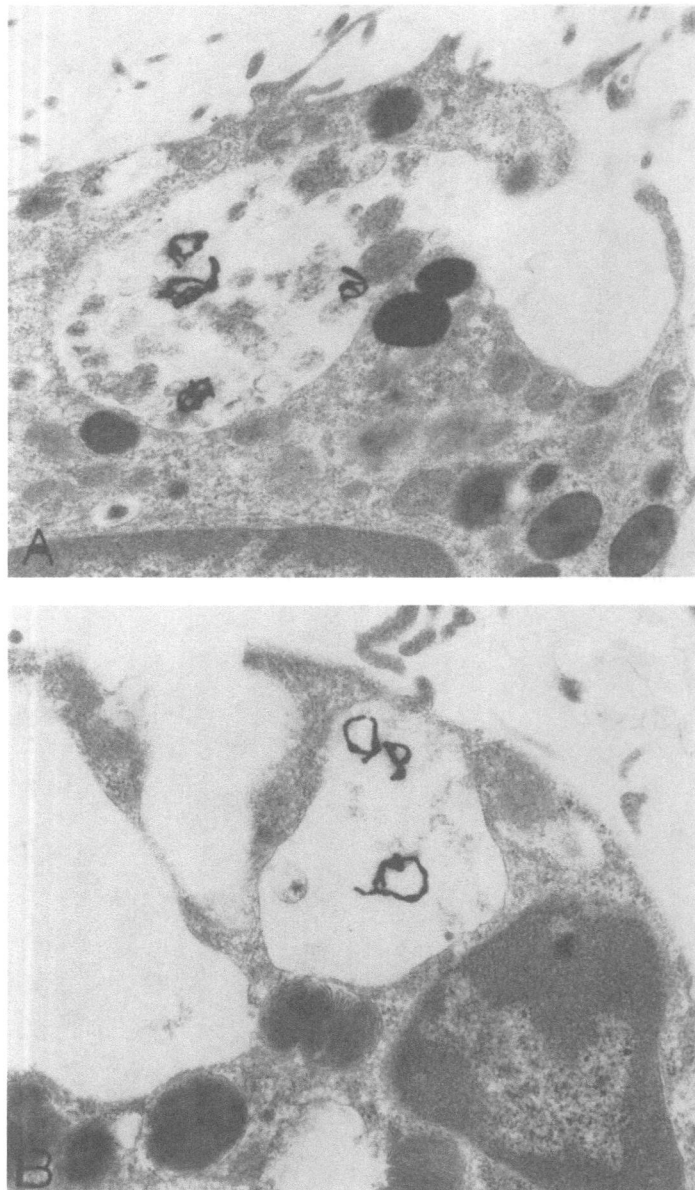

Figure 2.69   Isolated lung mast cells exposed to [³H]arachidonic acid and fixed 15 minutes after stimulation with anti-IgE show silver grains in cytoplasmic degranulation channels. OCUB, (**A**) ×17 000; (**B**) ×21 500

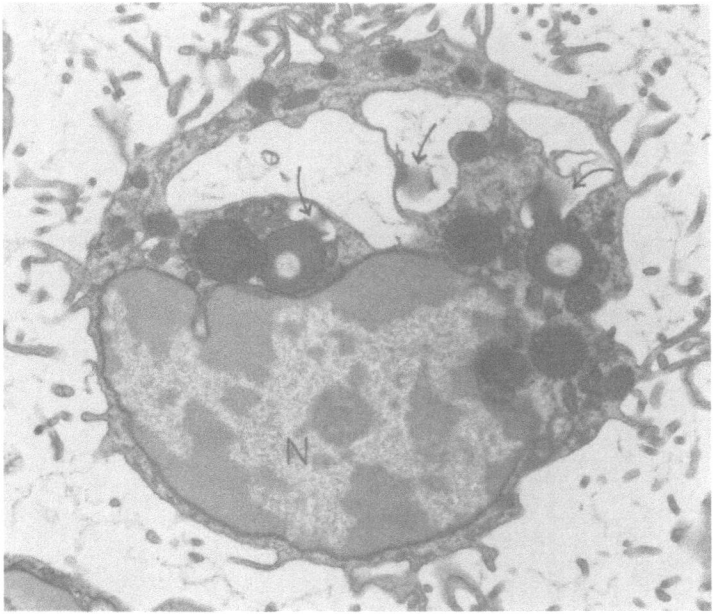

Figure 2.70 Isolated lung mast cell fixed 20 minutes after exposure to anti-IgE shows lipid bodies releasing contents into degranulation channels (arrows). N = nucleus (with permission, ref. 31). OPF, ×9000

Initially, large intercommunicating degranulation channels filled with altered matrix material were closed to the exterior, as determined by exclusion of various ultrastructural tracers (Fig. 2.65). These then opened to the cells' exterior through multiple narrow pores (Figure 2.66) throughout the circumference of the cell and released their solubilized granule materials. The empty channels now permeated the cells' cytoplasm, much like a sponge, and were accessible to extracellular electron-dense tracers (Figures 2.65, 67).

Lipid bodies (Figure 2.68), non-membrane-bound, homogeneously dense, rounded structures enmeshed in intermediate filaments adjacent to degranulation channels were rarely observed to release [3H]arachidonic acid ([3H]AA)-labelled lipid material (Figure 2.68) into degranulation channels (Figure 2.69). Although release of the contents of individual lipid bodies into degranulation channels was observed (Figure 2.70) and some individual cells displayed large numbers of lipid bodies, we found no significant change in the volume distribution of lipid bodies in the first 20 minutes following degranulation (Figure 2.71)[31]. By contrast, the volume distribution of cytoplasmic granules decreased 77% in the same time period (Figure 2.71). These morphometric data correlated with biochemical measurements of the release of [3H] lipids[43] and histamine[33].

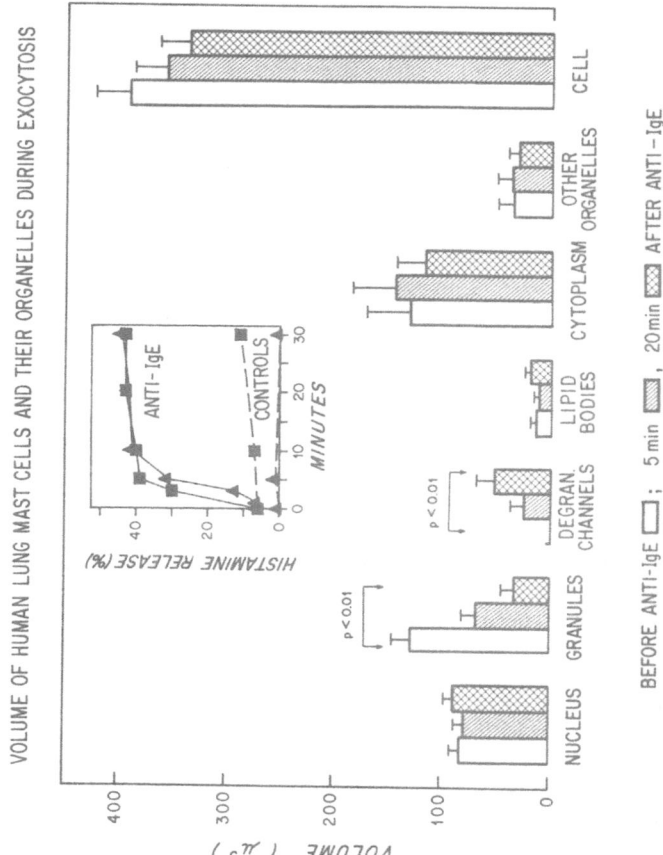

Figure 2.71 Quantitative analysis of human lung mast cell cellular and organelle volumes before and 5 or 20 minutes after stimulation with anti-IgE *in vitro*. Cells from two experiments that gave similar levels of histamine release (see inset) were analysed. Significant changes in organelle volume associated with degranulation are indicated (Student's *t*-test) (with permission, ref. 31).

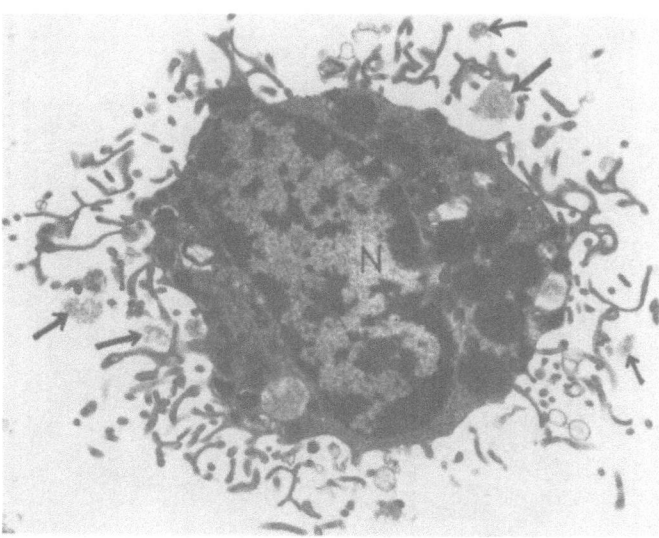

Figure 2.72 Isolated human lung mast cell fixed 20 minutes after exposure to anti-IgE shows extruded membrane-free, swollen granules (arrows) among markedly elongated and shed surface folds. N = nucleus. OCUB, ×7000

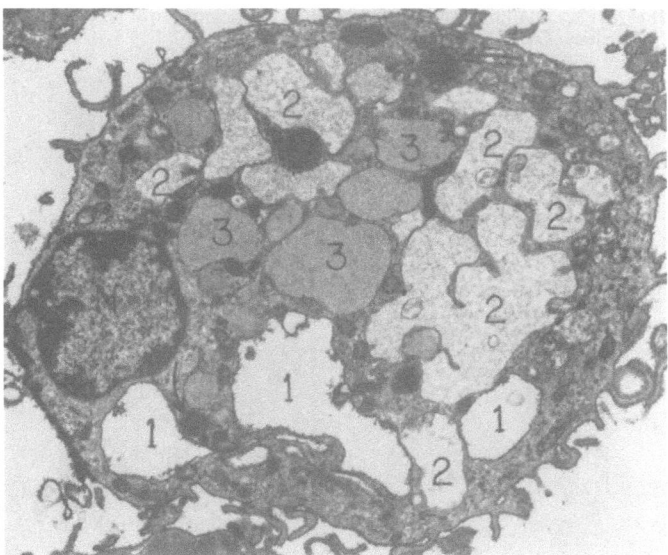

Figure 2.73 Isolated lung mast cell fixed 3 hours after stimulation with anti-IgE shows early recovery from degranulation. Some degranulation channels are empty and remain open as determined by the ability of cationized ferritin to stain their membranes (1); some degranulation channels show loosely structured contents and increased tortuosity (2); some degranulation channels have early condensation of contents and separation of new granule domains (3). Lipid bodies are present. N = nucleus (with permission, ref. 41). OCUB, CF, ×8100

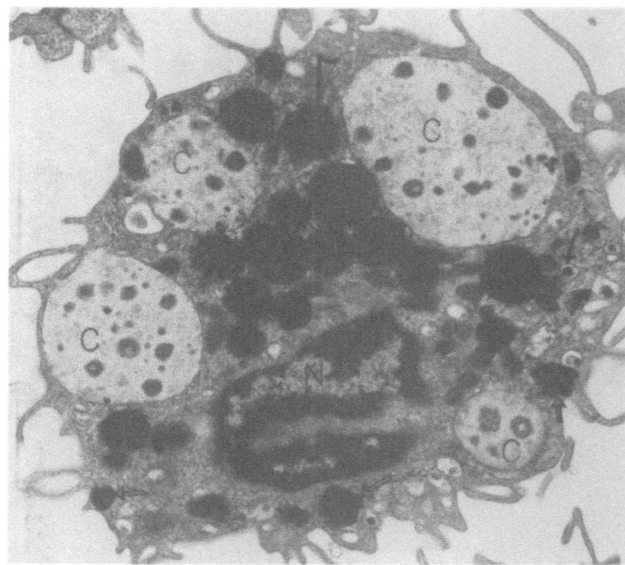

Figure 2.74 Isolated lung mast cell fixed 24 hours after stimulation with anti-IgE shows crystallization foci of dense granule contents in a less dense background matrix in large, resolving degranulation channels (C). Numerous large osmiophilic lipid bodies are present (arrowhead) as well as small progranules (arrows). Several new mature granules are seen (open arrows). N = nucleus. OCUB, ×7800

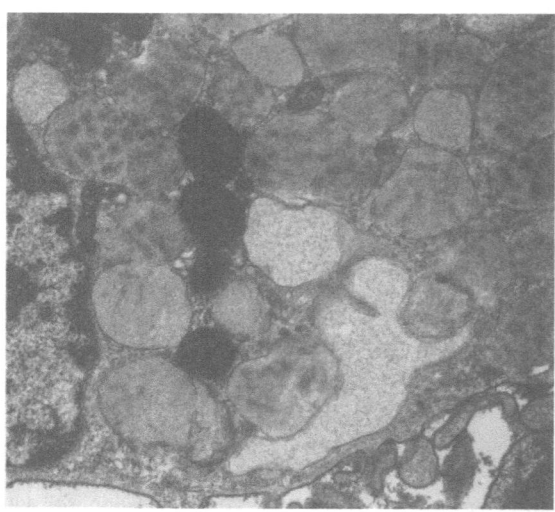

Figure 2.75 Isolated lung mast cell fixed 3 hours after exposure to anti-IgE shows progressive tortuosity, condensation, crystallization and separation of granule domains from recovering degranulation channels. Dense lipid bodies are adjacent to restructured granules (with permission, ref. 40). OCUB, CF, ×19 200

78

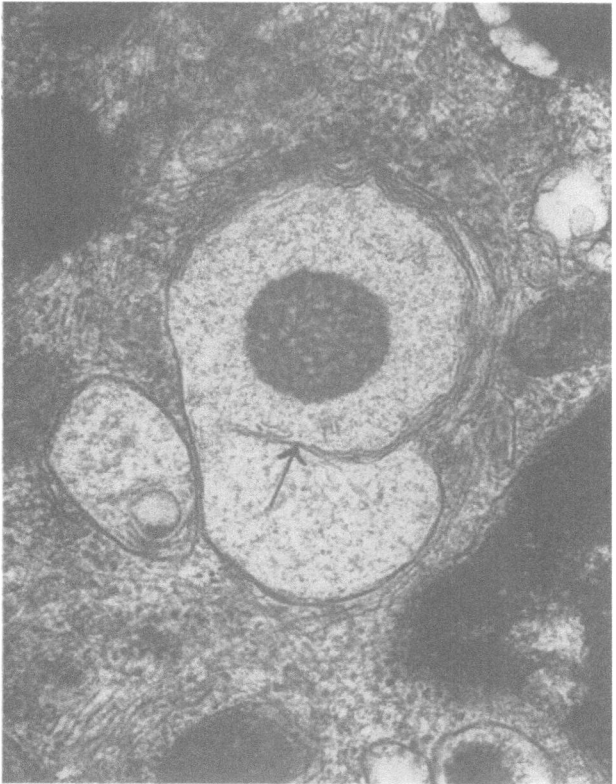

Figure 2.76 Isolated lung mast cell fixed 48 hours after exposure to anti-IgE shows condensation of a particulate nucleoid within less dense matrix in restructuring granules. Note the membrane which nearly separates two granules (arrow) (with permission, ref. 40). OCUB, ×49 700

Rarely, in one of a total of seven kinetic experiments, we observed extrusion of individual non-membrane-bound altered granule matrix material to the cells' exterior (Figure 2.72)

Early recovery period (3–24 hours)[40]: Although some overlap was evident, we were able to identify morphologic events characteristic of early recovery times and of late recovery intervals following degranulation. The initiating event for each of these patterns reflected the mechanism of resoluton of degranulation channels. Although individual cells preferentially entered one or the other recovery pathways, we also found cells with the simultaneous expression of both recovery pathway morphologies. These mixed patterns contributed considerable complexity to the analysis of recovery from anaphylactic degranulation of human mast cells.

Early recovery from anaphylactic degranulation of human mast cells was stimulated by the sealing of degranulation pores and channels (or their failure

79

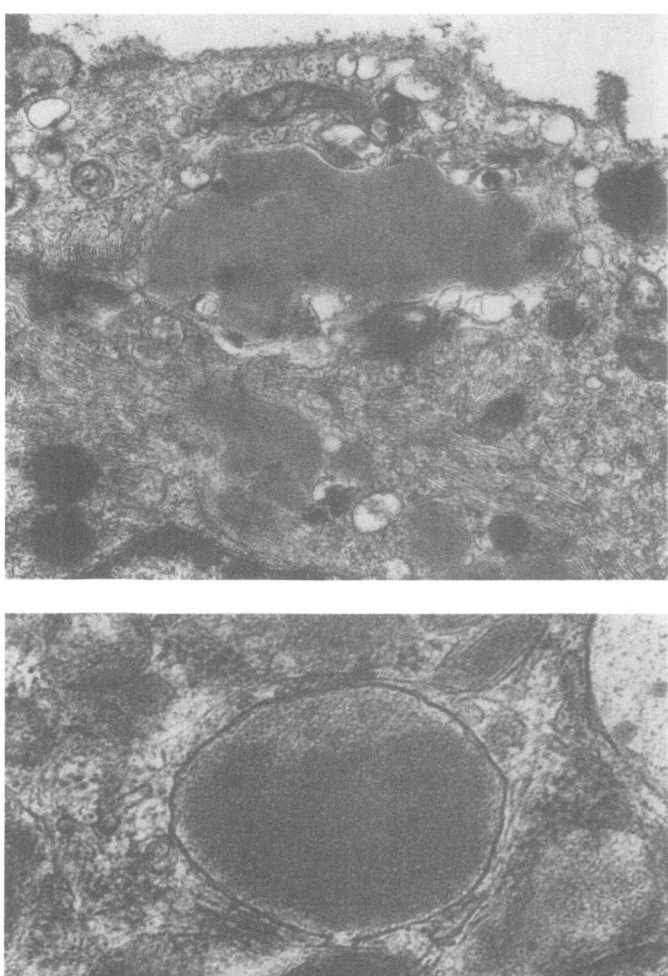

Figure 2.77 Isolated lung mast cells fixed 48 hours (**A**) and 12 hours (**B**) after stimulation with anti-IgE show newly-formed crystal granules. In (**A**), crystallization and condensation in a previous degranulation channel gives rise to a large irregularly-shaped structure; in (**B**), a separated crystallized single granule has formed. Note free ribosomes in adjacent cytoplasm (with permission, ref. 40). OCUB, CF, (**A**) ×23 100; (**B**) ×49 100

to open). We were also able to say that some channels, once open, had resealed, by observing completely empty channels within the cytoplasm which did not admit extracellular tracers. More frequently, closed channels in the recovery period did not admit tracers and did contain solubilized granule materials. Initially, these materials were unstructured and only lightly dense in vast, lucent backgrounds (Figure 2.73). Condensation of channel contents occurred as channels decreased in length and width and developed increased tortuosities (Figure 2.73). Some large channels displayed foci of dense granule materials in a less dense matrix (Figure 2.74). Eventually channel contents came to fill granule-sized domains (Figures 2.75, 76) within which condensation and crystallization of content materials was visible (Figures 2.75–77). Collections of minute lipid bodies, vesicles and cytoplasmic invaginations into channels (Figures 2.78–82) participated in

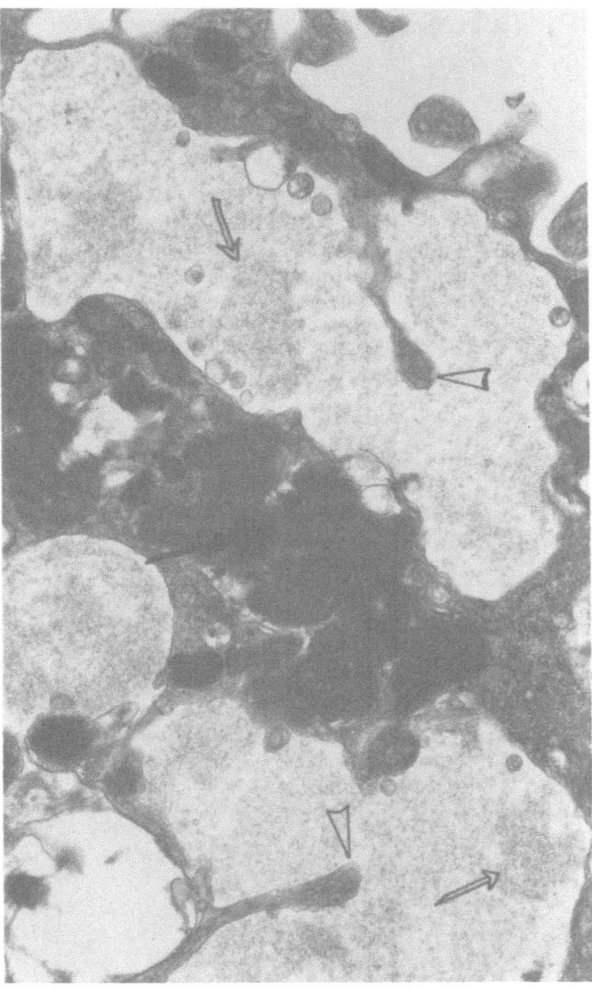

Figure 2.78 Isolated lung mast cell fixed 24 hours after stimulation with anti-IgE shows recovering degranulation channels. Channels with less condensed contents show focal granule-sized domains of increased condensation associated with vesicles (open arrows) and elongated invaginations of cytoplasmic processes (arrowheads). Channels with markedly condensed contents also contain small osmiophilic lipid bodies (arrow). OCUB, ×18 900

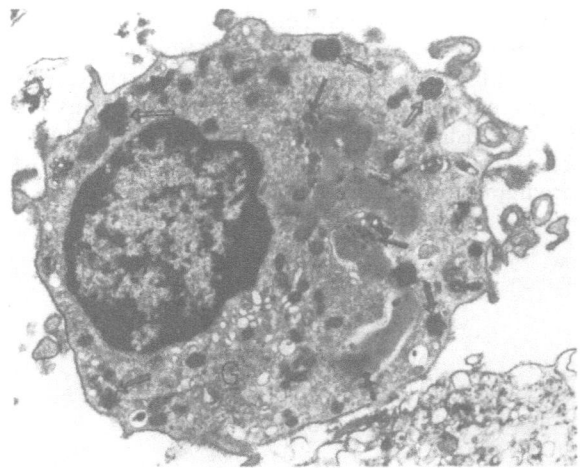

Figure 2.79 Isolated lung mast cell fixed 48 hours after stimulation with anti-IgE shows nearly complete condensation of contents in resolving degranulation channels. These channels also contain numerous small, dense lipid bodies (arrows) between condensed contents and overlying channel-granule membranes. Golgi area (G) contains numerous vesicles and vacuoles. Newly-formed mature granules are seen in increased numbers (open arrows) (with permission, ref. 40). OCUB, CF, ×8400

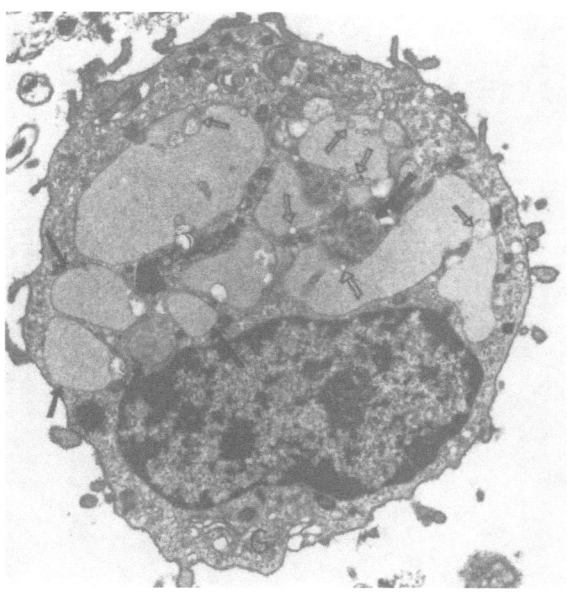

Figure 2.80 Isolated lung mast cell fixed 24 hours after stimulation with anti-IgE shows development of granule domains (arrows) with crystallization foci from recovering degranulation channels. These channels also contain numerous vesicles (open arrows). Golgi (G) area expansion is present. The immature nucleus contains a large nucleolus and chromatin is partially dispersed. OCUB, CF, ×7500

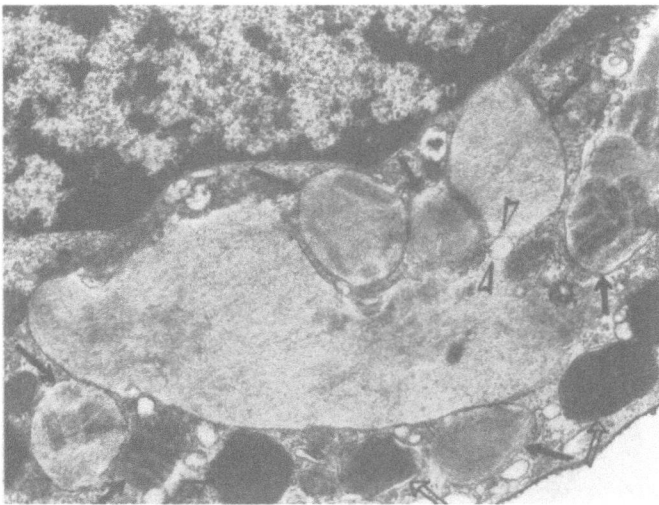

Figure 2.81 Isolated lung mast cell fixed 48 hours after stimulation shows partitioning of new granule domains (arrows) from recovering degranulation channels. Note the vesicle at one granule separation point (arrowheads). New mature granules are plentiful (open arrows). OCUB, CF, ×19 900

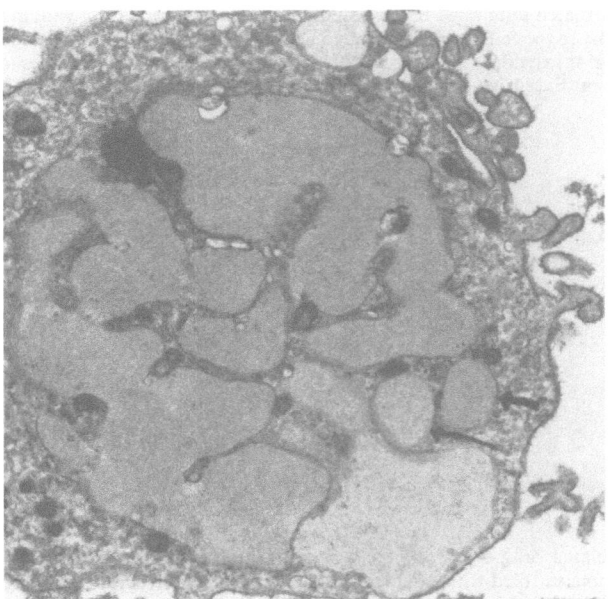

Figure 2.82 Isolated lung mast cell fixed 12 hours after stimulation with anti-IgE shows granules separating (arrows) from recovering degranulation channels. Increased cytoplasmic filaments and ribosomes are adjacent to resolving channel-granules. OCUB, CF, ×11 400

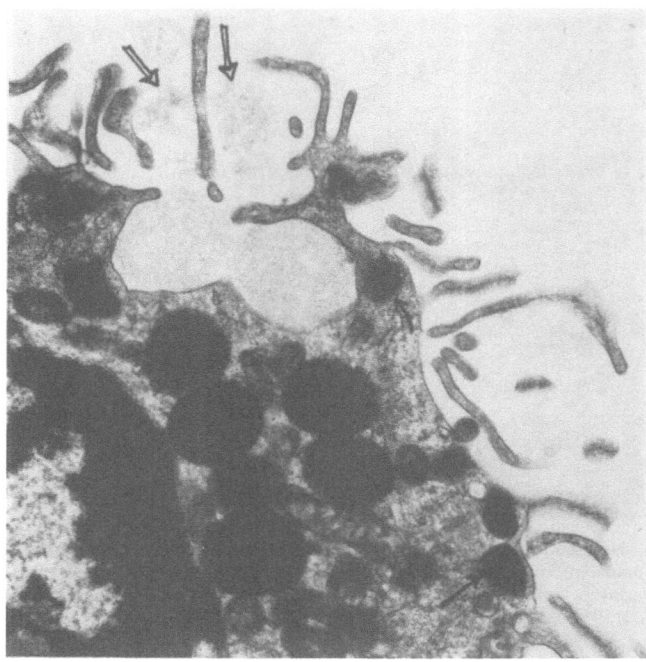

Figure 2.83 Isolated lung mast cell fixed 20 minutes after stimulation with anti-IgE shows a widely open pore to the cell's exterior through which rapidly solubilizing, altered granule matrix materials are being extruded (open arrows). Unaltered lipid bodies and granules (arrows) remain in the cytoplasm. Extensive elongated surface folds are present. OCUB, ×18 200

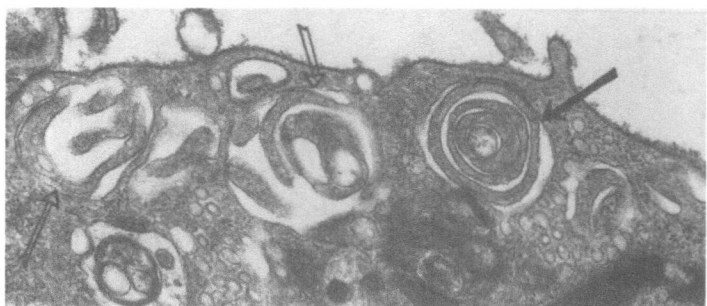

Figure 84 Isolated lung mast cell fixed 3 hours after stimulation with anti-IgE shows a peripheral cytoplasm filled with canalicular structures. These structures are filled with surface folds, some of which remain attached and some of which appear detached. Cationized ferritin binds to the cell surface and to the membranes of a surface fold-containing canaliculus (arrow) demonstrating surface continuity at another section plane. Two canaliculi are closed and do not stain with cationized ferritin (open arrows). OCUB, CF, ×22 100

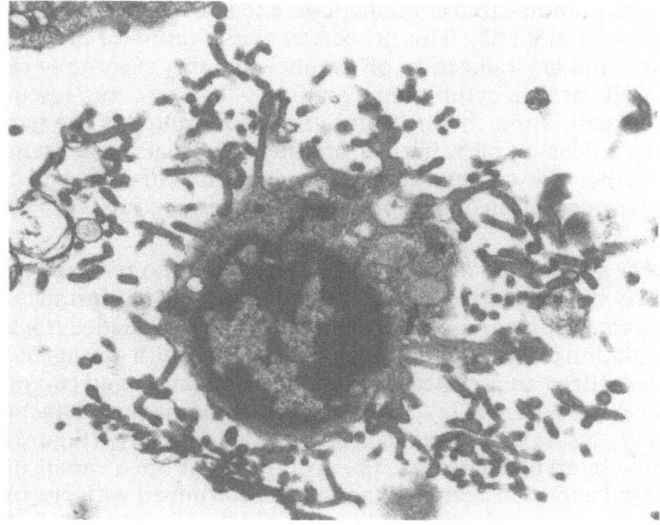

Figure 2.85 Isolated lung mast cell fixed 20 minutes after exposure to anti-IgE shows massive shedding of numerous elongated, cationized ferritin-stained surface folds. Several granules remain in the cytoplasm (arrows). OCUB, CF, ×10 900

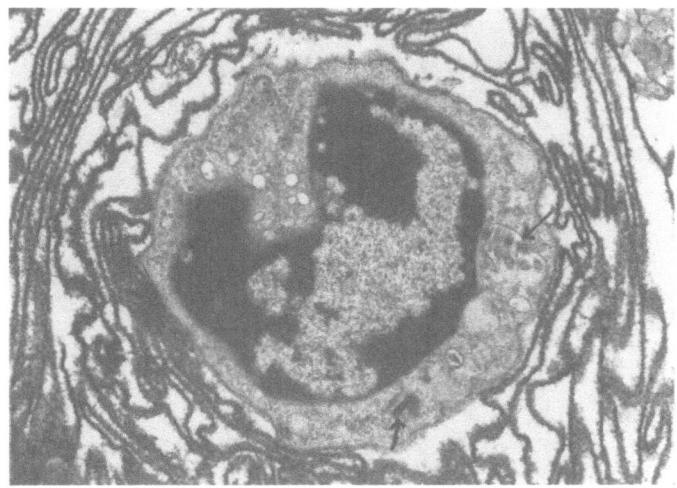

Figure 2.86 Isolated lung mast cell fixed 30 minutes after stimulation with anti-IgE is small and has a condensed nucleus, and a narrow rim of cytoplasm which contains vesicles and several scroll granules (arrows). The surface profile is smooth and the cell is surrounded by free, cationized ferritin-stained cellular membranes (with permission, ref. 33). OCUB, CF, ×10 500

partitioning as granule-sized containers were remodelled from degranulation channels (Figures 2.80, 82). This process of conservation of membranes and condensation and crystallization of channel contents eventually resulted in separated well-formed cytoplasmic granules. This process resembled the reverse of degranulation channel formation and resulted in the repackaging of materials, at least in part, in their original containers, e.g. granule membranes. Whether the contents represent a mixture of new and reutilized materials or condensation of only previous granule materials is not yet known.

Late recovery period (18–48 hours)[36, 41]: Mast cells also resolved degranulation channels by exteriorizing their membranes. In this instance, initially narrow degranulation pores open to the cells' exterior widened (Figure 2.83), and degranulation channel membranes in continuity with plasma membranes became externalized and created considerable elongation and complexities to surface processes (Figure 2.72). Recovery of membranes and detached as well as attached processes was observed in canalicular structures (Figure 2.84). As recovery time intervals increased, the proportion of open canalicular structures increased and then decreased again, as determined with electron-dense tracers. Also, many such canaliculi were initially peripherally located. As

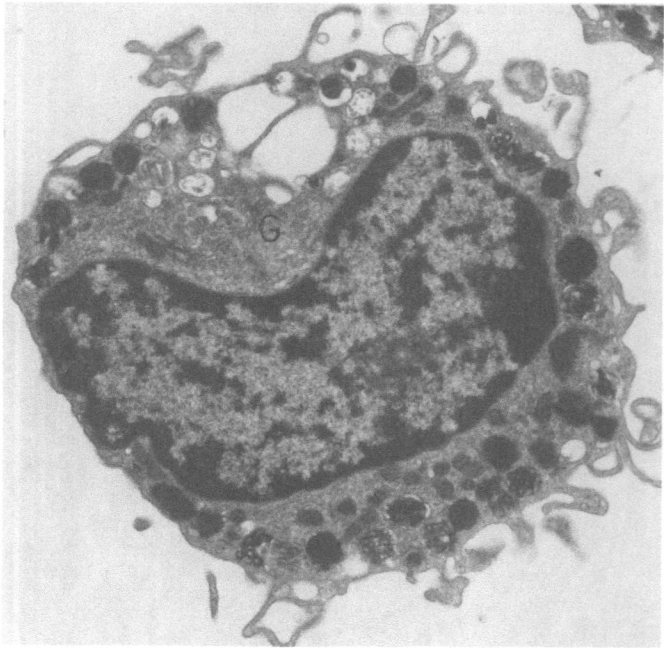

Figure 2.87 Isolated lung mast cell fixed 24 hours after exposure to anti-IgE shows blast transformation. The large nucleus is undergoing chromatin dispersion and a large nucleolus is present. Mature granules are present in the peripheral cytoplasm. An expanded Golgi (G) area has large vacuoles, vesicles, multivesicular bodies and progranules. OCUB, ×10 300

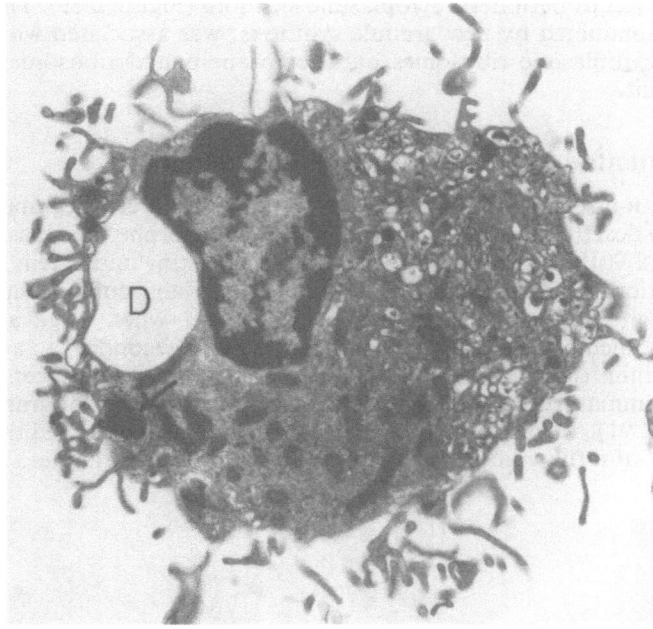

Figure 2.88 Isolated lung mast cell fixed 18 hours after stimulation with anti-IgE shows expanded Golgi area filled with vesicles and progranules. Several mature granules (arrow) and residual degranulation channel (D) remain. OCUB, ×10 500

these structures closed, they moved to occupy more central locations in the cytoplasm. These large, completely degranulated, recovering mast cells did not undergo appreciable size reductions prior to the onset of the synthesis of new granules.

Rather than endocytose expanded surface structures, some mast cells shed them completely (Figure 2.85). Thus, not only were all mast cell granules shed but large amounts of membranes and surface processes were simultaneously shed. This process resulted in considerable size reduction of viable mast cells which typically displayed smooth, shorn surfaces (Figure 2.86). Smooth mast cell surfaces, in our experience, are only seen following such a shedding process. These small mast cells (7 microns) had condensed nuclei surrounded by a very narrow cytoplasmic rim and were identifiable by the presence of at least one residual mast cell granule.

Later recovery events were characterized by two morphologic processes: (1) blastogenesis, and (2) synthesis of new granules. Morphologically, blast transformation of small mast cells was characterized by the appearance of nucleoli, dispersion of condensed chromatin and nuclear enlargement (Figure 2.87). Cytoplasm also expanded as Golgi structures enlarged and new progranules developed there (Figure 2.88). Widespread increases in cytoplasmic vesicles were noted and small progranules and immature granules came to occupy peripheral cytoplasmic locations (Figure 2.89). This recovery phase, dominated by new granule synthesis, was associated with increases in free cytoplasmic ribosomes but membrane-bound ribosomes remained infrequent.

Fine structure of human mast cell maturation

Observations obtained in the studies of human mast cell degranulation and recovery described above allowed us to identify morphologic mast cell cycles (Figure 2.90)[36]. We observed that mature, resting mast cells in control preparations maintained a fairly constant size and complement of cyto- plasmic granules. This size balance was upset when large amounts of granules, membranes and surface folds were shed secondary to a degranula- tion stimulus (Figures 2.85, 86, 90). The resultant small mast cells displayed signs of immaturity as nuclear blast changes and synthesis of granules began (Figure 2.91). Nuclear and cytoplasmic size increases preceded the re-estab- lishment of a full complement of mature cytoplasmic granules. These large

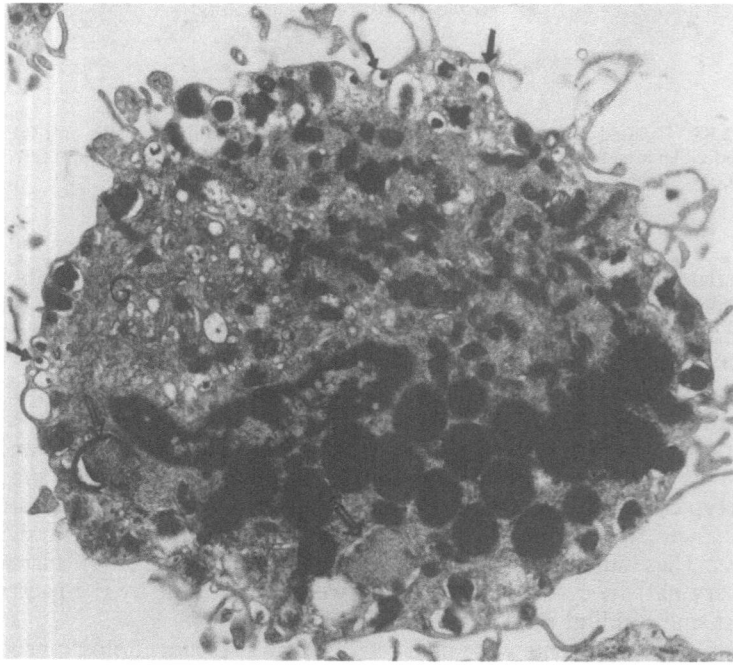

Figure 2.89 Isolated lung mast cell fixed 36 hours after stimulation with anti-IgE shows exten- sive increases in cytoplasmic vesicles, vacuoles and progranules (arrows). Many progranules occupy peripheral cytoplasmic areas. The Golgi area (G) is expanded. Several mature particle granules are present (open arrows). The remainder of the cytoplasm is filled with lipid bodies and mitochondria. Rough endoplasmic reticulum is conspicuously absent. Most surface folds now appear attached to the cell. OCUB, ×9500

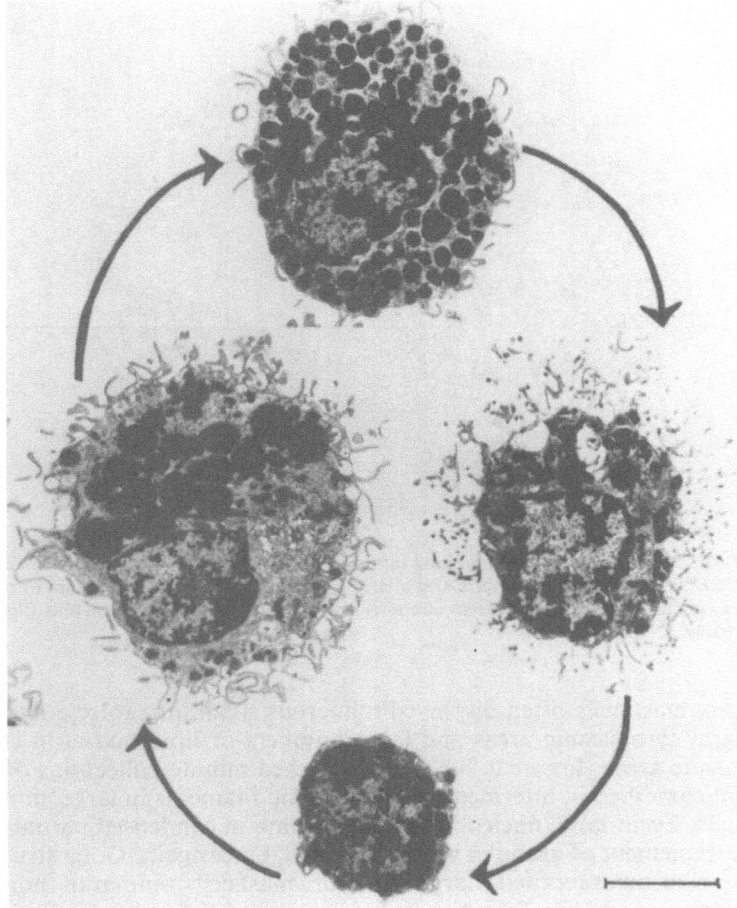

Figure 2.90 Montage of isolated, purified, cultured control and anti-IgE stimulated human lung mast cells. Clockwise starting at the top. Mature mast cell in culture for 18 hours shows a full complement of cytoplasmic granules and eight dense non-membrane-bound lipid bodies which cluster near the centrally-located, monolobed nucleus. The nucleus shows a partially condensed pattern. Nucleoli are absent. The surface is adorned with narrow surface folds.

At 20 minutes post-stimulus, this mast cell is actively shedding membranes and surface processes. Nearly all cytoplasmic granules have been released. Two lipid bodies and several mast cell granules remain.

Small, lymphocyte-sized mast cell recovered 6 hours after stimulation has five remaining cytoplasmic granules and a uniformly narrow rim of cytoplasm within which vesicles are located. The surface is free of processes and displays only a few angular protrusions. The single-lobed nucleus occupies nearly the entire area of the cell. The nuclear chromatin is completely condensed. A large nucleolus is present.

Large immature mast cell recovered 24 hours after stimulation. Nuclear chromatin is dispersed and a large nucleolus is seen. Numerous elongated narrow surface folds are present. These all display connections to the cell. The cytoplasm is filled with large dense lipid bodies. An expanded Golgi area is actively producing progranules which are moving to occupy distant cytoplasmic areas (with permission, ref. 36). OCUB, ×4100. Bar = 4 microns

89

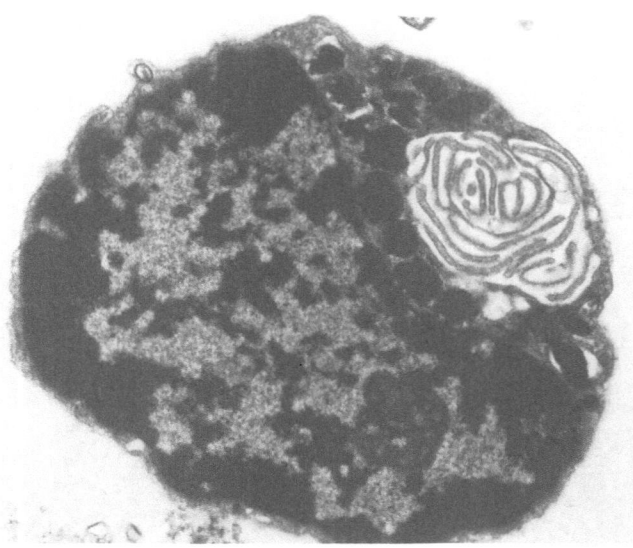

Figure 2.91 Small immature isolated lung mast cell fixed 18 hours after exposure to anti-IgE. The nucleus has condensed chromatin and a large nucleolus. The surface is devoid of folds or processes. A narrow rim of cytoplasm contains several granules and a canaliculus filled with surface folds. OCUB, ×12 900

immature mast cells often displayed numerous small immature granules in peripheral cytoplasmic areas and large numbers of lipid bodies in central cytoplasmic areas (Figure 2.90). We also noted minute collections of lipid material enmeshed in intermediate cytoplasmic filaments in large immature mast cells. Eventually, nucleoli receded, chromatin condensed partially and a full complement of granules was established. Once again, Golgi structures and free ribosomes receded. Large immature mast cells, similar to those described here, are readily found at sites of increased tissue mast cells *in vivo* (Figure 2.46). Mast cells can also divide *in vivo*. Such replicating mast cells also undergo cell size changes, thus providing another mechanism for mast cell size reduction and increase during replication and subsequent maturation of mast cells. The *in vitro* recovery intervals we examined were not characterized by cell division as a mechanism for producing small immature mast cells.

Large, immature mast cells (Figure 2.90) are similar in size to large, immature basophils or basophilic myelocytes (Figure 2.35)[14]. No other similarities exist, however, and comparison of these differences should allow one to differentiate large immature mast cells from large basophilic myelocytes. For example, mast cells have very small immature granules – much smaller than their mature granules – and do not display an extensive network of expanded cisternae of rough endoplasmic reticulum (Figure 2.90). Basophilic myelocytes characteristically display the latter and their immature granules are very large – much larger than their mature granules (Figure 2.35).

Human mast cell lipid bodies, the morphological hallmark of activation

Lipid bodies are spherical, variably dense, non-membrane-bound organelles found in many types of mammalian cells[30, 44], as well as in human mast cells (Figure 2.92)[30]. We have noted increases in these structures in mast cells examined in biopsies of various inflammatory (Figure 2.93) and neoplastic disorders. These mast cells *in vivo* may also, but not necessarily, show piecemeal degranulation. We have come to associate the presence of increased numbers of lipid bodies with mast cell activation *in vivo* and/or recovery from degranulation *in vitro*. Not only do mast cell lipid bodies differ morphologically from mast cell granules[30, 31], they are dissimilar in their postulated mode of generation[32], and in their behaviour during anaphylactic degranulation[31, 33] and recovery from degranulation[36, 40, 41]. We carried out ultrastructural autoradiographic experiments that also revealed differences in the contents of human mast cell lipid bodies (Figure 2.94) and granules (Figure 2.95)[30, 31]. We found that radiolabelled sulphur could be localized to granules (Figure 2.95), not lipid bodies, reflecting the presence of sulphur-containing glycosaminoglycans in granules, not lipid bodies. By contrast, tritium-labelled arachidonic acid ([³H]AA) was localized to lipid bodies (Figure 2.94), not granules, thereby implicating these enigmatic organelles in the storage and/or metabolism of arachidonic acid, the precursor of

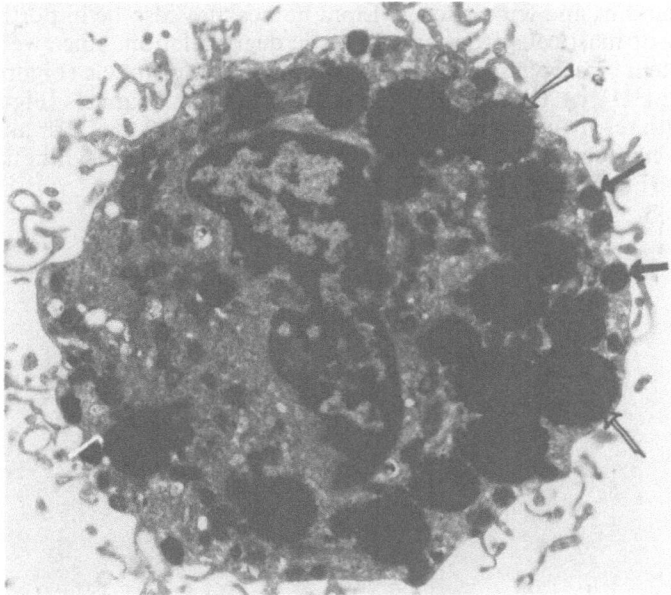

Figure 2.92 Isolated lung mast cell fixed 6 hours after stimulation with anti-IgE has large numbers of osmiophilic cytoplasmic lipid bodies (open arrows) and small numbers of mature granules (arrows). OCUB, ×9800

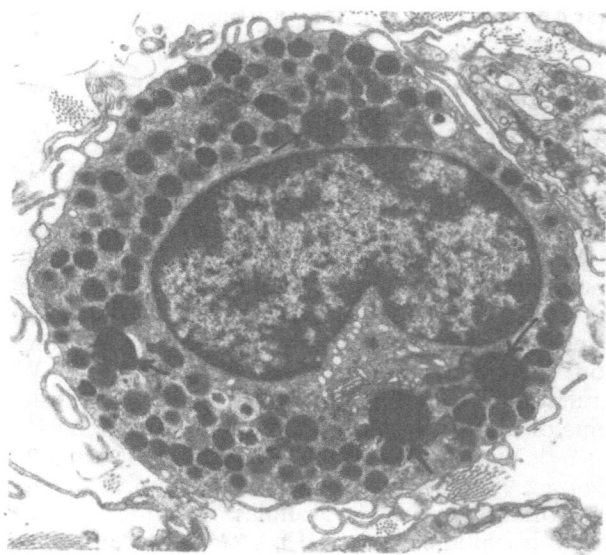

Figure 2.93 Gut mast cell *in vivo* from the resected ileal specimen from a patient with Crohn's disease has large lipid bodies (arrows) and many granules in the cytoplasm. OCUB, ×5900

prostaglandins and leukotrienes. Lipid bodies may also be important to the recovery of mast cells from anaphylactic degranulation, since we routinely found them closely associated with degranulation channels (Figure 2.96)[31], releasing [3H]AA-labelled lipids into degranulation channels (Figures 2.69, 97)[31], with resolving degranulation channels (Figures 2.78, 79)[40] and present in large numbers in large immature mast cells actively synthesizing new granules (Figure 2.98)[36,41].

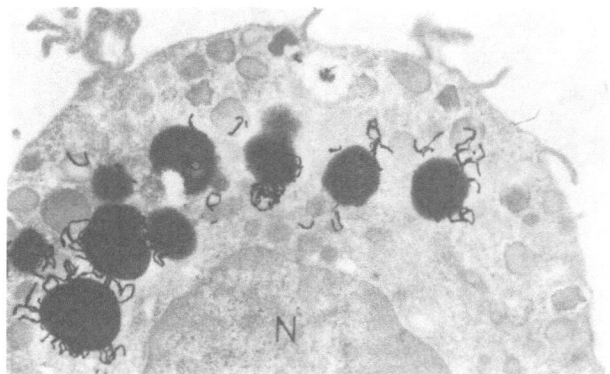

Figure 2.94 Autoradiograph of isolated lung mast cell fixed after exposure to tritium-labelled arachidonic acid shows numerous silver grains incorporated into large dense lipid bodies but not into smaller, less dense granules. N = nucleus. OCUB, [3H]AA, ×14000

92

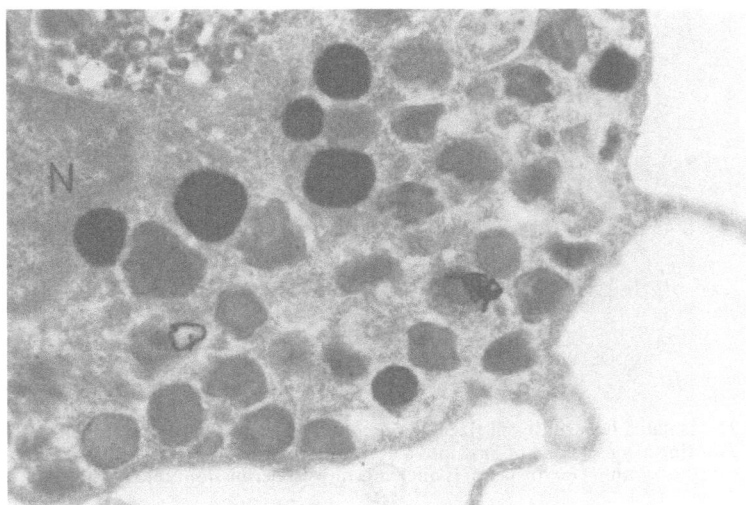

Figure 2.95 Autoradiograph of isolated lung mast cell fixed after exposure to radiclabelled sulphur shows silver grains overlying granules but not lipid bodies. N = nucleus. OCUB, ^{35}S, ×19 200

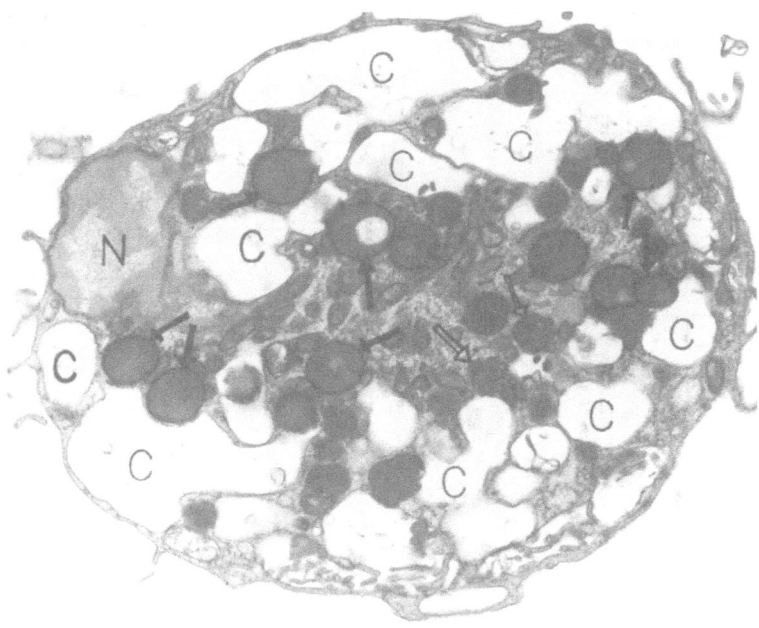

Figure 2.96 Isolated lung mast cell fixed 20 minutes after exposure to anti-IgE shows close associations of lipid bodies (arrows) and empty degranulation channels (C). Granules (open arrows). N = nucleus. OPF, ×11 200

93

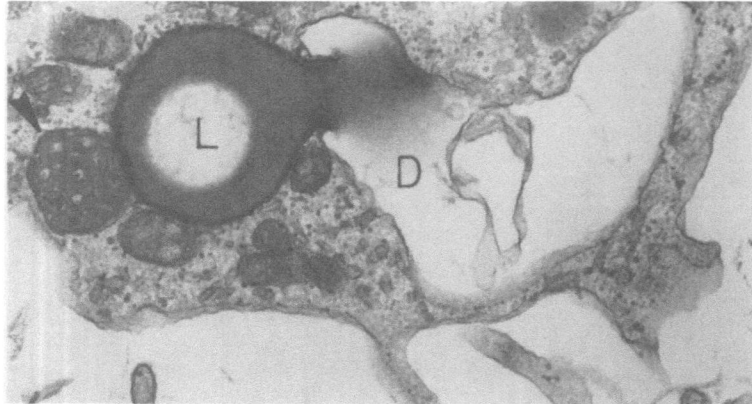

Figure 2.97 Isolated lung mast cell fixed 20 minutes after exposure to anti-IgE shows a lipid body (L) squirting a dense cloud of lipid into a degranulation channel (D) within the cytoplasm. An adjacent scroll granule (arrowhead) is unchanged (with permission, ref. 31). OPF, ×31 200

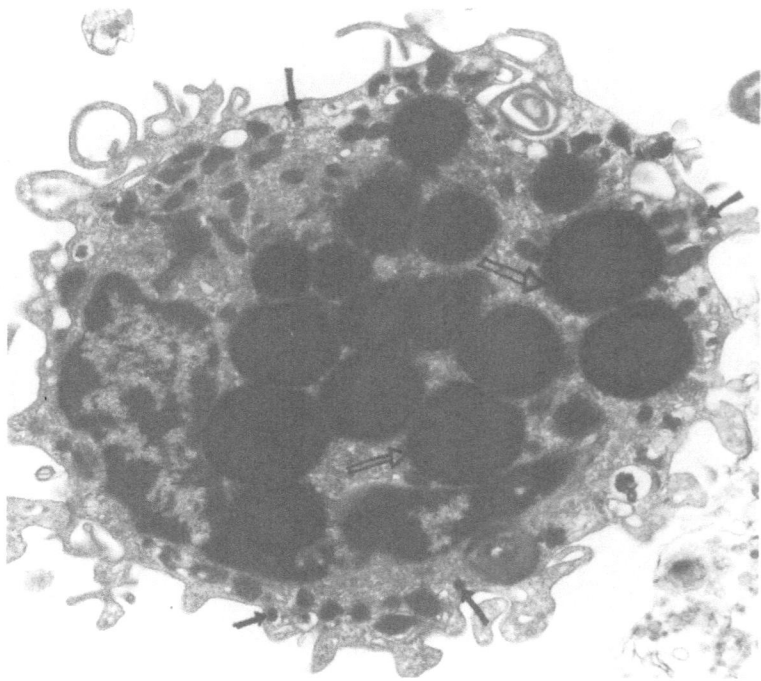

Figure 2.98 Large, immature, isolated lung mast cell fixed 24 hours after exposure to anti-IgE shows large numbers of lipid bodies (open arrows) and peripherally located immature granules and progranules (arrows). OCUB, ×11 200

94

CONCLUDING REMARKS

Human basophils and mast cells can be distinguished by applying ultrastructural criteria for doing so[37, 38, 45]. These criteria are stable for resting, mature basophils and mast cells. Both cells show considerable alteration of their fine structure during rapid and slow release reactions and recovery from them. The effect of these functional events on morphologic expression must also be considered in cell identification. Similarly, maturational events are characteristic for each cell, and knowledge of the fine structure of large and small immature mast cells, as well as of basophilic myelocytes, will facilitate the correct identification of mast cell and basophil lineages.

ACKNOWLEDGEMENTS

We thank P. Estrella, S. Kissell, and L. Letourneau for excellent photographic assistance. This work was supported by the Lillian Gong Memorial Research Fund and USPHS Grant 28834.

References

1. Ehrlich, P. (1877). Beiträge zur Kenntnis der Anilinfärbungen und ihrer Verwendung in der mikroskopischen Technik. *Archiv Mikrosk. Anatomie*, **13**, 263–77
2. Ehrlich, P. (1879). Beiträge zur Kenntnis der granulierten Bindegewebszellen und der eosinophilen Leukocythen. *Arch. Anat. Physiol.*, **3**, 166–9
3. Dvorak, A. M., Mihm, M. C., Jr. and Dvorak, H. F. (1976). Degranulation of basophilic leucocytes in allergic contact dermatitis reactions in man. *J. Immunol.*, **116**, 687–95
4. Dvorak, A. M., Newball, H. H., Dvorak, H. F. and Lichtenstein, L. M. (1980). Antigen-induced IgE-mediated degranulation of human basophils. *Lab. Invest.*, **43**, 126–39
5. Dvorak, A. M., Monahan, R. A., Osage, J. E. and Dickersin, G. R. (1980). Crohn's disease: Transmission electron microscopic studies. II. Immunologic inflammatory response. Alterations of mast cells, basophils, eosinophils, and the microvasculature. *Human Pathol.*, **11**, 606–19
6. Dvorak, A. M., Lett-Brown, M., Thueson, D. and Grant, J. A. (1981). Complement-induced degranulation of human basophils. *J. Immunol.*, **126**, 523–8
7. Findlay, S. R., Dvorak, A. M., Kagey-Sobotka, A. and Lichtenstein, L. M. (1981). Hyperosmolar triggering of histamine release from human basophils. *J. Clin. Invest.*, **67**, 1604–13
8. Dvorak, A. M. and Monahan, R. A. (1982). Crohn's disease. Ultrastructural studies showing basophil leukocyte granule changes and lymphocyte parallel tubular arrays in peripheral blood. *Arch. Pathol. Lab. Med.*, **106**, 145–9
9. Dvorak, A. M., Dvorak, H. F. and Galli, S. J. (1983). Ultrastructural criteria for identification of mast cells and basophils in humans, guinea pigs and mice. *Am. Rev. Resp. Disease, Supplement, Comparative Biology of the Lung*, **128**, S49–S52
10. Dvorak, A. M., Galli, S. J., Schulman, E. S., Lichtenstein, L. M. and Dvorak, H. F. (1983). Basophil and mast cell degranulation: ultrastructural analysis of mechanisms of mediator release. *Fed. Proc.*, **42**, 2510–15
11. Galli, S. J., Dvorak, A. M. and Dvorak, H. F. (1984). Basophils and mast cells: Morphologic insights into their biology, secretory patterns and function. In Ishizaka, K. (ed.) *Progress in Allergy. Mast Cell Activation and Mediator Release*. Vol. 34, pp 1–141. (Basel, Switzerland: S. Karger)
12. Dvorak, A. M., Lett-Brown, M. A., Thueson, D. O., Pyne, K., Raghuprasad, P. K., Galli, S. J. and Grant, J. A. (1984). Histamine-releasing activity (HRA). III. HRA induces human basophil histamine release by provoking noncytotoxic granule exocytosis. *Clin. Immun. Immunopathol.*, **32**, 142–50.

13. Ishizaka, T., Dvorak, A. M., Conrad, D. H., Niebyl, J. R., Marquette, J. P. and Ishizaka, K. (1985). Morphologic and immunologic characterization of human basophils developed in cultures of cord blood mononuclear cells. *J. Immunol.*, **134**, 532–40
14. Dvorak, A. M., Ishizaka, T. and Galli, S. J. (1985). Ultrastructure of human basophils developing *in vitro*. Evidence for the acquisition of peroxidase by basophils and for different effects of human and murine growth factors on human basophil and eosinophil maturation. *Lab. Invest.*, **53**, 57–71.
15. Dvorak, H. F., Mihm, M. C., Jr., Dvorak, A. M., Johnson, R. A., Manseau, E. J., Morgan, E. and Colvin, R. B. (1974). Morphology of delayed-type hypersensitivity reactions in man. I. Quantitative description of the inflammatory response. *Lab. Invest.*, **31**, 111–30
16. Dvorak, H. F. and Dvorak, A. M. (1975). Basophilic Leukocytes: Structure, Function, and Role in Disease. In Lichtman, M. A. (ed.) *Clinics in Haematology, Granulocyte and Monocyte Abnormalities*. Vol. 4, pp. 651–83. (London: W. B. Saunders Co.)
17. Dvorak, A. M. (1978). Biology and Morphology of Basophilic Leukocytes. In Bach, M. K. (ed.) *Immediate Hypersensitivity, Modern Concepts and Developments*. (Immunology Series) Vol. 7, pp. 369–405. (New York: Marcel Dekker, Inc.)
18. Galli, S. J., Dvorak, A. M. and Dvorak, H. F. (1983). Morphology, biochemistry, and function of basophils. In Williams, W. J., Beutler, E., Erslev, A. J. and Lichtman, M. A. (eds.) *Hematology*. 3rd Edn., pp. 820–5. (New York: McGraw-Hill)
19. Fox, C. C., Dvorak, A. M., MacGlashan, D. W., Jr. and Lichenstein, L. M. (1984). Histamine-containing cells in human peritoneal fluid. *J. Immunol.*, **132**, 2177–9
20. Galli, S. J., Dvorak, A. M., Hammond, M. E., Morgan, E., Galli, A. S. and Dvorak, H. F. (1981). Guinea pig basophil morphology *in vitro*. I. Ultrastructure of uropod-bearing (motile) basophils and modulation of motile structures by serum and substrate effects. *J. Immunol.*, **126**, 1066–74
21. Dvorak, A. M., Mihm, M. C., Jr., Osage, J. E., Kwan, T. H., Austen, K. F. and Wintroub, B. U. (1982). Bullous pemphigoid, an ultrastructural study of the inflammatory response: Eosinophil, basophil and mast cell granule changes in multiple biopsies from one patient. *J. Invest. Dermatol.*, **78**, 91–101
22. Dvorak, H. F., Mihm, M. C., Jr., Dvorak, A. M., Barnes, B. A., Manseau, M. J. and Galli, S. J. (1979). Rejection of first set skin allografts in man. The microvasculature is the critical target for the immune response. *J. Exp. med.*, **150**, 322–37
23. Dvorak, A. M., Dvorak, H. F. and Karnovsky, M. J. (1972). Uptake of horseradish peroxidase by guinea pig basophilic leukocytes. *Lab. Invest.*, **26**, 27–39
24. Dvorak, A. M., Hammond, M. E., Morgan, E., Orenstein, N. S., Galli, S. J. and Dvorak, H. F. (1980). Evidence for a vesicular transport mechanism in guinea pig basophilic leukocytes. *Lab. Invest.*, **42**, 263–76
25. Dvorak, A. M., Klebanoff, S. J., Henderson, W. R., Monahan, R. A., Pyne, K. and Galli, S. J. (1985). Vesicular uptake of eosinophil peroxidase by guinea pig basophils and by cloned mouse mast cells and granule-containing lymphoid cells. *Am. J. Pathol.*, **118**, 425–38
26. Dvorak, A. M., Dickersin, G. R., Connell, A. B., Carey, R. W. and Dvorak, H. F. (1976). Degranulation mechanisms in human leukemic basophils. *Clin. Immun. Immunopathol.*, **5**, 235–46
27. Dvorak, A. M., Monahan, R. A. and Dickersin, G. R. (1981). Diagnostic electron microscopy. I. Hematology: Differential diagnosis of acute lymphoblastic and acute myeloblastic leukemia. Use of ultrastructural peroxidase cytochemistry and routine electron microscopic technology. In Sommers, S. C. and Rosen, P. P. (eds.) *Pathology Annual, Part I*. pp. 101–37. (New York: Appleton-Century-Crofts)
28. Dvorak, A. M. and Monahan, R. A. (1985). Guinea pig bone marrow basophilopoiesis. *J. Exp. Pathol.*, **2**, 13–24
29. Dvorak, A. M., Nabel, G., Pyne, K., Cantor, H., Dvorak, H. F. and Galli, S. J. (1982). Ultrastructural identification of the mouse basophil. *Blood*, **59**, 1279–85
30. Dvorak, A. M., Dvorak, H. F., Peters, S. P., Schulman, E. S., MacGashan, D. W., Jr., Pyne, K., Harvey, V. S., Galli, S. J. and Lichtenstein, L. M. (1983). Lipid bodies: Cytoplasmic organelles important to arachidonate metabolism in macrophages and mast cells. *J. Immunol.*, **131**, 2965–76 (Republished (1984) *J. Immunol.*, **132**, 1586–97)

96

31. Dvorak, A. M., Hammel, I., Schulman, E. S., Peters, S. P., MacGlashan, D. W., Jr., Schleimer, R. P., Newball, H. H., Pyne, K., Dvorak, H. F., Lichtenstein, L. M. and Galli, S. J. (1984). Differences in the behavior of cytoplasmic granules and lipid bodies during human lung mast cell degranulation. *J. Cell Biol.*, **99**, 1678–87
32. Hammel, I., Dvorak, A. M., Peters, S. P., Schulman, E. S., Dvorak, H. F., Lichtenstein, L. M. and Galli, S. J. (1985). Differences in the volume distributions of human lung mast cell granules and lipid bodies: Evidence that the size of these organelles is regulated by distinct mechanisms. *J. Cell Biol.*, **100**, 1488–92
33. Dvorak, A. M., Schulman, E. S., Peters, S. P., MacGlashan, D. W., Jr., Newball, H. H., Schleimer, R. P. and Lichtenstein, L. M. (1985). Immunoglobulin E-mediated degranulation of isolated human lung mast cells. *Lab. Invest.*, **53**, 45–56
34. Fox, C. C., Dvorak, A. M., Peters, S. P., Kagey-Sobotka, A. and Lichtenstein, L. M. (1985). Isolation and characterization of human intestinal mucosal mast cells. *J. Immunol.*, **135**, 483–91
35. Dvorak, A. M. and Monahan, R. A. (1985). Abdominal pain, hepatomegaly and weight loss in a fifty-four-year-old man: Renal cell carcinoma and adenoma. *Norelco Reporter*, **32**, 61–6
36. Dvorak, A. M., Schleimer, R. P. and Lichtenstein, L. M. (1987). Morphologic mast cell cycles. *Cell. Immunol.*, **105**, 199–204.
37. Dvorak, A. M. (1988). Human mast cells. In Beck, F., Hild, W., Kritz, W., Ortmann, R., Pauly, J. E., Schiebler, T. H. (eds.) *Advances in Anatomy, Embryology and Cell Biology.* (Berlin: Springer-Verlag)
38. Dvorak, A. M. (1986). Morphologic expressions of maturation and function can affect the ability to identify mast cells and basophils in man, guinea pig and mouse. In Befus, A. D., Bienenstock, J. and Denburg, J. A. (eds.) *Mast Cell Differentiation and Heterogeneity.* pp. 95–114. (New York: Raven Press)
38a. Kopicky-Burd, J. A., Kagey-Sobotka, A., Peters, S. P., Dvorak, A. M., Lennox, D. W., Lichtenstein, L. M. and Wigley, F. M. (1988). Characterization of human synovial mast cells. *J. Rheumatol.* (In press)
39. Asboe-Hansen, G. (1971). Mast cells and the skin. *International Academy of Pathology – Monograph 10.* pp. 83–111. (Baltimore: Williams and Wilkins Co.)
40. Dvorak, A. M., Schleimer, R. P., Schulman, E. S. and Lichtenstein, L. M. (1986). Human mast cells use conservation and condensation mechanisms during recovery from degranulation. *In vitro* studies with mast cells purified from human lungs. *Lab. Invest.*, **54**, 663–78
41. Dvorak, A. M., Schleimer, R. P. and Lichtenstein, L. M. (1988). Human mast cells synthesise new granules during recovery from degranulation. *In vivo* studies with mast cells purified from human lungs. *Blood*, **71**, 76–85
42. Dvorak, A. M. (1986). Mast cell degranulation in human hearts. *N. Engl. J. Med.*, **315**, 969–70
43. Peters, S. P., MacGlashan, Jr., D. W., Schulman, E. S., Schleimer, R. P., Hayes, E. C., Rokach, J., Adkinson, J. R. N. F. and Lichtenstein, L. M. (1984). Arachidonic acid metabolism in purified human lung mast cells. *J. Immunol.*, **132**, 1972–9
44. Galli, S. J., Dvorak, A. M., Peters, S. J., Schulman, E. S., MacGlashan, Jr., D. W., Isomura, T., Pyne, K., Harvey, V. S., Hammel, I., Lichtenstein, L. M. and Dvorak, H. F. (1985). Lipid bodies: Widely distributed cytoplasmic structures that represent preferential non-membrane repositories of exogenous ^{3}H-arachidonic acid incorporated by mast cells, macrophages and other cell types. In Bailey, J. M. (ed.) *Prostaglandins, Leukotrienes, and Lipoxins.* pp. 221–39. (New York: Plenum)
45. Dvorak, A. M. (1986). Morphologic and immunologic characterization of human basophils (1879 to 1985). *J. Immunol. Immunopharmacol.*, **8**

3
The Receptor for Immunoglobulin E

D. H. CONRAD

INTRODUCTION

Cellular receptors for IgE are broadly divided into two major categories. The division is based primarily on the relative affinity for ligand, although it is noted that high affinity IgE receptors are found exclusively on mast cells and basophils, while low affinity receptors are found on a much broader range of haematopoietic cell types (see Table 3.1). This general review will focus on some of the relevant findings regarding the structure and functions of both of these receptors. This review is not meant to be exhaustive and the reader is referred to several extensive reviews on both the high[1-3] and low[4,5] affinity receptors for IgE for additional information. The nomenclature used

Table 3.1 Receptors for IgE*

	$Fc_\epsilon RI$	$Fc_\epsilon RII$
Distribution	mast cells basophils	macrophages, monocytes, eosinophils, platelets, B lymphocytes, ?T lymphocytes
Number/cell	10^4–10^6	10^3–10^5
Affinity	10^9–10^{12} mol/l	10^6–10^8 mol/l
Structure	tetramer α – 45–50 kD β – 31 kD 2τ – 9 kD	single polypeptide chain 45 kD – human 49 kD – murine
Modulation	stabilized by IgE	stabilized by IgE increased synthesis by IL-4
Cell activation	crosslinked IgE or crosslinked $Fc_\epsilon RI$	inflammatory cells – aggregated/ complexed IgE lymphocyte – unknown
Consequences of activation	allergic mediator release	inflammatory cells – mediator release lymphocytes – possible IgE response control

*See text for further explanations and references regarding listed details

99

is based on the recommendations of an *ad hoc* committee which met at the conference on Fc receptors and immunoglobulin binding factors at Saxton River, Vermont in June, 1987. Thus, high affinity receptors for IgE are designated as $Fc_\epsilon RI$ and low affinity IgE receptors as $Fc_\epsilon RII$.

HIGH AFFINITY RECEPTOR FOR IgE ($Fc_\epsilon RI$)

Discovery

The first discovery of receptors for IgE was made by Ishizaka *et al.*[6] who demonstrated, by autoradiographic techniques, that human myeloma IgE preferentially bound to basophils; subsequent studies demonstrated that monkey mast cells also bound human IgE[7]. Since the procedures employed used monomeric IgE and required extensive washing steps, high affinity $Fc_\epsilon RI$ were selectively discerned.

Just as the characterization of IgE itself was greatly aided by the acquisition of purified reagent, i.e. IgE producing myelomas; the discovery of clonal cell lines bearing high numbers of IgE receptors has been invaluable with respect to the characterization of IgE receptors. While to date, no such lines yet exist for the study of the human high affinity receptor, several do exist in rodents. The first and most extensively used, is the rat basophilic leukaemia (RBL) cell, initially described by Eccleston *et al.*[8] in 1973. Kulczycki *et al.*[9] adapted this cell line for tissue culture, and demonstrated that the cells have high levels of IgE receptors (10^5–10^6) per cell. Most of the receptor characterizations and many of the mechanisms of mediator release studies have utilized RBL cells because of the ease of maintenance and rapid growth characteristics. The neoplastic nature of RBL cells is always a matter of concern with regard to extrapolation of studies to 'normal' cell types, and whenever possible, studies have been, and should continue to be extended to normal cell counterparts. More recently, growth factor (interleukin-3) dependent and independent murine mast cell lines have been developed, and these also represent an alternative to RBL cells.

Structure of the $Fc_\epsilon RI$

Early studies identified a surface accessible IgE binding component on both RBL cells and rat peritoneal mast cells which was readily labelled by techniques that selectively labelled the cell membrane[10, 11]. This component migrated on SDS–PAGE gels at 55–60 kD, but the broad nature of the band suggested considerable molecular weight (MW) heterogeneity. Subsequent studies with tunicamycin, an inhibitor of N-linked glycosylation, demonstrated that the MW heterogeneity was due to carbohydrate[12]; both this study and a separate one using endoglycosidases found that ~30% of the surface exposed $Fc_\epsilon RI$ was carbohydrate[12, 13].

Component structure

This surface accessible component in highly purified form is capable of binding strongly to IgE, indeed for unknown reasons, the affinity of the solubilized receptors is higher than that estimated for the cell bound form

$(\sim 10^{12}\,M^{-1}$ vs $\sim 10^{10}\,M^{-1}$, respectively)[14]. However, MW differences estimated for the IgE receptor complex vs the free receptor had early on suggested that additional components, not readily accessible to the cell membrane, may also be present[14,15]. This indeed turned out to be true; Holowka et al.[16] and subsequently Perez-Montfort et al.[17] demonstrated, primarily via the use of crosslinking reagents that the surface accessible receptor (now termed α-component) was non-covalently associated with two other membrane components; a 31 kD component, termed β and an 18 kD disulphide linked dimer termed τ. The properties of the various polypeptides comprising the high affinity IgE receptor led to the working model[18] for the $Fc_\epsilon RI$ shown in Figure 3.1. Labelling studies of both detergent solubilized $Fc_\epsilon RI$[19] and the cytoplasmic face of the membrane[20] in conjunction with the use of membrane impermeant crosslinking reagents[21,22] support the concept, shown in the model, that β and τ are exposed at the cytoplasmic, but not at the exterior, face of the plasma membrane. The lack of glycosylation and the finding that β and τ on both RBL cells[17,23] and cloned murine mast cell lines[22] easily label with hydrophobic probes further support the concept that β and τ are intrinsic membrane proteins.

Lipid association

A rationale for the lack of observing significant quantities of these components in early biosynthetic labelling studies was seen in that β and τ dissociate from the α in detergent solutions[24]. Other studies have further supported the

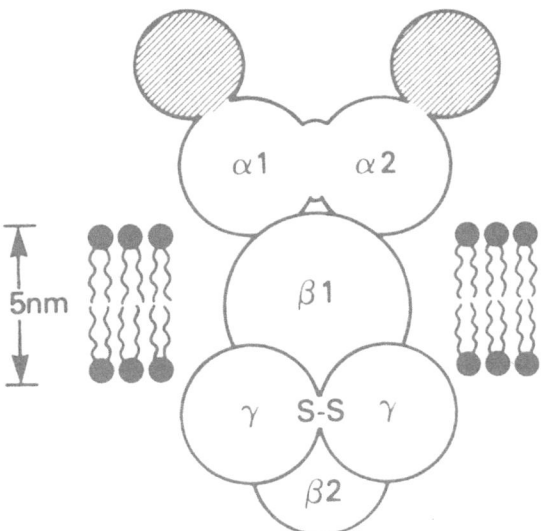

Figure 3.1 Model for the $Fc_\epsilon RI$. The subunits and domains are depicted as spheres and the columns are proportional to the size of the respective domains. Shaded areas represent carbohydrate. Modification of this model, as necessitated by the recent cloning of the α-chain[32] is discussed in the text. (Reprinted from Reference 18, with permission)

concept that specific lipid–receptor interactions occur; specifically maintenance of a critical ratio of phospholipid/detergent allowed co-isolation of all of the components without requiring crosslinking reagents[25]. Indeed, recent studies have indicated that certain phospholipid types, specifically sphingomyelin and phosphatidylcholine, are enriched when the lipids associated with purified $Fc_\epsilon RI$ are studied[26]. It is quite possible that the tightly associated lipid is important not only for the maintenance of $Fc_\epsilon RI$ structure, but also for the biologic function of the receptor, and in this regard, the recent finding that sphingolipids act as inhibitors of protein kinase C[27] is illustrative. Also of note is the observation that only the intact α, β, τ_2 structure is capable of significant reincorporation into lipid bilayers[28, 29]. The α-component alone which, as noted above, retains IgE binding capacity, gave essentially no bilayer reincorporation. In studies to date it has also not been possible to demonstrate reassociation of the α, β, τ_2 complex once disassociated by detergent, indicating that irreversible changes have occurred as a result of the disassociation[24].

Phosphate incorporation

Exposure to the cytoplasm is also consistent with phosphorylation studies which demonstrated some phosphate incorporation into both β and τ chains on RBL cells[30]. This activity would presumably be mediated at the cytoplasmic face of the membrane. Interestingly, triggering of RBL cells to release mediators caused an increase in β chain and a decrease in τ chain phosphorylation, respectively[31]. However, the finding that only a small percentage of β and/or τ was phosphorylated combined with the observation that the modifications occurred in both unoccupied and occupied receptors suggests that phosphorylation/dephosphorylation of the receptor is not important with regard to triggering the mediator release cascade[31]. The α-component on mast cells has also been shown to incorporate phosphate[32, 33], but the low levels of phosphate incorporation again suggest that phosphorylation of the $Fc_\epsilon RI$ is not important in the biologic function of the receptor. The data do indicate, however, that all of the $Fc_\epsilon RI$ components can function as substrates for protein kinases, and indeed a tyrosine kinase activity co-purifies to some extent with the $Fc_\epsilon RI$[34]. Although the kinase activity can be disassociated from the receptor itself, the results suggest that there is some interaction between the $Fc_\epsilon RI$ and a tyrosine kinase; further study will be required to determine what importance, if any, can be attached to this kinase.

α-Chain cloning

Protease digestion studies of the α-chain[13], combined with the finding of two epitopes per α-component for a monoclonal anti-receptor antibody[35] indicated that the α-chain has two potentially related domains. The recent reported cloning of the α-component[36] both supports the model shown in Figure 3.1, and indicates that revisions are necessary. Six tryptic peptides from the α-component were sequenced, and portions of that sequence were used to construct an oligonucleotide probe which was subsequently used to identify potential α-nucleotide sequences in the cDNA library. The deduced amino acid sequence has indicated a domain-like structure delineated by disulphide bonds, consistent with the model shown in Figure 3.1. However, a potential hydrophobic transmembrane region was also present which ended in a highly charged (presumably cytoplasmic) tail. Additional supportive evidence for the existence of this cytoplasmic 'α'-tail is seen in that one monoclonal anti-α has been developed that reacts only after cells have been disrupted and membrane vesicles are allowed to form; since the cytoplasmic surface would now be exposed, the anti-α is able to react (D. Holowka, personal communication). Re-expression of the cloned α-component has not yet been achieved and little, if any, binding of the non-glycosylated protein produced by the putative α-clone to either IgE or anti-receptor antibodies was seen. However, the complete sequences of all six tryptic peptides were found within the deduced sequence, and still more recent data indicate that anti-peptide antibodies, made using the derived sequence, will react on a Western blot analysis with the α-chain from RBL cells (J.-P. Kinet, personal communication). Thus, the overall data strongly indicate that the correct gene has been identified. These data suggest that β and τ, and possibly also carbohydrate, on the α-component are necessary for the correct 'folding' of the α to allow IgE binding. The lack of binding of anti-receptor antibodies is more difficult to explain, but the possibility that carbohydrate plays a role in the epitope(s) for these antibodies must be considered. In any case, it is clear that the cloning and sequence determination of the α-component, which will probably be quickly followed by the cloning of β and/or τ will necessitate revisions in Figure 3.1. An exciting possibility is that the sequence determination of β and τ will allow at least some clues as to their function, which is at present unknown. The α sequence demonstrates some homology with the Ig gene superfamily and, in some regions, exhibits very significant homology with the recently cloned murine Fc_τ receptor[37, 38]. Interestingly, no homology was seen with the lymphocyte IgE receptor ($Fc_\epsilon RII$) (discussed further below).

Structure in other species

Much less is known about the high affinity IgE receptor in other species. Crosslinking studies demonstrated the presence of α, β and τ-like structures using murine mast cell lines[22]; however, in humans, using leukaemic basophils[39, 40] or human cord blood basophils[41] only the surface accessible α-component has been identified. As noted above, this lack of progress is, in large part, due to the unavailability of appropriate human cell lines.

Specificity and affinity of the $Fc_\epsilon RI$

IgE will only bind to the receptor on the mast cells/basophils of the same or closely related species, thus, IgE is termed a 'homocytotropic' antibody. Exceptions do exist, making this term less correct than originally envisioned. Rat and mouse IgE bind to human basophil[39, 40] and human lung mast cell[42] IgE receptors. Although the affinity is about 10-fold lower than for human

IgE, the bound IgE, when crosslinked with antigen or anti-IgE, will cause mediator release[39, 42]. Even within related species, binding heterogeneity can exist. Thus, normal murine mast cells possess a set of high affinity receptors which bind rat and mouse IgE equally well, and additional receptors which bind only mouse IgE[43]. The significance of this fine specificity is unknown.

While in general, the high affinity IgE receptor is highly specific with respect to isotype, some loss of specificity is observed after non-ionic detergent solubilization of the $Fc_\epsilon R_I$. Some binding of ^{125}I-surface labelled receptor to rat IgG columns[44] and, in a later study, especially IgG_{2a} columns was observed[45]. Since rat IgG_{2a} is homocytotropic, it is possible that this activity is mediated through the IgE receptor. If so, the affinity of interaction is certainly much lower than for IgE, and thus, preformed aggregates (antigen/antibody complexes, etc.) would almost certainly be required in order to obtain significant ligand binding and subsequent mediator release.

Affinity

Early work using pH extremes[46] established that the receptor IgE interaction was reversible, and the RBL model[47] further established that the interaction could be described as a non-covalent reaction between a molecule of IgE and a single receptor. The affinity is the highest of all presently known Fc-receptor interactions. Depending upon the method, the affinity has been estimated to be at least 10^9 mol/l and possibly as high as 10^{12} mol/l in both the human[41, 48] and rodent systems[14, 43, 49]. This high affinity is primarily due to the very slow rate of disassociation ($k_{-1} < 10^{-5} \mathrm{sec}^{-1}$)[47]; this same slow disassociation, in combination with the stabilization effect that IgE has on the receptor halflife, presumably explains the known persistence of IgE in skin sites where it is bound to tissue mast cells.

Importance of receptor aggregation

Monomeric IgE remains at the cell surface for long periods of time and with the exception that increased receptor halflife is seen (see below), causes no known biochemical changes in the mast cell/basophil. Early classical studies demonstrated that receptor aggregation was necessary for mediator release[50, 51]. Work with either model dimeric haptens[52] or covalent IgE dimers[53] also indicated that the unit signal necessary for cell activation was two IgE molecules linked together. Indeed, further studies with a polyclonal anti-receptor demonstrated that IgE was necessary only to cause clustering of IgE receptors. Thus, divalent, but not monovalent (Fab) anti-receptor induced mediator release from mast cells[54] and RBL cells[55].

Even though a dimeric signal can clearly cause cell activation, other studies have indicated that higher degrees of receptor aggregation can cause both a quantitatively as well as a qualitatively different signal. Thus, RBL cells released mediators consistently better with trimers and higher oligomers (of IgE) than did dimers[56] and a monoclonal anti-IgE, termed A2[57], also caused poor mediator release at concentrations where primarily dimers were formed[58]. In addition, with RBL cells, IgE dimers demonstrated little decrease in lateral mobility within the membrane, while higher oligomers rapidly became immobilized[58, 59]. Qualitative differences in mediator release patterns were also seen in the human basophil system. Donor variability with respect to mediator release was seen, resulting in 'high and low' responders being identified[60]. Especially with low responders, dimeric IgE gave essentially no leukotriene release and very low histamine release, while trimeric IgE released both mediators[60].

Receptor–receptor associations

A full understanding of the aggregate size relationship to mediator release also requires an understanding of possible receptor–receptor associations, either directly, or via other cell membrane constituents. The valency of the receptor, at least after detergent solubilization is clearly one IgE molecule bound per receptor unit, as demonstrated by co-precipitation studies with rat and mouse IgE[14, 61]. The valency of the receptor, while in the membrane, is less clear. Co-capping studies with RBL cells also indicated monovalency[62], while studies with human basophils indicated that unoccupied receptor capped along with occupied (IgE) receptor[63]. The resolution of this overall issue will require a better understanding of the microenvironment of the IgE receptor in the membrane. Presently, it is clear that some association of receptors can occur. Receptor aggregation by antigen causes endocytosis of not only the occupied receptor, but a significant amount (up to 30%) of unoccupied receptors were found to 'co-endocytose'[64]. Other studies demonstrated that cell-bound small oligomers gradually coalesce into large clusters which are attached to the cytoskeleton[59, 65] and contain high numbers (perhaps 1000s) of molecules. Receptor–receptor association is also induced by mycoplasma infection of RBL cells; a new component of 71 kD that contains either dimeric disulphide linked receptor (α-component) or $Fc_\epsilon RI$ linked to an as yet unknown membrane component was observed[66, 67]. Thus, these studies indicate that the $Fc_\epsilon RI$, while in the membrane, is capable of interacting both with itself as well as other membrane constituents. The importance of these interactions with regard to cell activation and mediator release remains to be elucidated.

Effect of IgE on the halflife of $Fc_\epsilon RI$

As with the majority of the data concerning the $Fc_\epsilon RI$, the work involving the regulation of receptor expression has been performed on RBL cells. Culture of RBL cells in the presence of saturating concentrations of IgE results in a 2–3 fold increase in receptor levels[68]. This increase was not altered by inclusion of cycloheximide to the culture, which indicated that protein synthesis was not necessary to achieve the increased receptor levels. In additional experiments, Furuichi et al.[68] and Quarto et al.[69] demonstrated that ligand binding greatly slowed the loss of the $Fc_\epsilon RI$ from the cell surface. The latter study also demonstrated that the α, β and τ receptor components were coordinately regulated. Thus, this work demonstrated that the increase in IgE binding activity associated with the IgE-cultured cells resulted from a lower degradative rate for the $Fc_{\epsilon}R_I$. At present, there is no evidence that degradation of the $Fc_{\epsilon}R_I$ involves the release of a $Fc_{\epsilon}R_I$ fragment analogous to $Fc_{\epsilon}R_{II}$ degradation (see below); the degradation of $Fc_{\epsilon}R_I$ is thought to involve internalization of the receptor with subsequent lysosomal degradation[70].

Site on the IgE molecule that interacts with the Fc$_{\epsilon}$RI

Physicochemical studies

The site of interaction of the receptor with IgE is an area of considerable interest in view of the possible therapeutic potential of peptides that could interfere with the binding of IgE to the mast cell/basophil. Controlled proteolytic digestion of rodent IgE indicated that the receptor slowed digestion of the IgE at certain sites[71]; the most profound effect was at a site between the $C_{\epsilon}2:C_{\epsilon}3$ domains. Energy transfer techniques have also been employed for this problem; this technique determines the quenching of fluorescent donor probes by appropriate acceptor probes. This quenching can be interpreted to yield an average distance between acceptor and donor probes. By using this technique, acceptor probes were inserted into the lipid bilayer and the fluorescent probe was placed on different regions of the IgE molecule[72]. Alternatively, the donor and acceptor probes were placed on anti-IgE monoclonal antibodies that interact with the $C_{\epsilon}1$ and $C_{\epsilon}3$ or $C_{\epsilon}4$ regions[73]. The overall data obtained are consistent with the limited proteolysis study discussed above in that the receptor interaction was somewhere in the $C_{\epsilon}3$ region; interestingly, the data also suggest that IgE bends at the $C_{\epsilon}2$, $C_{\epsilon}3$ region upon binding to the receptor leading to the so-called 'reclining' model for the receptor bound IgE[72, 73].

Peptides from the IgE sequence

An additional approach to determining the site of interaction of the IgE and $Fc_{\epsilon}R_I$ is to use either small fragments of IgE (produced by controlled proteolysis) or to synthesize peptides representing appropriate sequences in the IgE Fc region. Proteolysis has not yet been effective; the smallest 'active' fragment is the intact Fc from human IgE[74], and with rodent IgE even an Fc fragment that retains binding activity has been difficult to produce. With regard to synthetic peptides, an early study with a pentapeptide which exhibited anti-allergic activity[75] was shown by a consortium of laboratories[76] not to be due to any interference with IgE binding. Recently Stanworth's laboratory has reported some success with several peptides mimicking regions in the rat IgE Fc region[77]. A 1000-fold excess of a peptide representing amino acids 414–428 ($C_{\epsilon}3$ domain) reduced IgE binding to mast cells by more than 50%. Interestingly, this inhibition remained even after washing the cells. Some inhibition of binding was also seen with some peptides mimicking regions of the $C_{\epsilon}4$ domain. These results are suggestive, however, unless these peptides can be shown to directly interact with the $Fc_{\epsilon}R_I$, the possibility that the peptides cause alterations in overall mast cell membrane architecture remains as an explanation for the binding results.

Recombinant IgE

A relatively new method for determining the site of interaction on the IgE is to use recombinant DNA technology to produce recombinant IgE molecules (rIgE). Two groups[78, 79] have isolated unglycosylated Fc fragments of human IgE obtained from bacteria that contained the appropriate plasmid. These fragments bound to mast cells and basophils and, indeed, in a more recent study using human basophils[80], the affinity and number of binding sites detected by the recombinant IgE was identical to native IgE. These initial studies used rIgE containing the $C_\epsilon 2$, $C_\epsilon 3$ and $C_\epsilon 4$ domains. Recently, Geha et al.[81] have examined rIgE in further detail and found that the $C_\epsilon 2$, $C_\epsilon 3$ recombinant peptide was sufficient for binding to $Fc_\epsilon RI$; neither domain was sufficient by itself, indicating the importance of sites in both domains, or alternatively the integrity of both domains to allow for proper folding of the molecule. In any case, these results are compatible with the biophysical approaches discussed above, indicating that the primary site(s) of $Fc_\epsilon RI$ interaction with IgE are distal to the $C_\epsilon 4$ domain.

Mediator release cascade

An eventual goal in the study of the $Fc_\epsilon RI$ is the elucidation of the biochemical events that lead to allergic mediator release. As discussed above, it is now very clear that aggregation of $Fc_\epsilon RI$ initiates this cascade. The sequence of events which occurs in between the receptor aggregation and mediator release has been, and continues to be, an area of active investigation. At present, while many enzyme systems, cell components, etc. have been implicated, the exact role of these systems is both unclear and, in many cases, controversial. Several systems in which a fair amount of recent work has been done regarding this 'cascade' will be discussed herein. Given the scope of this review, it is not possible to discuss this area in detail; reference is given especially to a recent review by Metzger et al.[1] where the putative early events in the mediator release cascade are given a careful (and critical) review.

Clearly of great interest is what are the cellular components with which the $Fc_\epsilon RI$ interacts after aggregation. The divalent cation calcium has for some time[82] been known to be crucial in the mediator release cascade, both from the point of view of an influx of Ca^{2+} across the membrane and a release of Ca^{2+} from internal stores. Depending upon the cell type, there is some variation between whether the calcium requirement can be met by release from internal stores or whether some influx of Ca^{2+} from the exterior of the cell is required. Studies with Ca^{2+} sensitive probes[83], and patch clamp studies[84] indicated that rat mast cells have sufficient intracellular Ca^{2+} stores to allow mediator release. RBL cells, however, clearly require extracellular Ca^{2+} for secretion[85]; other cell types may fall between these two extremes.

Involvement of poly-phosphoinositides

With regard to the release of Ca^{2+} from internal stores, evidence is accumulating that the phosphatidyl inositide system (PI) is involved. Classic studies[86, 87] have demonstrated that the PI system is involved in a number of calcium dependent activation-pathways. The general scenario involves receptor-mediated hydrolysis of membrane phospholipids; of primary importance in the PI system is the hydrolysis of phosphatidylinositol 4,5-bisphosphate to form inositol 1,4,5-tris-phosphate (IP_3) and diacylglycerol. The IP_3, which is released into the cytoplasm can then either be further phosphorylated or be broken down and recycled into the membrane phospholipid. Further studies have shown that the kinetics of PI hydrolysis vary with the type of IgE crosslinking agent used and, in addition, while some PI hydrolysis occurs in the absence of external calcium, with RBL cells the majority of PI hydrolysis and any significant histamine release required external Ca^{2+}. The evidence suggests that the released IP_3 and possibly also a tetra phosphorylated inositol (1,3,4,5-tetrakis-phosphate) are active with respect to releasing internal Ca^{2+} stores[88, 89]. The diacylglycerol is a potent activator of protein kinase C (PKC), and there is at least suggestive evidence that PKC is involved in mediator release. In RBL cells low concentrations of the calcium ionophore A23187 did not induce mediator release unless a PKC activator such as a phorbol ester was present[90]. Also, $Fc_\epsilon RI$ aggregation induced increased activity in the plasma membrane PKC of cloned mast cell lines[91]; this increased activity could not be completely explained by translocation from the cytoplasm, suggesting that some membrane PKC was in a non-active or proenzyme form that was susceptible to activation by $Fc_\epsilon RI$ aggregation.

It is clear that in both mast cells[92] and RBL cells[90, 93], $Fc_\epsilon RI$ aggregation is associated with PI breakdown. There is a good correlation between the amplitude of the calcium cytoplasmic signal and total inositol phosphate increase and, at early points, histamine release[90]. Increasing aggregation gives a continued increase in cytoplasmic PI and Ca^{2+} signals while mediator release plateaus suggesting that there is an excess capacity for signal generation. Maeyama et al.[90] also raises the possibility that the PI breakdown may also be involved in the Ca^{2+} ion channel activation, since as mentioned above, the RBL cells used in this study require extracellular Ca^{2+} for mediator release. This would indicate a new role for PI hydrolysis. At present, however, the most likely scenario would involve internal calcium release, induced by cytoplasmic PIs and external influx, mediated by a separate ion channel system.

GTP-binding protein involvement

In the IgE-system, the requirement would be for the aggregated receptor to activate a putative phospholipase C. This phospholipase C is yet to be identified and indeed, its method of activation remains uncertain. In some receptor systems, this activation is mediated by a GTP-binding regulatory protein, prompting a search for such a protein associated with allergic mediator release. Indeed, permealized RBL cells will initiate the above discussed PI hydrolysis when a non-hydrolysable GTP analogue, guanosine-5'-O-3-thiotriphosphate (GTP-τS), is added[94], further pointing to such an association. A frequently used indicator of GTP-binding protein involvement is pertussis toxin (PT), since this agent selectively blocks this activity via ADP-ribosylation of the GTP-binding protein complex[95]. Although some inhibition of IgE-mediated release of histamine by PT has been reported[96], a recent careful study found no significant effect of PT on mediator release induced by IgE[97]. Interestingly, this same study did find that PT did block, in a dose-dependent manner, histamine release induced by the polyamine, compound 48/80 (rat mast cells), or f–met–leu–phe (human basophils), indicating that a different mediator release pathway is involved for the latter two releasing agents[97].

Cromolyn binding protein as an ion channel

One potential candidate for the ion channel which allows Ca^{2+} fluxes across the membrane is the calcium channel forming protein described by Pecht and colleagues[98]. This protein was isolated by virtue of its binding to the drug cromolyn, hence the name cromolyn binding protein (CBP). Cromolyn is presently used in the treatment of allergic disease and is known to inhibit mediator release from mast cells. While the mechanism of its action is not yet clear, the structure of cromolyn has led to suggestions that it interferes with the $Fc_{\epsilon}RI$ mediated gating of calcium through the plasma membrane. Evidence indicates that CBP preparations can act as an ion (calcium) channel. In early studies, RBL cells which are deficient in CBP were shown not to respond to an IgE stimulus[99] unless CBP was restored (Sendai virus fusion) to the cell[100]. In more recent experiments, the channel activity and interaction with $Fc_{\epsilon}RI$ was directly demonstrated by using reconstitution studies with model lipid bilayers. Thus, with bilayers that had *both* CBP and $Fc_{\epsilon}RI$, channel opening was evident by aggregating $Fc_{\epsilon}RI$ with IgE and the appropriate antigen[101]. Importantly, no channel opening was seen with bilayers containing only $Fc_{\epsilon}RI$, and with bilayers containing only CBP, a response was seen with anti-CBP but not IgE/antigen[101, 102]. Finally, in agreement with degranulation studies, the channels primarily transported calcium and the channel opening was blocked by cromolyn[101, 102]. Thus, the overall data suggest that aggregation of $Fc_{\epsilon}RI$ induces (possibly by co-aggregation) CBP dependent channel activity, and that this activity is responsible for calcium influx into cells.

The biochemical characterization of CBP is less clear. It was initially reported to be a surface protein of ~60 kD MW, and present at essentially the same level as $Fc_{\epsilon}RI$/cell[103]. However, more recent data (B. Rivney, personal communication) indicate that the 60 kD protein was a contaminant, and the protein responsible for the channel activity is thought to be present in considerably lower numbers per cell than the $Fc_{\epsilon}RI$. The development of stable monoclonal anti-CBP, in conjunction with scaled up preparative CBP isolations should, in the near future, allow sequencing and/or cloning of this very interesting protein and/or complex of proteins.

Desensitization of $Fc_{\epsilon}RI$ mediated cell activation

When $Fc_{\epsilon}RI$ aggregation occurs in the absence of calcium, the mediator release cascade is inactivated, in that restoring Ca^{2+} does not lead to degranulation. The inactivation can be either specific, at low aggregation values, or non-specific in the sense that at higher $Fc_{\epsilon}RI$ aggregation values in the absence of calcium, the cell becomes refractory to any $Fc_\epsilon R_I$ mediated degranulation stimulus[104]. The mechanism of this intriguing phenomena is unclear. The desensitization does not involve loss of $Fc_\epsilon R_I$ from the cell surface[105]. While there is a disparity as to whether no internalization or significant internalization occurs, depending on whether human basophils[105] or RBL cells[106] were studied, clearly sufficient receptor remains at the surface to initiate mediator release. The serine protease inhibitor diisopropyl-fluorophosphate (DFP) blocks desensitization in mouse mast cells[107] and human basophils[108] at 10–40 nmol/l and 100–500 nmol/l, respectively. Since higher concentrations of DFP and, as well, other serine protease inhibitors were early on[109] shown to block the activation pathway (i.e. mediator release) (reviewed in Reference 3), this work demonstrates that desensitization is an active process and may have parallels with the activation pathway. Recent work with human lung mast cells also demonstrated both specific and non-specific desensitization phenomena[110]. Intriguingly, this desensitization in mast cells was not blocked by DFP, indicating that the DFP inhibitable step either is not always crucial or that mast cells desensitize via a different mechanism than do basophils. In any case, the total degree of mediator release is a balance between sensitization and desensitization pathways. As the biochemical events occurring in both become clearer it may be possible to influence mediator release by tipping this balance in favour of desensitization.

LOW AFFINITY IgE RECEPTORS (Fc$_\epsilon$RII)

Discovery

The first demonstration of a cell type other than the mast cell/basophil which had specific receptors of IgE was by Lawrence et al.[111]. These investigators measured the ability of ^{125}I-labelled immunoglobulin to bind to various cell types isolated from human peripheral blood. Myeloma IgE which had been aggregated with $F(ab')_2$ anti-human Fab' bound to human lymphocytes. This finding was confirmed and extended by Gonzalez-Molina and Spiegelberg[112] in which it was shown both by $[^{125}I]IgE$ binding and rosette analysis that several human B lymphoblastoid lines and human peripheral blood B lymphocytes possessed $Fc_\epsilon R_{II}$.

Cells bearing Fc$_\epsilon$RII

Although much of the structural work to be subsequently discussed involves the B-lymphocyte $Fc_\epsilon R_{II}$, it is clear that the $Fc_\epsilon R_{II}$ is expressed on a number of cell types. In man $Fc_\epsilon R_{II}^+$ T cells[113] and even $Fc_\epsilon R_{II}^+$ T cell lines[114, 115] have been described by some workers, although it is generally agreed that normal individuals have very low $Fc_\epsilon R_{II}$ levels on their T cells and the function, if any, of this low $Fc_\epsilon R_{II}$ level is unknown. Also, cells of the monocyte/macrophage series[116], eosinophils[117] and platelets[118] express to variable extents the $Fc_\epsilon R_{II}$. Indeed, work, especially from Capron and colleagues (see References 5, 119 for review), has shown $Fc_\epsilon R_{II}$ involvement in parasitic immunity.

110

IgE specific killing of parasites, especially by $Fc_\epsilon R_{II}^+$ macrophages[116], platelets[120] and eosinophils[121] has been described. The structure of the $Fc_\epsilon R_{II}$ on these cell types is less well studied than the B cell $Fc_\epsilon R_{II}$, however, the observation that oligonucleotide probes from the B cell also react with the macrophage $Fc_\epsilon R_{II}$[122] underscores the similarities and indicates that detailed structural comparisons should soon be available.

Structure of the $Fc_\epsilon R_{II}$

The $Fc_\epsilon R_{II}^+$ lymphoblastoid cell lines have been used for structural characterizations in man. Vectorial surface iodination, followed by detergent solubilization and affinity chromatography on IgE-Sepharose gel indicated the presence of two major radioactive bands, a broad band centered at 86 kD and another intense band at 47 kD[123, 124]. In these studies, an additional band at 23 kD was variably seen, however, its presence was diminished by the addition of protease inhibitors indicating it was a proteolysed fragment of the larger components. The 47 kD protein possesses the IgE binding site, as evidenced by the observation that the highly purified 47 kD component rebound to IgE absorbents[125]. Indeed the higher MW component (~ 86 kD) is related to the 47 kD component in that both have identical tryptic peptide maps when surface iodinatable residues are compared. This, combined with the observation that the 86 kD component is more difficult to elute from IgE absorbents, led to the suggestion that the 86 kD component is a dimer of the 47 kD $Fc_\epsilon R_{II}$[125]. The $Fc_\epsilon R_{II}$ spontaneously degrades in both the human and murine (see below) systems. In man, a series of similar sized fragments with an average MW of 25 kD can be isolated from the cell-free supernatant[126]. These fragments have no N-linked glycosylation sites, however, in contrast to the murine system (see below), IgE binding activity is retained[127] in that the $Fc_\epsilon R_{II}$ fragments bind to, and can be eluted from, an IgE affinity column. In addition, via a radioimmunoassay, $Fc_\epsilon R_{II}$ immunoreactivity has been found in the supernatants of $Fc_\epsilon R_{II}^+$ macrophage and T cell lines, as well as B cell lines and even in human serum[127].

Cloning of the human $Fc_\epsilon R_{II}$

Taking advantage of mabs developed against the human $Fc_\epsilon R_{II}$[128-130], several groups have reported cloning the gene for the human $Fc_\epsilon R_{II}$[122, 131, 132]. The three groups used somewhat different cloning strategies, however, the deduced amino acid sequence was essentially identical in all cases. This, combined with the capability to transfect the gene and to get re-expression (and IgE binding) of the cloned $Fc_\epsilon R_{II}$ indicates that the correct gene has been cloned. Several interesting details have emerged from examining the sequence. There is no N-terminal signal sequence and the membrane spanning domain is very close to the amino-terminus, indicating that analogous to a minority of other membrane proteins, the carboxy terminus is exposed to the cell exterior and the amino-terminus is cytoplasmic. Second, the amount of N-linked glycosylation is quite small (one-site) and third, there is no homology of this receptor with the previously cloned[133] rodent IgE-binding factors (IgE-BF); this combined with the observation that in humans an IgE-BF comes from this receptor (see above), suggests that at least two distinct families of IgE-BF exist. Also of note is the lack of homology with $Fc_\epsilon RI$[36], further confirming that these receptors are distinct entities. Finally, significant homology with animal lectins, especially towards the carboxy terminus, was observed. The highest homology was with chicken hepatic lectin, but homology was also seen with other related proteins such as asialoglyco-protein receptor from both rat and human and rat mannose binding protein. The significance of this unexpected finding remains to be elucidated. The overall structural data have led to the following model (Figure 3.2) for the human $Fc_\epsilon RII$, which as expected, bears no similarity to the $Fc_\epsilon RI$ model (Figure 3.1).

Murine lymphocyte $Fc_\epsilon RII$

Initial studies used B lymphocytes from *Nippostrongylus brasiliensis* (Nb) infected mice, taking advantage of the elevated $Fc_\epsilon RII$ expression seen after helminth infection[134]. A single surface iodinatable component of 49 kD and a pI of 4.5 was isolated by affinity chromatography on IgE-affinity absorbents[135]. In subsequent studies, $Fc_\epsilon RII^+$ cell lines were established[136] by fusing B cells from Nb infected mice with the B cell lymphoma M12.4.5[137]. The resulting fusion partners were all $Fc_\epsilon RII^+$, albeit with different levels of $Fc_\epsilon RII$ expression[136]. Using the $Fc_\epsilon RII$ from these cells as immunogen, both poly- and monoclonal anti-$Fc_\epsilon RII$ have been produced[138], and these antibodies have aided in the characterization of $Fc_\epsilon RII$ post-translational processing events. A single chain precursor of 44 kD was found; this precursor had N-linked carbohydrate added co-translationally. The precursor was found only intracellularly, and fully processed active receptors began to appear at the cell surface at about 60 min. Once at the surface the $Fc_\epsilon RII$ degrades, presumably via a protease located at the cell surface, into a 38 kD soluble $Fc_\epsilon RII$ fragment and ~ 10 kD fragment that remains cell associated[138-140]. The soluble $Fc_\epsilon RII$ has essentially lost all IgE binding activity[140] in contrast to the human $Fc_\epsilon RII$ fragment[127]. Exposure to serum protease results in further breakdown and a ~ 28 kD non-glycosylated $Fc_\epsilon RII$ fragment is seen[139].

Modulation of the $Fc_\epsilon RII$

Ligand-dependent upregulation – rodent system

The important observation in the rodent system, that helminth-infection, such as Nb, caused a dramatic increase in IgE levels[141] allowed a system where $Fc_\epsilon RII^+$ cells could be studied under conditions of heightened IgE formation. Examination of Nb infected rats[142] or mice[134] demonstrated an accompanying increase in $Fc_\epsilon RII^+$ lymphocytes. Elevated levels of $Fc_\epsilon RII$ were also seen after injections of myeloma IgE into rats[143] or simply overnight culture of lymphocyte preparations with homologous IgE[144, 145]. While it is now clear that lymphokines such as IL-4 (see below) are also important in

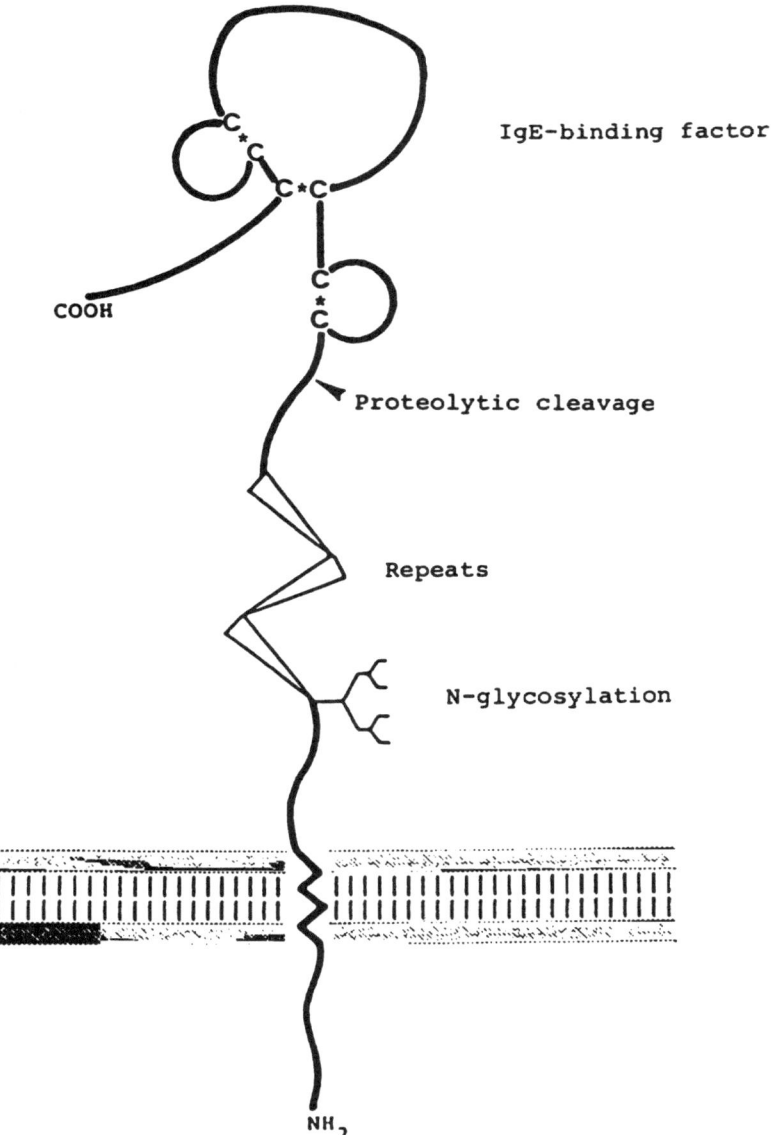

Figure 3.2 Model for the Fc$_\epsilon$R$_{II}$. Based on the recent cloning of the Fc$_\epsilon$R$_{II}$[122, 131, 132], the Fc$_\epsilon$R$_{II}$ is shown as a single chain polypeptide with the amino-terminus cytoplasmic. The 'Cs' represent conserved cysteines (see Reference 132) and the approximate site of proteolytic cleavage, which yields the soluble Fc$_\epsilon$R$_{II}$ fragment is also shown. The 'repeats' seen in the sequence result from a triplicated exon (H. Hofstetter, personal communication). See text for additional information. (Figure is courtesy of H. Hofstetter, Ciba Geigy Corp., Basel, Switzerland, and is based on Reference 132 and additional unpublished work)

$Fc_\epsilon R_{II}$ upregulation, these studies demonstrated that the ligand alone was sufficient for the induction of $Fc_\epsilon R_{II}$.

The recent development of murine B cell lines which bear ligand inducible $Fc_\epsilon R_{II}$[136] has allowed a detailed investigation of the mechanism of this induction. The observation that IgE-induced upregulation occurred only if saturating concentrations of ligand were present, suggested that IgE was protecting the receptor from degradation[136]. Further studies showed that this was indeed true; the halflife of $Fc_\epsilon R_{II}$ was extended 2–3 fold by IgE[140]. The degradation of the $Fc_\epsilon R_{II}$ was shown to involve the proteolytic release of the 38 kD $Fc_\epsilon R_{II}$ fragment, presumably at the cell surface, into the extracellular environment. Using a specific radioimmunoassay developed for solubilized $Fc_\epsilon R_{II}$ fragments[140], IgE was shown to directly inhibit the release of the fragment from both $Fc_\epsilon R_{II}^+$ hybridoma cells as well as murine splenic B cells. In contrast, no evidence was found to indicate that IgE increased the rate of $Fc_\epsilon R_{II}$ synthesis. Thus, the ligand specific upregulation observed in the murine system is due to a slowdown of $Fc_\epsilon R_{II}$ decay, the resulting new equilibrium between the synthesis and the decay rate results in a higher surface $Fc_\epsilon R_{II}$ expression. One final note on this is that these studies utilized $Fc_\epsilon R_{II}^+$ hybridoma cells. Previous studies which had concluded that $Fc_\epsilon R_{II}$ synthesis was elevated by IgE, used B lymphocytes[144]. While IgE mediated protection is operative in B lymphocytes, synthesis rate experiments have not been performed with these cells.

Ligand specific $Fc_\epsilon R_{II}$ upregulation – human system

This type of upregulation is more controversial with human lymphocytes. Early studies demonstrated that there was a correlation between serum IgE levels and the degree of $Fc_\epsilon R_{II}^+$ lymphocytes (reviewed in Reference 4). However, in contrast to the rodent system, simple addition of IgE to the culture media does not induce an increase in IgE-specific rosettes[146]. However, cell activation, in combination with the addition of IgE, does cause an increase in $Fc_\epsilon R_{II}$ levels[147]. In addition, Delespesse et al.[113] have shown that culture with IgE will cause maintenance of $Fc_\epsilon R_{II}$ levels which, in the controls (no IgE) will drop substantially after overnight culture. This data, combined with the observation that the human $Fc_\epsilon R_{II}$ also decays by releasing $Fc_\epsilon R_{II}$ fragment[126, 127], indicate that a 'protection' mechanism similar to that described above for the murine system, also operates in humans. The fact that K_a for the IgE–$Fc_\epsilon R_{II}$ interaction in humans is 10-fold less than in the rodent system (10^7 mol/l vs 10^8 mol/l) probably explains the lower IgE mediated protection in that receptor saturation is more difficult to maintain.

Lymphokine mediated $Fc_\epsilon R_{II}$ upregulation

A number of studies in rodent model systems have indicated that the $Fc_\epsilon R_{II}$ can be modulated by lymphokines. For a detailed discussion of these systems, the reviews by Ishizaka[148] and Katz[149] are recommended. Recent work has concentrated on interleukin 4 (IL-4) (formerly B-cell stimulatory factor-1). In man, Kikutani et al.[150] demonstrated that supernatants from PHA activated human T cells caused a dramatic increase in $Fc_\epsilon R_{II}$ levels and in a note added in proof, the activity causing this phenomena was indicated to be Il-4. DeFrance et al.[151] using purified recombinant human Il-4, confirmed that the $Fc_\epsilon R_{II}$ directly increased on small resting B cells. Subsequently, it was also demonstrated that IL-4, in conjunction with human IgE, caused an increase in $Fc_\epsilon R_{II}$ messenger RNA[122].

Hudak et al.[152] demonstrated that recombinant murine IL-4 caused $Fc_\epsilon R_{II}$ upregulation on murine B lymphocytes. Specificity for IL-4 was shown in that 11B11, a monoclonal anti-IL-4 known to block IL-4 actions[153], blocked the $Fc_\epsilon R_{II}$ upregulation, and in addition, τ-interferon blocked the IL-4 action. The latter agent blocks a number of IL-4 actions on B cells including Class II upregulation[154], anti-Ig co-stimulation[155] and the enhancement of IgE and IgG_1 synthesis[156].

Additional studies have demonstrated that the highest $Fc_\epsilon R_{II}$ levels are seen when both IgE and IL-4 are added simultaneously and, as shown with both $Fc_\epsilon R_{II}^+$ hybridoma clones and normal B lymphocytes, the increase with both agents together is additive[157]. As was the case with human lymphocytes, this increase was due to an increase in the $Fc_\epsilon R_{II}$ synthetic rate, demonstrated by metabolic labelling studies. Finally, the early increase in B cell $Fc_\epsilon R_{II}$ levels, seen after Nb infection of mice, was shown to be due to IL-4[157]. Thus, present knowledge indicates that B cell $Fc_\epsilon R_{II}$ elevated levels result from two distinct mechanisms; increased synthesis rates (IL-4) and decreased decay rates (IgE). Of note here is the observation that IL-4 is involved in the increase in IgE synthesis observed after a parasite infection. Nb infected mice that were also injected with high levels of the anti-IL-4 mab 11B11 failed to develop an IgE response; interestingly the IgG1 levels were not significantly affected[158]. Thus, 11B11 blocks both the increase in $Fc_\epsilon R_{II}$ as well as the IgE increase seen after helminth infections. As mentioned above, human IL-4 has also been cloned, and evidence was recently presented that human IL-4 would cause IgE synthesis in peripheral blood cultures[159].

Relationship between IgE-BF and the $Fc_\epsilon R_{II}$

Work extending over several years has demonstrated the existence and involvement in IgE immunoregulation of a differentially glycosylated polypeptide known as IgE-Binding Factor (IgE-BF). Ishizaka[148] summarizes recent knowledge of IgE-BF with regard to structure and mechanism of action. In this review, only details pertaining to the potential relationship between IgE-BF and the $Fc_\epsilon R_{II}$ will be discussed. This relationship has been a point of considerable interest. Huff et al.[160] demonstrated that poly- and monoclonal anti-IgE-BF would block IgE specific rosettes and stain the same percentage of splenic cells as were capable of rosetting with IgE. In recent work using human IgE-BF and both a monoclonal antibody against human IgE-BF and monoclonal anti-$Fc_\epsilon R_{II}$, limited cross-reactivity was found in that the anti-$Fc_\epsilon R_{II}$ reacted with the 60 kD, but not the lower MW IgE-BF forms[161]. There was, however, no reactivity seen between the monoclonal anti-IgE-BF and the B lymphocyte $Fc_\epsilon R_{II}$[161]. There is no evident homology between the cloned human $Fc_\epsilon R_{II}$[122, 131, 132] and rodent IgE-BF[133]. While the amino acid sequence of the rodent Fc$_\epsilon$RII is not yet available, the similar physicochemical properties of human and murine Fc$_\epsilon$RII suggests that a similar structure will be found. The rodent IgE-BF is essentially identical with a portion of a non-infective retroviral agent known as intracisternal A particles (IAP)[162, 163]. These IAP are found in essentially all murine cell lines in high copy number and the homology results have indicated a potential function for IAP. In contrast, as mentioned earlier, the only homologies for Fc$_\epsilon$RII were with certain animal lectins. Thus, the antigen cross-reactivities contrast with the apparent differences seen by structural analyses. One possible explanation for this paradox is that the antigenic cross-reactivity is with a conformational determinant not evident in the primary sequence; both IgE-BF and Fc$_\epsilon$RII share a common ligand, and if the binding site on the IgE is similar, such a conformational determinant could be anticipated.

Fc$_\epsilon$RII is a B cell differentiation antigen

Two observations suggest that the Fc$_\epsilon$RII may have functions not naturally exclusive but certainly outside its role as an Fc$_\epsilon$R. The first observation was that Fc$_\epsilon$RII both in mice[164] and humans[150] are apparently on a very high percentage of, if not all, B cells, and IL-4 causes Fc$_\epsilon$RII upregulation on all of these cells[152]. However, only a small percentage of these cells ever produce IgE, and, in addition, the Fc$_\epsilon$RII is actually lost after isotype switching[150]. Secondly, the Fc$_\epsilon$RII is apparently identical, as evidenced by mab studies, with a human B cell differentiation antigen known as CD23 or Blast 2[165, 166]. CD23 is especially prominent after Epstein–Barr virus (EBV) infection of B cells[167].

The finding of identity between CD23 and Fc$_\epsilon$RII is especially interesting when combined with recent observations indicating that CD23 may be important in B cell activation. Gordon et al.[168] found that MHM6, a mab against CD23, will, in the presence of phorbol esters, induce the progression of B cells through the G$_1$ stage of the cell cycle. In subsequent work it was noted that some, but not all, anti-CD23 mabs have this property[169], suggesting that a very specific type of interaction with the CD23/Fc$_\epsilon$RII is required in order to induce B cell proliferation. Interestingly, the anti-CD23 activating mabs also enhance the release of the CD23 fragment into the media[170]. Since the recently cloned[171] 12 kD human B cell growth factor (BCGF) also enhances CD23 fragment release[170], it is suggested that this property is responsible for the activating capacities of the respective anti-CD23 mabs. Agents that increase CD23 levels such as IgE or IL-4 provide more material for interaction with BCGF, and this potentially increases the action of BCGF with respect to more CD23 fragment being released. In early work, Gordon and colleagues had indicated that human B cells produce an autocrine growth factor[172, 173], and the CD23/Fc$_\epsilon$RII fragment is a potential candidate for such an activity. In support of this hypothesis, Swendeman and Thorley-Lawson[174] have reported that the CD23/Fc$_\epsilon$RII fragment does exhibit B cell growth factor properties for EBV-infected B lymphoblasts and receptor stimulated B blasts. Additionally, the purified CD23 fragment acted as a co-mitogen for PHA stimulated thymocytes. Since this is a property of interleukin-1, this further led to the suggestion that the intact CD23/Fc$_\epsilon$RII is a membrane form of interleukin-1. This intriguing suggestion would require a completely new form of IL-1 since CD23 has no homology with the known forms of IL-1 and, in addition, anti-IL-1 was not able to interact with the soluble CD23 molecule[174]. Finally, the correlation between high CD23 expression and EBV-infection[167] has been further studied by Wang et al.[175]. Expression of the EBV gene known as EBV nuclear antigen-2 (EBNA-2) in human lymphocytes resulted in very high expression of CD23, and the CD23 expressing cells now grew in large clumps. This probably explains why many EBV transformed B cell lines are so strongly Fc$_\epsilon$RII. In addition, together with the above data suggesting that CD23 is involved in B cell proliferation and/or differentiation, the data suggest that an increase in CD23 may play a central role in cell transformation. Thus, in conclusion of this section, it is clear that while much of this work is at a very early stage, the data clearly point to previously unsuspected roles for the Fc$_\epsilon$RII.

Fc$_\epsilon$RII – role in IgE synthesis modulation

There is little present information regarding the possible role of Fc$_\epsilon$RII, if any, in the control of IgE synthesis. In rodent model systems, IgE-BF have been known for some time to play such a role[148, 149], additionally human IgE-BF which modulate the IgE response have been demonstrated, and the glycosylation of human IgE-BF is apparently under the same regulatory constraints as the rodent counterparts[176, 177]. In addition, Young et al. have also identified Fc$_\epsilon$RII$^+$ T cell clones that produce IgE-potentiating factors[115]. The latter is similar in molecular size and lectin binding properties to the aforementioned rodent IgE-BF[178], and have suggested importance with regard to the control of IgE synthesis in man[179]. Although these IgE-BF come from Fc$_\epsilon$RII positive and not Fc$_\epsilon$RII negative cell lines, the exact relationship with the T cell Fc$_\epsilon$RII is not yet known.

The immunoregulatory properties of either intact B lymphocyte Fc$_\epsilon$RII or the Fc$_\epsilon$RI fragment(s) is also not yet clear. Initial work from Delepesse's laboratory indicated that Fc$_\epsilon$RII$^+$ human B cell lines released factors capable of potentiating IgE synthesis[180]. In addition, analogous to the more well studied rodent IgE-BF (reviewed in Reference 148), culture of the cells with tunicamycin resulted in a switch of biologic activity from potentiation to suppression[181]. In view of the finding that the human Fc$_\epsilon$RII fragment has no N-linked glycosylation sites[122, 126], the above data with tunicamycin are difficult to explain. It has not been formally shown that the 25 kD Fc$_\epsilon$RII fragment is responsible for the immunoregulatory activity seen, thus, possibly other factors, perhaps more analogous to the rodent IgE-BF, are responsible for the immunoregulatory activity seen with supernatants from Fc$_\epsilon$RII$^+$ B[180] and T[115, 182] cells.

CONCLUSIONS AND FUTURE PERSPECTIVES

As indicated herein, three apparently different IgE binding proteins are now known to exist. The highest in affinity is the mast cell Fc$_\epsilon$RI; the IgE binding portion of which (α-chain) is a member of the immunoglobulin gene superfamily and thus, is also related to the murine $Fc_\tau R$. This receptor is clearly involved in mediator release from mast cells and basophils, although the mechanisms of that involvement remain unclear. The soon to be determined amino acid composition and sequence of the receptor associated β and τ components will, in all probability, give further clues to the function of the $Fc_\epsilon RI$.

The $Fc_\epsilon RII$, defined rather simply as the 'low affinity' receptor for IgE exists on a variety of cell types. Present evidence from the cloning of the human lymphocyte $Fc_\epsilon RII$ combined with additional biochemical data involving the site of interaction of the $Fc_\epsilon RI$ vs $Fc_\epsilon RII$ with IgE indicate that the two receptors represent a different gene product that interacts with different sites on the IgE molecule. The lymphocyte receptor also sheds an $Fc_\epsilon RII$ fragment into the media; in the human, but not murine, system this fragment retains IgE binding activity, and has been termed an IgE-BF. This IgE-BF is different from the third class of IgE binding proteins, that being the classically studied IgE-BF of the rodent model systems; no sequence homology was seen between the two molecules. The possible immunoregulatory activity of the $Fc_\epsilon RII$ fragment is an area of active investigation, however, at present the function is unclear. Recent evidence pointing to growth factor-like activities of the lymphocyte $Fc_\epsilon RII$ is pointing to new previously unsuspected roles for this molecule. The $Fc_\epsilon RII$ on macrophages, platelets and eosinophils is not as well structurally characterized, however, functional studies point to a role in parasitic immunity. The exact relationship between the $Fc_\epsilon RII$ on the various cell types, via the use of molecular probes, should soon be available.

Overall, the progress especially in the past several years, has been most impressive, and the combined effort from a number of laboratories has greatly improved our understanding of IgE binding proteins. The rapid development of molecular techniques will serve to further increase future progress, and, in the near future, may allow new protocols for the treatment of human allergy.

ACKNOWLEDGEMENTS

Work performed in the author's laboratory was funded by grants AI18697 and AI22600. Preprints from H. Metzger, M. Beaven, T. Ishizaka and J. Gorden and the $Fc_\epsilon RII$ model from H. Hofstetter are gratefully acknowledged. Thanks are extended to K. Ishizaka, W. Lee, M. Rao and A. Keegan for assistance in final revisions and D. Schott for the preparation of the manuscript.

References

1. Metzger, H., Alcaraz, G., Hohman, R., Kinet, J.-P., Pribluda, B. and Quarto, R. (1986). The receptor with high affinity for immunoglobulin E. *Annu. Rev. Immunol.*, **4**, 419–70
2. Froese, A. (1984). Receptors for IgE on mast cells and basophils. *Prog. Allergy*, **34**, 142–87

3. Ishizaka, T. and Ishizaka, K. (1984). Activation of mast cells for mediator release through IgE receptors. *Prog. Allergy*, **34**, 188–235
4. Spiegelberg, H. L. (1984). Structure and function of Fc receptors for IgE on lymphocytes, monocytes, and macrophages. *Adv. Immunol.*, **35**, 61–88
5. Capron, A., Dessaint, J. P., Capron, M., Joseph, M., Ameisen, J. C. and Tonnel, A. B. (1986). From parasites to allergy: a second receptor for IgE. *Immunol. Today*, **7**, 15–18
6. Ishizaka, K., Tomioka, H. and Ishizaka, T. (1970). Mechanisms of passive sensitization. I. Presence of IgE and IgG molecules on human leukocytes. *J. Immunol.*, **105**, 1459–67
7. Tomioka, H. and Ishizaka, K. (1971). Mechanisms of passive sensitization. II. Presence of receptors for IgE on monkey mast cells. *J. Immunol.*, **107**, 971–8
8. Eccleston, E., Leonard, B. J., Lowe, J. S. and Welford, H. J. (1973). Basophilic leukaemia in the albino rat and a demonstration of the basopoietin. *Nature New Biol.*, **244**, 73–6
9. Kulczycki, A. Jr., Isersky, C. and Metzger, H. (1974). The interaction of IgE with rat basophilic leukemia cells. I. evidence for specific binding of IgE. *J. Exp. Med.*, **139**, 600–16
10. Conrad, D. H. and Froese, A. (1976). Characterization of the target cell receptor for IgE. II. Polyacrylamide gel analysis of the surface IgE receptor from normal rat mast cells and rat basophilic leukemia cells. *J. Immunol.*, **116**, 319
11. Pecoud, A. R., Ruddy, S. and Conrad, D. H. (1981). Functional and partial chemical characterization of the carbohydrate moieties of the IgE receptor on rat basophilic leukemia cells and rat mast cells. *J. Immunol.*, **126**, 1624–9
12. Hempstead, B. L., Parker, C. W. and Kulczyki, A. Jr. (1981). The cell surface receptor for immunoglobulin E. Effect of tunicamycin on molecular properties of receptor from rat basophilic leukemia cells. *J. Biol. Chem.*, **256**, 10717–23
13. Goetze, A., Kanellopoulos, J., Rice, D. and Metzger, H. (1981). Enzymatic cleavage products of the alpha subunit of the receptor for immunoglobulin E. *Biochemistry*, **20**, 6341–9
14. Rossi, G., Newman, S. A. and Metzger, H. (1977). Assay and partial characterization of the solubilized cell surface receptor for immunoglobulin. *J. Biol. Chem.*, **252**, 704–11
15. Conrad, D. H., Berczi, I. and Froese, A. (1976). Characterization of the target cell receptor for IgE. I. Solubilization of IgE-receptor complexes from rat mast cells and rat basophilic leukemia cells. *Immunochemistry*, **13**, 329–32
16. Holowka, D., Hartmann, H., Kannellopoulos, J. and Metzger, H. (1980). Association of the receptor for immunoglobulin E with an endogenous polypeptide on rat basophilic leukemia cells. *J. Receptor Res.*, **1**, 41–68
17. Perez-Montford, R., Kinet, J.-P. and Metzger, H. (1983). A previously unrecognized subunit of the receptor for immunoglobulin E. *Biochemistry*, **22**, 5722–8
18. Metzger, H., Kinet, J.-P., Perez-Montfort, R., Rivnay, B. and Wank, S. A. (1983). A tetrameric model for the structure of the mast cell receptor with high affinity for IgE. *Prog. Immunol.*, **5**, 493–501
19. Pecoud, A. R. and Conrad, D. H. (1981). Characterization of the IgE receptor by tryptic mapping. *J. Immunol.*, **127**, 2209–14
20. Holowka, D. and Baird, B. (1984). Lactoperoxidase-catalyzed iodination of the receptor for immunoglobulin E at the cytoplasmic side of the plasma membrane. *J. Biol. Chem.*, **259**, 3720–8
21. Lee, W. T. and Conrad, D. H. (1985). The murine lymphocyte receptor for IgE. III. Use of chemical cross-linking reagents to further characterize the B lymphocyte Fc epsilon receptor. *J. Immunol.*, **134**, 518–25
22. Staros, J. V., Lee, W. T. and Conrad, D. H. (1987). Membrane-impermeant cross-linking reagents: Application to the study of the cell surface receptor for IgE. In Disabato, G., Langone, J. J. and Vunakis, H. V. (eds.) *Methods in Enzymology*, Vol. 150, pp. 503–12. (NY: Academic Press)
23. Holowka, D., Gitler, C., Bercovici, T. and Metzger, H. (1981). Reaction of 5-iodonaphthyl-1-nitrene with the receptor for IgE on normal and tumor mast cells. *Nature*, **289**, 806–8
24. Kinet, J.-P., Alcaraz, G., Leonard, A., Wank, S. and Metzger, H. (1985). Dissociation of the receptor for immunoglubulin E in mild detergents. *Biochemistry*, **24**, 4117–24
25. Rivnay, B., Wank, S., Poy, G. and Metzger, H. (1982). Phospholipids stabilize the interaction between the alpha and beta subunits of the solubilized receptor for immunoglobulin E. *Biochemistry*, **21**, 6922–7

119

26. Rivnay, B. and Fischer, G. (1986). Phospholipid distribution in the microenvironment of the immunoglobulin E-receptor from rat basophilic leukemia cell membrane. *Biochemistry*, **25**, 5686–93
27. Hannun, Y. A., Loomis, C. R., Merrill, A. H., Jr. and Bell, R. M. (1986). Sphingosine inhibition of protein kinase C activity and of phorbol dibutyrate binding *in vitro* and in human platelets. *J. Biol. Chem.*, **261**, 12604–9
28. Rivnay, B., Rossi, G., Henkart, M. and Metzger, H. (1984). Reconstitution of the receptor for immunoglobulin E into liposomes. Reincorporation of purified receptors. *J. Biol. Chem.*, **259**, 1212–17
29. Rivnay, G. and Metzger, H. (1982). Reconstitution of the receptor for immunoglobulin E into liposomes: Conditions for incorporation of the receptor into vesicles. *J. Biol. Chem.*, **257**, 12800–8
30. Fewtrell, C., Goetze, A. and Metzger, H. (1982). Phosphorylation of the receptor for immunoglobulin E. *Biochemistry*, **21**, 2004–10
31. Perez-Montford, R., Fewtrell, C. and Metzger, H. (1983). Changes in the receptor for immunoglobulin E coincident with receptor-mediated stimulation of basophilic leukemia cells. *Biochemistry*, **22**, 5733–7
32. Hempstead, B. L., Kulczycki, A. Jr. and Parker, C. W. (1981). Phosphorylation of the IgE receptor from ionophore A23187 stimulated intact rat mast cells. *Biochem. Biophys. Res. Commun.*, **98**, 815–22
33. Hempstead, B. L., Parker, C. W. and Kulczycki, A. Jr. (1983). Selective phosphorylation of the IgE receptor in antigen-stimulated rat mast cells. *Proc. Natl. Acad. Sci., USA*, **80**, 3050–3
34. Quarto, R. and Metzger, H. (1986). The receptor for immunoglobulin E: examination for kinase activity and as a substrate for kinases. *Mol. Immunol.*, **23**, 1215–23
35. Basciano, L. K., Berenstein, E. H., Kmak, L. and Siraganian, R. P. (1986). Monoclonal antibodies that inhibit IgE binding. *J. Biol. Chem.*, **261**, 11823–31
36. Kinet, J.-P., Metzger, H., Hakimi, J. and Kochan, J. (1987). A cDNA presumptively clones coding for the α-subunit of the receptor with high affinity for immunoglobulin E. *Biochemistry*, **26**, 4605–10
37. Revetch, J. V., Luster, A. D., Weinschank, R., Kochran, J. Pavlovec, A., Portnoy, D. A., Hulmes, J., Pan, Y. C. E. and Unkeless, J. C. (1986). Structural heterogeneity and functional domains of murine immunoglobulin G Fc receptors. *Science*, **234**, 718–25
38. Lewis, V. A., Koch, T., Plutner, H. and Mellman, I. (1986). A complementary DNA clone for a macrophage–lymphocyte Fc receptor. *Nature*, **324**, 372–5
39. Conrad, D., Wingard, J. R. and Ishizaka, T. (1983). The interaction of human and rodent IgE with the human basophil IgE receptor. *J. Immunol.*, **130**, 327–33
40. Hempstead, B. L., Parker, C. W. and Kulczycki, A. Jr. (1979). Characterization of the IgE receptor isolated from human basophils. *J. Immunol.*, **123**, 2283–91
41. Ishizaka, T., Dvorak, A. M., Conrad, D. H., Niebyl, J. R., Marquette, J. P. and Ishizaka, K. (1985). Morphologic and immunologic characterization of human basophils developed in cultures of cord blood mononuclear cells. *J. Immunol.*, **134**, 532–40
42. Ishizaka, T., Conrad, D. H., Schulman, E. S., Sterk, A. R. and Ishizaka, K. (1983). Biochemical analysis of initial triggering events of IgE-mediated histamine release from human lung mast cells. *J. Immunol.*, **130**, 2357–62
43. Sterk, A. R. and Ishizaka, T. (1982). Binding properties of IgE receptors on normal mouse mast cells. *J. Immunol.*, **128**, 838–43
44. Kepron, M. R., Conrad, D. H. and Froese, A. (1982). The cross-reactivity of rat IgE and IgG with solubilized receptors of rat basophilic leukemia cells. *Mol. Immunol.*, **19**, 1631–9
45. Kepron, M. R. and Froese, A. (1987). A microassay for studies of the interaction between Fc receptors and low affinity ligands. *J. Immunol. Meth.*, **98**, 209–17
46. Ishizaka, T. and Ishizaka, K. (1974). Mechanisms of passive sensitization. IV. Dissociation of IgE molecules from basophil receptors at acid pH. *J. Immunol.*, **112**, 1078–84
47. Kulczycki, A. Jr. and Metzger, H. (1974). The interaction of IgE with rat basophilic leukemia cells. II. Quantitative aspects of the binding reaction. *J. Exp. Med.*, **140**, 1676–95
48. Pruzansky, J. J. and Patterson, R. (1986). Binding constants of IgE receptors on human blood basophils for IgE. *Immunology*, **58**, 257–62

49. Conrad, D. H., Bazin, H., Sehon, A. H. and Froese, A. (1975). Binding parameters of the interaction between rat IgE and rat mast cell receptors. *J. Immunol.*, **114**, 1688–91
50. Ishizaka, K. and Ishizaka, T. (1969). Immune mechanisms of reversed type reaginic hypersensitivity. *J. Immunol.*, **103**, 588–95
51. Ishizaka, T., Ishizaka, K. and Tomioka, H. (1972). Release of histamine and slow reacting substance of anaphylaxis (SRS-A) by IgE-anti-IgE reactions on monkey mast cells. *J. Immunol.*, **108**, 513–20
52. Siraganian, R. P., Hook, W. A. and Levine, B. B. (1975). Specific *in vitro* histamine release from basophils by divalent haptens: Evidence for activation by simple bridging of membrane-bound antibody. *Immunochemistry*, **12**, 149–57
53. Segal, D. M., Taurog, J. D. and Metzger, H. (1977). Dimeric immunoglobin E serves as a unit signal for mast cell degranulation. *Proc. Natl. Acad. Sci., USA*, **74**, 2993–7
54. Ishizaka, T. and Ishizaka, K. (1978). Triggering of histamine release from rat mast cells by divalent antibodies against IgE receptors. *J. Immunol.*, **120**, 800
55. Isersky, C., Taurog, J. D., Poy, G. and Metzger, H. (1978). Triggering of cultured neoplastic mast cells by antibodies to the receptor for IgE. *J. Immunol.*, **121**, 549–58
56. Fewtrell, C. and Metzger, H. (1980). Larger oligomers of IgE are more effective than dimers in stimulating rat basophilic leukemia cells. *J. Immunol.*, **125**, 701–10
57. Conrad, D. H., Studer, E., Gervasoni, J. and Mohanakumar, T. (1983). Properties of two monoclonal antibodies directed against the Fc and Fab' regions of rat IgE. *Int. Arch. Allergy Appl. Immunol.*, **70**, 352–60
58. Menon, A. K., Holowka, D., Webb, W. W. and Baird, B. (1986). Cross-linking of receptor-bound IgE to aggregates larger than dimers leads to rapid immobilization. *J. Cell Biol.*, **102**, 541–50
59. Menon, A. K., Holowka, D., Webb, W. W. and Baird, B. (1986). Clustering, mobility, and triggering activity of small oligomers of immunoglobulin E on rat basophilic leukemia cells. *J. Cell Biol.*, **102**, 534–40
60. MacGlashan, D. W. and Lichtenstein, L. M. (1985). Characteristics of human basophil sulfidopeptide leukotriene release: Releasability defined as the the ability of the basophil to respond to dimeric cross-links. *J. Immunol.*, **136**, 2231–9
61. Lee, W. T. and Conrad, D. H. (1984). The murine lymphocyte receptor for IgE. II. Characterization of the multivalent nature of the B lymphocyte receptor for IgE. *J. Exp. Med.*, **159**, 1790–5
62. Schlessinger, J., Webb, W. W., Elson, E. L. and Metzger, H. (1976). Lateral motion and valence of Fc receptors on rat peritoneal mast cells. *Nature*, **264**, 550–2
63. Ishizaka, T. and Ishizaka, K. (1975). Cell-surface IgE on human basophil granulocytes. *Ann. NY Acad. Sci.*, **254**, 462–75
64. Furuichi, K., Rivera, J. and Isersky, C. (1985). The fate of IgE bound to rat basophilic cells. IV. Functional relationship between the receptors for IgE. *J. Immunol.*, **134**, 1766–73
65. Menon, A. K., Holowka, D. and Baird, B. (1984). Small oligomers of immunoglobulin E (IgE) cause large-scale clustering of IgE receptors on the surface of rat basophilic leukemia cells. *J. Cell Biol*, **98**, 577–83
66. Chan, B. M. C., McNeill, K., Berczi, I. and Froese, A. (1986). Effects of mycoplasma infection of Fc receptors for IgE of rat basophilic leukemia cells. *Eur. J. Immunol.*, **16**, 1319–24
67. Roth, P. A., Rao, M. and Froese, A. (1986). Disulphide-linked receptors for IgE on rat basophilic leukaemia cells. *Immunology*, **58**, 671–6
68. Furuichi, K., Rivera, J. and Isersky, C. (1985). The receptor for immunoglobulin E on rat basophilic leukemia cells: effect of ligand binding on receptor expression. *Proc. Natl. Acad. Sci. USA*, **82**, 1522–5
69. Quarto, R., Kinet, J.-P. and Metzger, H. (1985). Coordinate synthesis and degradation of the alpha-, beta- and gamma-subunits of the receptor for immunoglobulin E. *Mol. Immunol.*, **22**, 1045–51
70. Isersky, C., Rivera, J., Segal, D. M. and Triche, T. (1975). The fate of IgE bound to rat basophilic leukemia cells. II. Endocytosis of IgE oligomers and effect on receptor turnover. *J. Immunol.*, **131**, 388–96
71. Perez-Montford, R. and Metzger, H. (1982). Proteolysis of soluble IgE-receptor complexes: Localisation of sites on IgE which interact with the Fc receptor. *Mol. Immunol.*, **19**, 1113–25

72. Baird, B. and Holowka, D. (1985). Structural mapping of Fc receptor bound immuno-globulin E: proximity to the membrane surface of the antibody combining site and another site in the Fab segments. *Biochemistry*, **24**, 6252–9
73. Holowka, D., Conrad, D. H. and Baird, B. (1985). Structural mapping of membrane-bound immunoglobulin E-receptor complexes: Use of monoclonal anti-IgE antibodies to probe the conformation of receptor-bound IgE. *Biochemistry*, **25**, 6260–7
74. Ishizaka, K., Ishizaka, T. and Lee, E. H. (1970). Biologic function of the Fc fragments of E myeloma protein. *Immunochemistry*, **7**, 687–702
75. Hamburger, R. N. (1975). Peptide inhibition of the Prausnitz–Kustner reaction. *Science*, **189**, 389–90
76. Bennich, H., Ragnarsson, U., Johansson, S. G., Ishizaka, K., Ishizaka, T., Levy, D. A. and Lichtenstein, L. M. (1977). Failure of the putative IgE pentapeptide to compete with IgE for receptors on basophils and mast cells. *Int. Arch. Allergy. Appl. Immunol.*, **53**, 459–68
77. Burt, D. S. and Stanworth, D. R. (1987). Inhibition of binding of rat IgE to rat mast cells by synthetic IgE peptides. *Eur. J. Immunol.*, **17**, 437–40
78. Kenten, J., Helm, B., Ishizaka, T., Cantini, P. and Gould, H. (1984). Properties of a human immunoglobulin E-chain fragment synthesized in *Escherichia coli*. *Proc. Natl. Acad. Sci. USA*, **81**, 2955–9
79. Liu, F.-T., Albrandt, K. A., Bry, C. G. and Ishizaka, T. (1984). Expression of a biologically active fragment of human IgE epsilon chain in *Escherichia coli*. *Proc. Natl. Acad. Sci. USA*, **81**, 5369–73
80. Ishizaka, T., Helm, B., Hakimi, J., Niebyl, J., Ishizaka, K. and Gould, H. (1986). Biological properties of a recombinant human immunoglobulin epsilon-chain fragment. *Proc. Natl. Acad. Sci. USA*, **83**, 8323–7
81. Helm, B., Marsh, P., Vercelli, D., Padlan, E., Gould, H. and Geha, R. (1988). The mast cell binding site on human immunoglobulin E. *Nature*, **331**, 180–3
82. Mongar, J. L. and Schild, H. O. (1958). The effect of calcium and pH on the anaphylactic reaction. *J. Physiol.*, **140**, 272–84
83. White, J. R., Ishizaka, T., Ishizaka, K. and Sha'afi, R. I. (1984). Direct demonstration of increased cellular concentration of free calcium as measured by quin-2 in stimulated rat peri-toneal mast cells. *Proc. Natl. Acad. Sci. USA*, **81**, 3978–82
84. Lindau, M. and Fernandez, J. M. (1986). IgE-mediated degranulation of mast cells does not require opening of ion channels. *Nature*, **319**, 150–3
85. Beaven, M. A., Rogers, J., Moore, J. P., Hesketh, T. R., Smith, G. A. and Metcalfe, J. C. (1984). The mechanism of the calcium signal and correlation with histamine release in 2H3 cells. *J. Biol. Chem.*, **259**, 7129–36
86. Berridge, M. J. and Irvine, R. F. (1984). Inositol triphosphate, a novel second messenger in cellular signal transduction. *Nature*, **312**, 315–21
87. Berridge, M. J. (1984). Inositol triphosphate and diacylglycerol as second messengers. *Biochem. J.*, **220**, 345–60
88. Cunha-Melo, J. R., Dean, N. M., Moyer, J. D., Maeyama, K. and Beaven, M. A. (1987). The kinetics of phosphoinositide hydrolysis in rat basophilic leukemia (RBL-2H3) cells varies with the type of IgE receptor crosslinking agent used. *J. Biol. Chem.*, **262**, 11455–63
89. Cunha-Melo, J. R., Dean, N. M. and Beaven, M. A. (1987). Formation of inositol 1,4,5-triphosphate and inositol 1,3,4-triphosphate from inositol 1,3,4,5-tetrakisphosphate and their pathways of degradation in RBL-2H3 cells. (*Submitted*)
90. Maeyama, K., Hohman, R. J., Metzger, H. and Beaven, M. (1986). Quantitative relation-ships between aggregation of IgE receptors, generation of intracellular signals, and histamine secretion in rat basophilic leukemia (2H3) cells. *J. Biol. Chem.*, **261**, 2583–92
91. White, J. R., Pluznik, D. H., Ishizaka, K. and Ishizaka, T. (1985). Antigen-induced increase in protein kinase C activity in plasma membrane of mast cells. *Proc. Natl. Acad. Sci. USA*, **82**, 8193–7
92. Musch, M. W. and Siegel, M. I. (1986). Antigen-stimulated metabolism of inositol phospholipids in the cloned murine mast-cell line MC9. *Biochem. J.*, **234**, 205–12
93. Beaven, M. A., Moore, J. P., Smith, G. A., Hesketh, T. R. and Metcalfe, J. C. (1984). The calcium signal and phosphatidylinositol breakdown in 2H3 cells. *J. Biol. Chem.*, **259**, 7137–42

94. Ali, H., Cunha-Melo, J. R. and Beaven, M. A. (1987). Receptor-mediated release of inositol 1,4,5-trisphosphate in basophilic RBL-2H3 cells permealized with streptolysin O: Evidence for simultaneous production of inositol 1,4-bisphosphate and inositol 1,4,5-trisphosphate. (*Submitted*)
95. Katada, T. and Ui, M. (1982). Direct modification of the membrane adenylate cyclase system by islet-activating protein due to ADP-ribosylation of a membrane protein. *Proc. Natl. Acad. Sci. USA*, **79**, 3129–33
96. Nakamura, T. and Ui, M. (1984). Islet activating protein, pertussis toxin, inhibits Ca^{+2}-induced and guanine nucleotide-dependent releases of histamine and arachidonic acid from rat mast cells. *FEBS Lett.*, **173**, 414–18
97. Saito, H., Okajima, F., Molski, T. F. P., Sha'afi, R. I., Ui, M. and Ishizaka, T. (1987). Effects of ADP-ribosylation of GTP-binding protein by pertussis toxin on immunoglobulin E-dependent and -independent histamine release from mast cells and basophils. *J. Immunol.*, **138**, 3927–34
98. Mazurek, N., Schindler, H., Schurholz, T. L. and Pecht, I. (1984). The cromolyn binding protein constitutes the Ca^{++} channel of basophils opening upon immunological stimulus. *Proc. Natl. Acad. Sci. USA*, **81**, 6841–5
99. Mazurek, N., Bashkin, P., Pertrauk, A. and Pecht, I. (1983). Basophil variants with impaired cromoglycate binding do not respond to an immunological degranulation stimulus. *Nature*, **303**, 528–30
100. Mazurek, N., Bashkin, P., Loyter, A. and Pecht, I. (1983). Restoration of Ca^{++} influx and degranulation capacity of variant RBL-2H3 cells upon implantation of isolated cromolyn binding protein. *Proc. Natl. Acad. Sci. USA*, **80**, 6014–18
101. Mazurek, N., Dulic, V., Pecht, I., Schindler, H. G. and Rivnay, B. (1986). The role of the Fc_ϵ receptor in calcium channel opening in rat basophilic leukemia cells. *Immunol. Lett.*, **12**, 31–5
102. Pecht, I., Schweitzer-Stenner, R., Rivnay, B. and Corcia, A. (1986). Characterization of the ion channel activity in planar bilayers containing IgE-Fc_ϵ receptor and the cromolyn-binding protein. *EMBO J.*, **5**, 849–54
103. Mazurek, N., Bashkin, P. and Pecht, I. (1982). Isolation of a basophilic membrane protein binding the anti-allergic drug cromolyn. *EMBO J.*, **1**, 585–90
104. MacGlashan, D. W., Jr. and Lichtenstein, L. M. (1981). The transition from specific to non-specific desensitation in human basophils. *J. Immunol.*, **127**, 2410–14
105. MacGlashan, D. W. Jr., Mogowski, M. and Lichtenstein, L. M. (1983). Studies of antigen binding on human basophils. II. Continued expression of antigen-specific IgE during antigen-induced desensitization. *J. Immunol.*, **130**, 2337–42
106. Furuichi, K., Rivera, J. and Isersky, C. (1984). The fate of IgE bound to rat basophilic cells. III. Relationship between antigen induced endocytosis and serotonin release. *J. Immunol.*, **133**, 1513–20
107. Ishizaka, T., Sterk, A. R., Daeron, M., Becker, E. and Ishizaka, K. (1985). Biochemical analysis of desensitization of mouse mast cells. *J. Immunol.*, **135**, 491–501
108. Kazimierczak, W., Meier, H. L., MacGlashan, D. W. Jr. and Lichtenstein, L. M. (1984). An antigen-activated, DFP-inhibitable enzyme controls basophil desensitization. *J. Immunol.*, **132**, 399–405
109. Austen, K. F. and Brocklehurst, W. E. (1960). Anaphylaxis in chopped guinea pig lung. Effect of peptidase substrates and inhibitors. *J. Exp. Med.*, **113**, 521–39
110. MacGlashan, D., Jr. and Lichtenstein, L. M. (1987). Basic characteristics of human lung mast cell desensitization. *J. Immunol.*, **139**, 501–5
111. Lawrence, D. A., Weigle, W. O. and Spiegelberg, H. L. (1975). Immunoglobulins cytophilic for human lymphocytes, monocytes, and neutrophils. *J. Clin. Invest.*, **55**, 268
112. Gonzalez-Molina, A. and Spiegelberg, H. L. (1976). Binding of IgE myeloma proteins to human cultured lymphoblastoid cells. *J. Immunol.*, **117**, 1838
113. Delespesse, G., Sarfati, M., Rubio-Truijillo, M. and Wolowiec, T. (1986). IgE receptors on human lymphocytes. III. Expression of IgE receptors on mitogen-stimulated human mononuclear cells. *Eur. J. Immunol.*, **16**, 1043–7
114. Nutman, T. B., Volkman, D. S., Hussain, R., Fauci, A. S. and Ottesen, E. A. (1985). Filarial parasite-specific T cell lines: Induction of IgE synthesis. *J. Immunol.*, **134**, 1178

115. Young, M. C., Leung, D. Y. and Geha, R. S. (1984). Production of IgE-potentiating factor in man by T cell lines bearing Fc receptors for IgE. *Eur. J. Immunol.*, **14**, 871–8
116. Capron, A., Dessaint, J.-P., Joseph, M., Rousseaux, R., Capron, M. and Bazin, H. (1977). Interaction between IgE complexes and macrophages in the rat: a new mechanism of macrophage activation. *Eur. J. Immunol.*, **7**, 315–30
117. Capron, M., Kusnierz, J. P., Prin, L., Spiegelberg, H. L., Ovlaque, G., Gosset, P., Tonnel, A. B. and Capron, A. (1985). Cytophilic IgE on human blood and tissue eosinophils: detection by flow microfluorometry. *J. Immunol.*, **134**, 3013–18
118. Joseph, M., Capron, A., Ameisen, J. C., Capron, M., Vorng, H., Pancre, V., Kusnierz, J. P. and Auriault, C. (1986). The receptor for IgE on blood platelets. *Eur. J. Immunol.*, **16**, 306–12
119. Capron, A. and Dessaint, J. P. (1985). Effector and regulatory mechanisms in immunity to schistosomes: A heuristic view. *Annu. Rev. Immunol.*, **3**, 455–76
120. Joseph, M., Auriault, C., Capron, A., Vorng, H. and Viens, P. (1983). A new function for platelets: IgE-dependent killing of schistosomes. *Nature*, **303**, 810–12
121. Capron, M., Spiegelberg, H. L., Prin, L., Bennich, H., Butterworth, A. E., Pierce, R. J., Ouaissi, M. A. and Capron, A. (1984). Role of IgE receptors in effector function of human eosinophils. *J. Immunol.*, **132**, 462–8
122. Kikutani, H., Inui, S., Sato, R., Barsumian, E. L., Owaki, H., Yamasaki, K., Kaisho, T., Uchibayashi, N., Hardy, R. R., Hirano, T., Tsumasawa, S., Sakiyama, F., Suemura, M. and Kishimoto, T. (1986). Molecular structure of human lymphocyte receptor for immunoglobulin E. *Cell*, **47**, 657–65
123. Meinke, G. C., Magro, A. M., Lawrence, D. A. and Spiegelberg, H. L. (1978). Characterization of an IgE receptor isolated from cultured B type lymphoblastoid cells. *J. Immunol.*, **121**, 1321–6
124. Melewicz, F. M., Plummer, J. M. and Spiegelberg, H. L. (1982). Comparison of the Fc receptors for IgE on human lymphocytes and monocytes. *J. Immunol.*, **129**, 563–9
125. Peterson, L. H. and Conrad, D. H. (1985). Fine specificity, structure, and proteolytic susceptibility of the human lymphocyte receptor for IgE. *J. Immunol.*, **135**, 2654–60
126. Sarfati, M., Nakajima, T., Frost, H., Kilccherr, E. and Delespesse, G. (1987). Purification and partial biochemical characterization of IgE-binding factors secreted by a human B lymphoblastoid cell line. *Immunology*, **60**, 539–45
127. Sarfati, M., Nutman, T., Fonteyn, C. and Delespesse, G. (1986). Presence of antigenic determinants common to IgE Fc receptors on human macrophages, T and B lymphocytes and IgE-binding factors. *Immunology*, **59**, 569–75
128. Rector, E., Nakajima, T., Rocha, C., Duncan, D., Lestourgeon, D., Mitchell, R. S., Fischer, J., Sehon, A. H. and Delespesse, G. (1985). Detection and characterization of monoclonal antibodies specific to IgE receptors on human lymphocytes by flow cytometry. *Immunology*, **55**, 481–8
129. Suemura, M., Kikutani, H., Barsumian, E. L., Hattori, Y., Kishimoto, S., Sato, R., Maeda, A., Nakamura, H., Owaki, H., Hardy, R. R. and Kishimoto, T. (1986). Monoclonal anti-Fc$_\epsilon$ receptor antibodies with different specificities and studies on the expression of Fc$_\epsilon$ receptors on human B and T cells. *J. Immunol.*, **137**, 1214–20
130. Noro, N., Yoshioka, A., Adache, M., Yasuker, K., Masuda, T. and Yodoi, J. (1986). Monoclonal antibody (H107) inhibiting IgE binding to Fc$_\epsilon$R(+) human lymphocytes. *J. Immunol.*, **137**, 1258–63
131. Ikuta, K., Takami, M., Kim, L. W., Honjo, T., Miyoshi, T., Tagaya, Y., Kawabe, T. and Yodoi, J. (1987). Human lymphocyte Fc receptor for IgE: Sequence homology of its cloned cDNA with animal lectins. *Proc. Natl. Acad. Sci.*, **84**, 819–23
132. Ludin, C., Hofstetter, H., Sarfati, M., Levy, C. A., Suter, U., Alaimo, D., Kelchherr, E., Frost, H. and Delespesse, G. (1987). Cloning and expression of the cDNA coding for a human lymphocyte IgE receptor. *EMBO J.*, **6**, 109–14
133. Martens, L. L., Huff, T., Jardieu, P., Trounstine, M. L., Coffman, R. L., Ishizaka, K. and Moore, K. W. (1985). cDNA clones encoding IgE-binding factors from a rat–mouse T cell hybridoma. *Proc. Natl. Acad. Sci. USA*, **82**, 2460–4
134. Vander-Mallie, R., Ishizaka, T. and Ishizaka, K. (1982). Lymphocytes bearing receptors for IgE. VIII. Affinity of mouse IgE for Fc-epsilon receptor on mouse B lymphocytes. *J. Immunol.*, **128**, 2306

135. Conrad, D. H. and Peterson, L. H. (1984). The murine lymphocyte receptor for IgE. I. Isolation and characterization of the murine B cell Fc$_\epsilon$ receptor and comparison with Fc$_\epsilon$ receptors from rat and human. *J. Immunol.*, **132**, 796–803

136. Lee, W. T. and Conrad, D. H. (1986). Murine B cell hybridomas bearing ligand-inducible Fc receptors for IgE. *J. Immunol.*, **136**, 4573–80

137. Kim, K. J., Kannellopoulos-Langevin, C., Merwin, R. M., Sachs, D. H. and Ascfsky, R. (1979). Establishment and characterization of Balb/c lymphoma lines with B cell properties. *J. Immunol.*, **122**, 549–54

138. Rao, M., Lee, W. T. and Conrad, D. H. (1987). Characterization of a monoclonal antibody directed against the murine B lymphocyte receptor for IgE. *J. Immunol.*, **138**, 1845–51

139. Keegan, A. D. and Conrad, D. H. (1987). The murine lymphocyte receptor for IgE V. Biosynthesis, transport, and maturation of the B cell Fc$_\epsilon$ receptor. *J. Immunol.*, **139**, 1199–205

140. Lee, W. T., Rao, M. and Conrad, D. H. (1987). The murine lymphocyte receptor for IgE IV. The mechanism of ligand-specific receptor upregulation on B Cells. *J. Immunol.*, **139**, 1191–8

141. Jarrett, E. E. and Stewart, D. C. (1972). Potentiation of rat reaginic (IgE) antibody by helminth infection. Simultaneous potentiation of separate reagins. *Immunology*, **23**, 749–55

142. Yodoi, J. and Ishizaka, K. (1979). Lymphocytes bearing Fc receptors for IgE. I. Presence of human and rat T lymphocytes with Fc$_\epsilon$ receptors. *J. Immunol.*, **122**, 2577–83

143. Bazin, H. and Beckers, A. (1976). IgE myelomas in rats. In Johansson, S. G. O., Strandberg, K. and Uvnas, B. (eds.) *Molecular and Biological Aspects of the Acute Allergic Reaction.* pp. 125–52. (NY: Plenum Press)

144. Yodoi, J., Ishizaka, T. and Ishizaka, K. (1979). Lymphocytes bearing Fc receptors for IgE. II. Induction of Fc$_\epsilon$-receptor bearing rat lymphocytes by IgE. *J. Immunol.*, **123**, 455–62

145. Chen, S. S., Bohn, J. A., Liu, F.-T. and Katz, D. H. (1981). Murine lymphocytes expressing Fc receptors for IgE (Fc$_\epsilon$R). I. Conditions for inducing FceR$^+$ lymphocytes and inhibition of the inductive events by suppressive factor of allergy (SFA). *J. Immunol.*, **127**, 166–73

146. Ishizaka, K. and Sandberg, K. (1981). Formation of IgE binding factors by human T lymphocytes. *J. Immunol.*, **126**, 1692–6

147. Yodoi, J. and Ishizaka, K. (1980). Induction of Fc$_\epsilon$-receptor bearing cells *in vitro* in human peripheral lymphocytes. *J. Immunol.*, **124**, 934–8

148. Ishizaka, K. (1984). Regulation of IgE synthesis. *Annu. Rev. Immunol.*, **2**, 159–82

149. Katz, D. and Marcelletti, J. F. (1984). Regulation of the IgE antibody system in human and experimental animals. In Yamamura, Y. and Tada, T. (eds.) *Progress in Immunology, Volume V.* page 465. (NY: Academic Press)

150. Kikutani, H., Suemura, M., Owaki, H., Nakamura, H., Sato, R., Yamasaki, K., Barsumian, E. L., Hardy, R. R. and Kishimoto, T. (1986). Fc$_\epsilon$ receptor, a specific differentiation marker transiently expressed on mature B cells prior to isotype switching. *J. Exp. Med.*, **164**, 1455–69

151. DeFrance, T., Aubry, J. P., Rousset, F., Vanbervliet, B., Bonnefoy, J. Y., Arai, N., Takebe, Y., Yokota, T., Lee, F., Arai, K., DeVries, J. and Banchereau, J. (1987). Human recombinant interleukin 4 induces Fc$_\epsilon$ receptors (CD23) on normal human B lymphocytes. *J. Exp. Med.*, **165**, 1459–67

152. Hudak, S. A., Gollmick, S. O., Conrad, D. H. and Kehry, M. R. (1987). Murine B cell stimulatory factor 1 (interleukin 4) increases expression of the Fc receptor for IgE on mouse B cells. *Proc. Natl. Acad. Sci. USA*, **84**, 4606–10

153. Ohara, J. and Paul, W. E. (1985). Production of a monoclonal antibody to and molecular characterization of B-cell stimulatory factor-1. *Nature*, **315**, 333–6

154. Mond, J. J., Carmen, J., Sarma, C., Ohara, J. and Finkelman, F. D. (1986). Interferon-gamma suppresses B cell stimulation factor (BSF-1) induction of Class II MHC determinants on B cells. *J. Immunol.*, **137**, 3534–7

155. Rabin, E. M., Mond, J. J., Ohara, J. and Paul, W. E. (1986). Interferon-gamma inhibits the action of B cell stimulatory factor (BSF)-1 on resting B cells. *J. Immunol.*, **137**, 1573–6

156. Coffman, R. L. and Carty, J. (1986). A T cell activity that enhances polyclonal IgE production and its inhibition by interferon-gamma. *J. Immunol.*, **136**, 949–54
157. Conrad, D. H., Waldschmidt, T. J., Lee, W. T., Rao, M., Keegan, A. D., Noelle, R. J., Lynch, R. G. and Kehry, M. R. (1987). Effect of B cell stimulatory factor-1 (Interleukin 4) on Fc, and Fc, receptor expression on murine B lymphocytes and B cell lines. *J. Immunol.*, **139**, 2290–6
158. Finkelman, F. D., Katona, I. M., Urban, J. F., Jr., Snapper, C. M., Ohara, J. and Paul, W. E. (1986). Suppression of *in vivo* polyclonal IgE responses by monoclonal antibody to the lymphokine B-cell stimulatory factor 1. *Proc. Natl. Acad. Sci. USA*, **83**, 9675–8
159. Arai, K., Yokota, T., Takebe, Y., Arai, M., Otsuka, T., Miyajima, A., Kastelein, R., Coffman, R., Banchereau, J., DeVries, J. and Lee, F. (1987). Isolation and characterization of Il-4 and IgA inducing factor genes and their products. *Fed. Proc.*, **46**, 1498 (Abstr. 6895)
160. Huff, T. F., Yodoi, J., Uede, T. and Ishizaka, K. (1984). Presence of an antigenic determinant common to rat IgE-potentiating factor and, IgE-suppressive factor and Fc epsilon receptors on T and B lymphocytes. *J. Immunol.*, **122**, 406–12
161. Kisaki, T., Huff, T. F., Conrad, D. H., Yodoi, J. and Ishizaka, K. (1987). Monoclonal antibody specific for T cell-derived human IgE binding factors. *J. Immunol.*, **138**, 3345–51
162. Moore, K. W., Jardieu, P., Mietz, J. A., Trounstine, M. L., Kuff, E. L., Ishizaka, K. and Martens, D. L. (1986). Rodent IgE-binding factor genes are members of an endogenous, retrovirus-like gene family. *J. Immunol.*, **136**, 4283–90
163. Kuff, E. L., Mietz, J. A., Troustine, M. L., Moore, K. W. and Martens, C. L. (1986). cDNA clones encoding murine IgE-binding factors represent multiple structural variants of intracisternal A-particle genes. *Proc. Natl. Acad. Sci. USA*, **83**, 6583–7
164. Katona, I. M., Urban, J. F., Jr., Titus, J. A., Stephany, D. A., Segal, D. M. and Finkelman, F. D. (1984). Characterization of murine lymphocyte IgE receptors by flow microfluorometry. *J. Immunol.*, **133**, 1521–8
165. Yukawa, K., Kikutani, H., Owaki, H., Yamasaki, K., Yokota, A., Nakamura, H., Barsumian, E. L., Hardy, R. R., Suemura, M. and Kishimoto, T. (1987). A B cell-specific differentiation antigen CD23, is a receptor for IgE (Fc, R) on lymphocytes. *J. Immunol.*, **138**, 2576–80
166. Bonnefoy, J.-Y., Aubry, J.-P., Peronne, C., Wijdenes, J. and Banchereau, J. (1987). Production and chararacterization of a monoclonal antibody specific for the human lymphocyte low affinity receptor for IgE: CD23 is a low affinity receptor for IgE. *J. Immunol.*, **138**, 2970–8
167. Thorley-Lawson, D. A., Nadler, L. M., Bhan, A. K. and Schooley, R. T. (1985). BLAST-2 [EBVCS], an early cell surface marker of human B cell activation, is superinduced by Epstein Barr virus. *J. Immunol.*, **134**, 3007–12
168. Gordon, J., Rowe, M., Walker, L. and Guy, G. (1986). Ligation of the CD23, p45 (BLAST-2, EBVCS) antigen triggers the cell-cycle progression of activated B lymphocytes. *Eur. J. Immunol.*, **16**, 1075–80
169. Gordon, J., Webb, A. J., Guy, G. R. and Walker, L. (1987). Triggering of B lymphocytes through CD23: epitope mapping and studies using antibody derivatives indicate an allosteric mechanism of signaling. *Immunology*, **60**, 517–21
170. Guy, G. R. and Gordon, J. (1987). Coordinated action of IgE and a B-cell stimulatory factor on the CD23 receptor molecule upregulates B-lymphocyte growth. *Proc. Natl. Acad. Sci. USA*, **84**, 6239–43
171. Sharma, S., Mehta, S., Morgan, J. and Maizel, A. (1987). Molecular cloning and expression of a human B-cell growth factor gene in *Escherichia coli*. *Science*, **235**, 1489–92
172. Gordon, J., Ley, S. C., Melamed, M. D., English, L. S. and Hughes, Jones, N. C. (1984). Immortalized B lymphocytes produce B-cell growth factor. *Nature*, **310**, 145–7
173. Gordon, J., Guy, G. and Walker, L. (1985). Autocrine models of B-lymphocyte growth. I. Role of cell contact and soluble factors in T-independent B-cell responses. *Immunology*, **56**, 329–35
174. Swendeman, S. and Thorley-Lawson, D. A. (1987). The activation antigen BLAST-2, when shed, is an autocrine BCGF for normal and transformed B cells. *EMBO J.*, **6**, 1637–42

175. Wang, F., Gregory, C. D., Rowe, M., Rickinson, A. B., Wang, D., Birkenbach, M., Kikutani, H., Kishimoto, T. and Kieff, E. (1987). Epstein–Barr virus nuclear antigen 2 specifically induces expression of the B-cell activation antigen CD23. *Proc. Natl. Acad. Sci. USA*, **84**, 3452–6

176. Huff, T. F. and Ishizaka, K. (1984). Formation of IgE-binding factors by human T-cell hybridomas. *Proc. Natl. Acad. Sci. USA*, **81**, 1514–18

177. Huff, T. F., Jardieu, P. and Ishizaka, K. (1986). Regulatory effects of human IgE-binding factors on the IgE response of rat lymphocytes. *J. Immunol.*, **136**, 955–62

178. Young, M., Geha, R. S., Maksad, K. N. and Leung, D. Y. M. (1986). Characterization of human T cell-derived IgE-potentiating factor. *Eur. J. Immunol.*, **16**, 985–91

179. Leung, D. Y. M. and Geha, R. S. (1986). Control of IgE synthesis in man. *J. Clin. Immunol.*, **6**, 273–83

180. Sarfati, M., Rector, E., Wong, K., Rubio-Trujillo, M., Sehon, A. H. and Delespesse, G. (1984). *In vitro* synthesis of IgE by human lymphocytes. II. Enhancement of the spontaneous IgE synthesis by IgE-binding factors secreted by RPMI 8866 lymphoblastoid B cells. *Immunology*, **53**, 197–205

181. Sarfati, M., Rector, E., Sehon, A. H. and Delespesse, G. (1984). *In vitro* synthesis of IgE by human lymphocytes. IV. Suppression of the spontaneous IgE synthesis by IgE-binding factors secreted by tunicamycin-treated RPMI 8866 cells. *Immunology*, **53**, 783–90

182. Saryan, J. A., Leung, D. Y. and Geha, R. S. (1983). Induction of human IgE synthesis by a factor derived from T cells of patients with hyper-IgE states. *J. Immunol.*, **130**, 242–7

4
Preformed Mediators of
Human Mast Cells and Basophils

L. B. SCHWARTZ

Immediate hypersensitivity reactions occur following release of mediators from mast cells and basophils. These cell types each possess high affinity receptors for IgE in their plasma membrane and contain histamine inside the secretory granules in their cytoplasmic compartment. They differ from one another by morphologic criteria and by the production of distinct proteoglycan, enzyme and lipid mediators. Mature mast cells reside in tissues; basophils normally are found in the circulation, but may migrate into tissues at sites of delayed-type hypersensitivity reactions or ectoparasitic infestation. The highest concentrations of mature mast cells in normal tissues are found in the intestine (mucosa and submucosa), upper and lower respiratory tract (alveoli, bronchiolar/bronchial subepithelial and nasal mucosal regions) and skin (dermis)[1], where signs and symptoms of allergic reactions are often noted. In addition, two types of human mast cells with distinct neutral protease compositions have been described (see below)[2]. These mast cell types differ in their tissue distributions, dependence on functional T lymphocytes and secretory response to certain activating agents. Little is known of the differential contribution of each mast cell type or of basophils to various allergic conditions as well as the biologic activities of mast cells (and basophils) in those 80% of individuals who are not atopic.

Mast cells contain preformed mediators which are stored in the secretory granules and which are released into the extracellular space following either immunologic (IgE-dependent) or non-immunologic-induced exocytosis. In contrast, newly generated mediators (discussed in Chapter 5), such as prostaglandin D_2 and leukotriene C_4, are present in negligible amounts in resting mast cells, but are synthesized *de novo* and secreted after mast cell activation. The secretion of preformed and newly-generated mediators appear to occur independently of one another, at least in activated rodent mast cells. Neither inhibition of prostaglandin D_2 production with indomethacin[3] nor inhibition of leukotriene production with various antagonists[4] blocks histamine release from mast cells. Furthermore, adenosine reportedly augments IgE-dependent histamine release without affecting the production of newly-generated mediators[5].

This chapter will focus on the major preformed mediators of human mast cells, which include histamine, proteoglycans (heparin and chondroitin sulphate E) and neutral proteases (tryptase and chymase). Acid hydrolases and oxidative enzymes, small quantities (on a weight basis) of which have been observed in human mast cells, and chemotactic activities, will not be addressed in this review. The potential biologic role of each mast cell mediator under consideration will be explored. The ability of these mediators, particularly the neutral proteases, to perform as clinically useful markers of mast cell activation and to delineate two types of human mast cells will be reviewed.

HISTAMINE

Histamine is measured either by a radioenzyme assay[6], whereby histamine methyltransferase transfers a radiolabelled methyl group from s-adenosyl methionine to histamine, or by a fluorescence assay[7], whereby o-phthalaldehyde forms a fluorescent product with histamine. Partial purification of histamine or methyl histamine may be performed in order to increase sensitivity and specificity, e.g. by organic/aqueous extractions[6], thin layer chromatography[8, 9] or high performance liquid chromatography[10]. In general, the radioenzyme techniques, though more expensive and technically involved, are more sensitive than fluorescence procedures and are subject to less interference from substances in plasma.

Histamine appears to be the only biogenic amine present in human mast cells and basophils. Serotonin, present in rodent mast cells[11], is found in human platelets. Dopamine, present in bovine mast cells[12], is a human neurotransmitter. Histamine is also found in certain gastrointestinal and neurologic tissues[13, 14].

Normal concentrations of histamine are 100–300 pg per ml of plasma[15] and 1–2 pg per human basophil[16, 17] or mast cell[18]. Histamine is synthesized from histidine by histidine decarboxylase in these cell types (Figure 4.1) and is stored in cytoplasmic secretory granules at acid pH[19]. Under these conditions histamine exhibits a positive charge and appears to be bound to negatively charged carboxyl or sulphate groups in the proteoglycan–protein matrix[20]. After release into a neutral pH environment histamine becomes less positively charged, dissociates from the complex and is freely soluble.

Histamine is best-suited to act locally near its site of release, because greater than 90% is metabolized by histamine N-methyl transferase and diamine oxidase (histaminase) after one pass through the circulation (Figure 4.1). Further metabolism of methyl histamine to methyl imidazole acetic acid and ribosylation of imidazole acetic acid may occur. Consequently, acute allergic reactions only result in transient elevations of plasma histamine concentrations. Even after systemic anaphylaxis, histamine levels return to normal by 30 min[21, 22]. In some cases evidence for the release of histamine *in vivo* may be better appreciated in urine, where a small fraction of

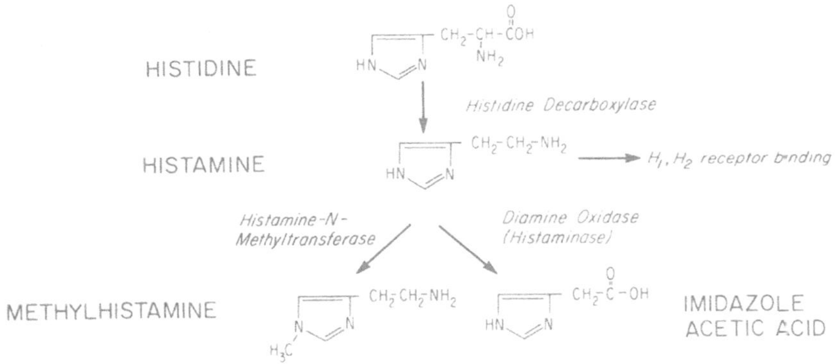

Figure 4.1 Histamine synthesis and degradation

histamine appears intact[23]. Plasma N^t-methylhistamine[24], a histamine metabolite, has a somewhat longer halflife than histamine and may be a useful marker. However, its measurement is technically difficult. Neither histamine, nor histamine metabolites, distinguish mast cell from basophil activation. Thus, histamine is of limited diagnostic value for acute allergic reactions due to its rapid metabolism. In contrast, plasma histamine concentrations are a sensitive indicator of systemic mastocytosis, even in the absence of acute symptoms, and presumably reflect the increase in mast cell concentration rather than an increase in mast cell activation[25, 26].

Histamine-dependent biologic activities are expressed by binding to H_1 and H_2 receptors on cell surfaces[27]. These activities are summarized in Table 4.1. Many biologic responses, though predominantly H_1 receptor- or H_2 receptor-mediated, result from their combined effects. Subcutaneous injection of

Table 4.1 Biologic activities of histamine

H_1 *Receptor*
  Bronchial and intestinal smooth muscle contraction
  Vascular permeability
  Elevate cGMP

H_2 *Receptor*
  Gastric acid and pepsin secretion
  Permeability through bronchial epithelium
  Suppress lymphocyte-mediated cytotoxicity and granule secretion from neutrophils and
    basophils
  Elevate cAMP

H_1 *and* H_2 *Receptors*
  Chemokinesis of eosinophils and neutrophils
  C3b receptor expression on eosinophils
  Prostaglandin I_2 production by endothelial cells
  Wheal and flare cutaneous response
  Hypotension, headache, flushing and tachycardia
  Vasodilation

131

histamine elicits a triple response consisting of local erythema (arteriolar vasodilation), circumferential erythema (axon reflex-induced vasodilation) and later a central oedematous wheal (enhanced venular permeability). Both H_1 and H_2 receptors appear to be involved, because a combination of H_1 and H_2 antagonists are more effective at blocking the reaction than either antagonist alone[28]. Dilatation of arterioles and enhancement of venular permeability presumably facilitate the tissue deposition of plasma components, which conceivably could include tissue nutrient factors needed for beneficial tissue repair as well as immune complexes[29] that result in a harmful inflammatory response.

The effect of raising plasma histamine levels by continuous intravenous infusion of histamine was studied in normal subjects[30]. Elevated plasma histamine levels (0.6 to 6 ng/ml) resulted in tachycardia, widened pulse pressure together with diastolic hypotension, flushing and headaches, all of which returned to baseline within 1–2 min after discontinuation of the histamine infusion. Each histamine-induced response was mediated through a combination of H_1 and H_2 receptors, because a combination of H_1 and H_2 receptor antagonists raised the plasma concentration of histamine required to elicit each response more than either class of antagonist alone.

Histamine also causes bronchial and gastrointestinal smooth muscle to contract via H_1 receptors[31], and gastric parietal cells to secrete acid via H_2 receptors[27]. H_1 antagonists can block almost completely the decrease in FEV1 following histamine inhalation. However, after allergen broncho-provocation the decrease in FEV1 occurring during the initial phase of the early response is only slightly attenuated by H_1 antagonists[32]; the late phase response is not affected. In addition, enhanced permeability through bronchial epithelium occurs after allergen challenge and is blocked, in part, by H_2 antagonists[33]. Nevertheless, the clinical effectiveness of antihistamines in asthma has not been convincingly demonstrated.

Histamine *in vitro* exhibits a number of interesting activities that, in general, occur at higher concentrations than those mentioned above[34]. These include an H_2 receptor-induced suppression of T lymphocyte-mediated cytotoxicity and release of lymphokines, proliferation of lymphocytes, and secretion of granule mediators by neutrophils, basophils and mast cells. In addition, T lymphocyte suppressor activity is enhanced. Chemokinesis of eosinophils and neutrophils is enhanced by H_1- and H_2-receptor mechanisms. The expression of C3b receptors on eosinophils (not monocytes and neutrophils) is increased[35] as is the complement-dependent killing of schistosomula by eosinophils *in vitro*[36]. In addition, histamine activates endothelial cells to generate prostaglandin I_2 (prostacycline)[37], a potent inhibitor of platelet aggregation.

The concentration of mast cells (containing 1–2 pg histamine/cell) in skin ($3000/mm^3$), intestinal mucosa ($20\,000/mm^3$), and lung (15–$25\,000/mm^3$) indicate that local tissue concentrations of histamine, after extensive degranulation, could be as high as 5–30 μg/ml ($10\,000$–$60\,000$ higher than normally present in plasma), enough to elicit the responses noted above. Indeed, one study showed histamine concentration in nasal lavage fluid after allergen challenge averaged 2 ng/ml in atopics and 0.5 ng/ml in non-atopics[38], even without taking into account the dilution of endogenous secretions by the lavage fluid. In another study histamine was released into skin chamber fluid overlying sites of exposed dermis after cutaneous allergen challenge and levels up to 1.6 ng/ml were found[39].

PROTEOGLYCANS

The characteristic staining properties of mast cells with basic dyes permitted the initial detection of mast cells by Ehrlich in 1879. This remains today the principal method of their detection, and which depends on the presence of highly sulphated (negatively charged) proteoglycans present in mast cell secretory granules. Proteoglycans are composed of glycosaminoglycan side chains (repeating unbranched disaccharide units of a uronic acid and hexosamine moieties that are variably sulphated) covalently linked to a single-chain protein core via a specific trisaccharide-protein linkage region of gal–gal–xyl–ser. Two classes of proteoglycan, heparin and chondroitin sulphate E have been associated with human mast cells in lung[40], skin[41] and intestine[42] (Table 4.2). The distribution of these proteoglycans between the human TC (connective tissue-like) and T (mucosal-like) mast cells has not yet been clarified.

Heparin disaccharides have the structure shown in Figure 4.2 with an average of 2.5 sulphate groups per disaccharide. The disaccharide consists of either glucuronic acid without a sulphate residue or iduronic acid containing

Table 4.2 Proteoglycans of mast cells and basophils

Cell source	Proteoglycan
Human	
Mast cells	
lung (dispersed cells; T > TC[a])	heparin[40]
skin (mastocytosis tissue; TC > T)	heparin[41]
colon (tissue fragments; T > TC)	chondroitin sulphate E[42]
Basophils (chronic myelogenous leukaemia)	chondroitin sulphate A[51]
Rat	
peritoneal lavage (CTMC[b])	heparin[43, 54]
skin (CTMC)	heparin[44]
intestine (dispersed cells, *N. brasiliensis*	
infested, MMC[c])	chondroitin sulphate di-B
basophil leukaemia tumour (?MMC)	chondroitin sulphate di-B and heparin[49, 56]
Mouse	
peritoneal lavage (CTMC)	heparin[47]
bone marrow-derived (MCC, tissue culture)	chondroitin sulphate E[47, 48]

[a] T: tryptase positive, chymase negative mast cell; TC: tryptase positive, chymase positive mast cell
[b] CTMC: connective tissue mast cell
[c] MMC: mucosal mast cell

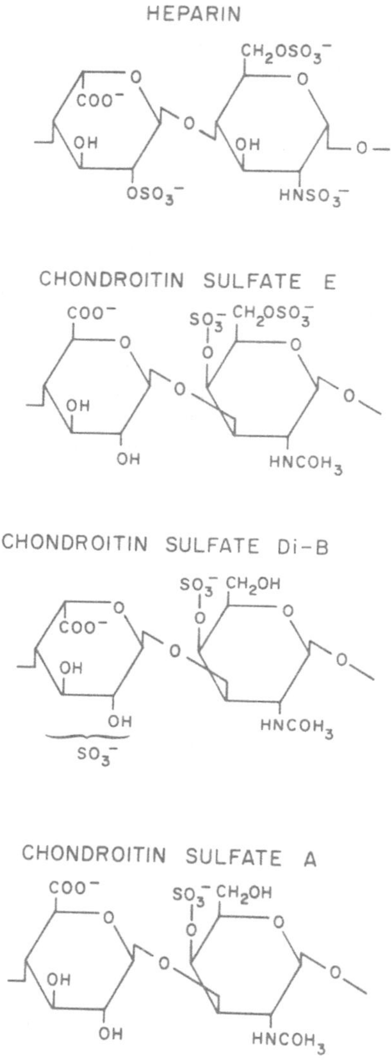

HEPARIN

CHONDROITIN SULFATE E

CHONDROITIN SULFATE Di-B

CHONDROITIN SULFATE A

Figure 4.2 Glycosaminoglycans of mast cells and basophils: structures of the characteristic disaccharides

2-O-sulphate, that is linked to a glucosamine containing a 4-O-sulphate and 2-N-sulphate. Rarely, one finds a 2-N-acetyl rather than N-sulphate. The N-sulphate is particularly susceptible to nitrous acid; treatment with nitrous acid results in the destruction of heparin, but not chondroitin sulphate glycosaminoglycans which lack the N-sulphate. The protein core for rat and mouse heparin proteoglycan consists predominantly of (−gly−ser−)$_n$ (43% gly,

39% ser)[43,44] and, like the protein cores for the chondroitin disulphates E[45] and diB[46], is resistant to digestion by proteases.

The disaccharide structures for chondroitin sulphate A, chondroitin sulphate E and chondroitin sulphate di-B are shown in Figure 4.2. Each contains a galactosamine with a 4-O-sulphate. In addition, type E has a 6-O-sulphate on the galactosamine and type di-B has a 2- or 3-O-sulphate on iduronic acid. Type E was the predominant glycosaminoglycan synthesized *in vitro* by mouse bone marrow-derived mucosal mast cells in culture[47,48], and was synthesized *in vitro* (presumably by mast cells) by a preparation of human colon tissue fragments[42]. Type di-B is synthesized *in vitro* by the rat basophil leukaemia tumour[49] (RBL-1, now thought to be a rat mucosal mast cell tumour) and *in vivo* by rat mucosal mast cells[50], but has not been reported to be made by human or mouse cells. Chondroitin sulphate A is the intracellular proteoglycan of human basophils[51], as well as an extracellular proteoglycan constituent of connective tissue.

The evidence for two types of mast cells, particularly in rodents, is based, in part, on the type of proteoglycan synthesized by different types of mast cells[52,53]. Normally, rat and mouse connective tissue mast cells contain predominantly heparin proteoglycan of about 750 000 apparent MW[54]; in the presence of p-nitrophenyl-B-D-xyloside, a substitute for the protein core onto which glycosaminoglycans can be synthesized, rat connective tissue mast cells synthesize predominantly a chondroitin disulphate[55]. Mouse mucosal mast cells synthesize the chondroitin disulphate, type E, with an apparent Mr of 200 000[48]. RBL-1 cells (probably a mucosal mast cell) synthesize predominantly the di-B type of chondroitin disulphate (apparent Mr of 100 000–300 000) as well as heparin[49,56]. Heparin proteoglycan synthesized by human skin and lung mast cells, most likely representing a mixture of the human T and TC types, has an apparent Mr of 60 000[40,41]. Chondroitin disulphate E has been associated in humans with mast cells obtained from the colon[42], and chondroitin monosulphates with basophils from patients with chronic myelogenous leukaemia[51]. Although the type of proteoglycan may be helpful in distinguishing between different types of mast cells, the ability of rat peritoneal mast cells and RBL-1 cells to synthesize more than one class of proteoglycan *in vitro* suggests the likelihood that more than one class of proteoglycan might be synthesized by and reside in a single mast cell *in vivo*.

The functions of mast cell proteoglycans, both intragranular and extragranular, have not been clearly established. These proteoglycans bind to histamine, neutral proteases and acid hydrolases at the acid pH within secretory granules, and may facilitate uptake and packaging of these preformed mediators into secretory granules. Mast cell proteoglycans also regulate the stability and enzymatic activities of many of the enzymes present.

After release from mast cells the proteoglycans may continue to exert a regulatory effect on those substances that remain associated, particularly the neutral proteases. The stabilizing effect of heparin and, to a lesser extent, chondroitin disulphate E, on human tryptase activity[57,58] may be crucial for the full expression of mast cell-mediated events. In addition, heparin (and to a lesser degree, chondroitin disulphate E) may express anticoagulant[59,60], anticomplement[61,62] and Hageman factor autoactivation[63] activities.

NEUTRAL PROTEASES

Neutral proteases are enzymes that catalyse the cleavage of peptide bonds and perform optimally at neutral pH. Those present in human mast cells, particularly chymase[68] and tryptase[65, 66] (Table 4.3), are important to consider for two reasons. First they are the major protein constituents of the secretory granules and probably account for 20–50% of the total cellular protein. Second, they appear to be specific markers for human mast cells[1, 2, 67], being present in negligible amounts in basophils[68]. Finally, tryptase and chymase serve as markers that distinguish the two types of human mast cells, termed T and TC. They most certainly will play an important role in mast cell biology and, in addition, have the capability of serving as specific and sensitive markers for mast cell activation *in vivo*.

Tryptase

Trypsin-like activity was first detected in human mast cells by histochemical techniques employing tryptic substrates[69]. The principal enzyme accounting for this activity was later purified to homogeneity, termed tryptase and specifically localized to human mast cell secretory granules[65, 66, 70]. Other cell types in normal lung, small intestine, and skin[1, 2, 67] as well as eosinophils, neutrophils, monocytes and lymphocytes from peripheral blood[68] do not have detectable tryptase. Basophils contain negligible amounts of tryptase (0.04–0.05 pg/cell)[68] compared to the two human mast cell types, T (12 pg/cell) and TC (35 pg/cell) mast cells (see below)[18]. Thus, the enzyme is a discriminating marker for mast cells, and logically should be found in complex biologic fluids after mast cell activation.

A sensitive and specific sandwich ELISA was developed utilizing mouse

Table 4.3 Tryptase and chymase from human mast cells

	Tryptase	*Chymase*
Molecular weight (daltons)	134 000	30 000
Subunit structure	tetramer	monomer
Protease type	serine endoprotease, trypsin-like specificity	serine endoprotease, chymotrypsin-like specificity
pg per mast cell		
T (lung)	10	0.05
TC (skin)	35	4.5
Heparin	bound and stabilized	bound
Regulation	insensitive to plasma protease inhibitors; dissociation from heparin by divalent cations and conversion to inactive monomers	sensitive to plasma protease inhibitors

136

IgG monoclonal and goat IgG polyclonal anti-tryptase antibodies[71] that permits quantification of tryptase in buffer, serum or plasma. This has enabled the measurement of tryptase released *in vivo*. Tryptase was first assessed in a cutaneous allergen challenge system[72]. The peak appearance of released histamine (30 min) occurred somewhat earlier than for tryptase (60 min), but the allergen dose-response relationships were analogous, as expected for two mediators being exocytosed from the same granules. The delayed appearance of tryptase relative to histamine in the chamber fluid, most likely reflects slower diffusion through tissue of the large tryptase–proteoglycan complex than of free histamine. No peak of histamine or tryptase was found during late phase cutaneous reactions, 4–9 hours after onset of allergen challenge[73].

Tryptase has also been examined as a marker of mast cell participation in subjects with systemic mastocytosis and anaphylaxis[74]. In both cases elevated concentrations of tryptase were detected in plasma and/or serum compared to control subjects and those with septic shock or myocardial infarction. The potential usefulness of tryptase as a clinical marker of mast cell activation results from being able to measure it in serum as well as plasma, its apparent prolonged halflife (hours) in plasma and its selective presence in mast cells over basophils and other cell types. Clinicians may soon have the capability of objectively determining mast cell involvement in a variety of clinical situations.

Tryptase is a tetrameric serine endoprotease of 134 000 daltons with subunits of 31 500 daltons and 33 000 daltons, each with an active enzymatic site[57, 65, 66]. The subunits also share antigenic sites[67]. The apparent difference in molecular weight between these subunits probably reflects differences in the post-translational processing of identical gene products, although distinct primary amino acid sequences have not been ruled out. Tryptase obtained from skin mast cells initially was reported to be distinct from lung tryptase[75]; however, they now appear to be identical based on immunologic, physicochemical and enzymatic criteria[1, 18, 76]. Tryptase, like all other rat and human mast cell proteases thus far examined, is stored in secretory granules fully active; no inactive tryptase has been found. Furthermore, tryptase is not inhibited by incubation with plasma[57] or urine[77], or by concentrated preparations of purified inhibitors such as α_1 trypsin inhibitor[66, 70], α_2 macroglobulin[66], nexin (Johnson, Schwartz and Baker, unpublished work) and human lung-derived anti-leukoprotease[78] and elastase-specific inhibitor[79] (and Alter, Kramps and Schwartz, unpublished work). Instead, the enzyme is uniquely stabilized in its active tetrameric form by association with heparin proteoglycan; when free in solution tryptase subunits rapidly dissociate from one another into inactive monomers[57]. Chondroitin disulphate E stabilizes tryptase somewhat less well than heparin, whereas chondroitin monosulphates are little better than buffer alone under physiologic conditions[58]. The primary physiologic means of dissociating tryptase from heparin, and thereby down-regulating its activity, appears to occur via divalent cations (Figure 4.3). Physiologic concentrations of calcium and magnesium decrease the apparent halflife of heparin-bound tryptase to almost 1 hour[54], seemingly by dissociating the enzyme from the sulphate moieties.

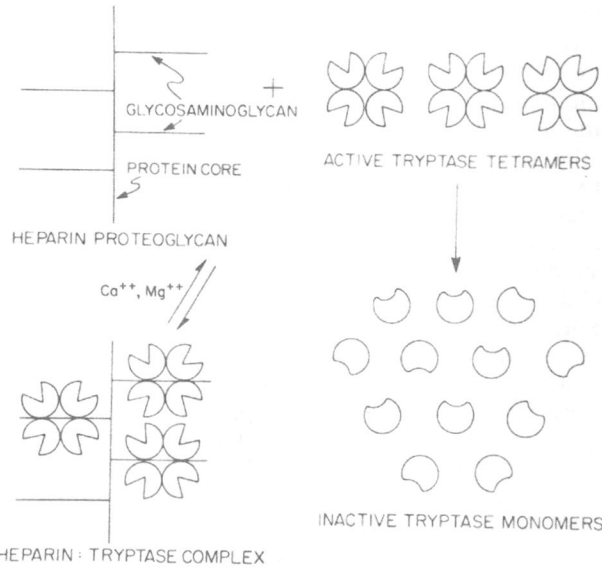

Figure 4.3 Regulation of tryptase by heparin and divalent cations

In spite of the abundant content of tryptase in mast cells, its biologic role has not been convincingly demonstrated. Several potential sites of action have been investigated *in vitro*. For example, tryptase generates the anaphylatoxin C3a from C3[80], but has no effect on C5 (Schwartz and Hugli, unpublished material). It is possible that C3a, locally generated in tissues, could produce smooth muscle contraction and increased vasopermeability. Tryptase activates procollagenase isolated from cultured rheumatoid synovial cells[81]. The increased concentration of mast cells in rheumatoid synovium[82] and destruction of synovial connective tissue in rheumatoid arthritis suggest a possible role for mast cell tryptase in this disease. Tryptase rapidly inactivates fibrinogen as a coagulable substrate for thrombin[83]. The lack of fibrin deposition and the rapid resolution of urticarial lesions may, in part, reflect the action of this fibrinogenolytic protease. Finally, tryptase does not appear to promote bradykinin generation; it has no detectable kallikrein activity with high[84] and low[85] molecular weight kininogens and no urinary (tissue)[77] or plasma[86] prekallikrein activating activity. The bradykinin or lysylbradykinin generated *in vivo* after IgE-dependent events[87], therefore, is not due to tryptase.

Chymase

Chymotryptic activity in mast cells was also detected first by histochemical techniques in sections of human gingiva and skin[88]. An enzyme termed chymase (Table 4.3) was later purified from human skin[64] and selectively localized to mast cells in normal human lung, small intestine and skin by immunohistochemical techniques[2, 89]. However, unlike tryptase, chymase is not present in all mast cells, but only in the TC mast cell type that is preferentially present in skin and small bowel submucosa[2] (see below). In dispersed preparations of foreskin mast cells, almost all of which are of the TC phenotype, there are 4.5 pg of chymase/mast cell by immunoassay compared to 35 pg of tryptase/mast cell[18]. Analysis of dispersed lung mast cells (93% T, 7% TC) indicates that all immunologic and enzymatic chymase activity might be accounted for by the minor presence of TC mast cells. Thus it appears that the T mast cell lacks immunoreactive chymase. They also appear to lack an antigenically distinct form of chymase with similar chymotryptic activity. However, a recent histochemical study indicates the presence of chymotryptic activity in human mast cells residing in intestinal lamina propria[90], presumably of the T type, suggesting the presence of distinct chymotryptic proteinases in each human mast cell type (similar to the situation in rats). Further studies will be necessary to identify the source of chymotryptic histochemical activity in T mast cells.

Human chymase, a serine endoprotease, is a monomer of $30\,000\,Mr$[64]. It is antigenically unrelated to cathepsin G from human neutrophils, bovine chymotrypsin, or rat mast cell chymase (rat mast cell protease I)[91]. Like tryptase, human chymase is stored in mast cell secretory granules fully active, and is presumably bound to the negatively-charged granular proteoglycan. Unlike tryptase, chymase is inhibited by plasma proteinase inhibitors and is presumably down-regulated after release by this mechanism.

Human chymase converts angiotensin I to angiotensin II as well, if not better, than the classical plasma dipeptidase termed angiotensin converting enzyme[91-93]. Whether this vasoconstrictor is generated *in vivo* during activation of the TC type of mast cell needs to be clarified. In addition, chymase has the capacity to degrade basement membrane components at the dermal : epidermal junction and facilitate separation of these cutaneous regions[94]. Although blister formation does not occur in classical mast-cell dependent urticarial reactions, it has been reported to occur in systemic cutaneous mastocytosis and, therefore, may be of pathobiologic importance.

Additional proteases

Protease activities with Hageman factor-cleaving, Hageman factor-activating, kallikrein, prekallikrein activating, elastase, and cathepsin G activities have also been reported as being associated with human mast cells[95-97]. As yet, none have been purified from human mast cells. In addition, a carboxypeptidase activity has been associated preferentially with the TC type of mast cell[98]. It is sensitive to inhibition by potato carboxypeptidase inhibitor as well as EDTA and O-phenanthroline, thereby distinguishing it from tryptase, chymase, and the carboxypeptidase activity found in human cultured keratinocytes. The presence of chymase and carboxypeptidase together in human TC mast cells is strikingly similar to the presence in rat connective tissue mast cells of chymase and carboxypeptidase A[99].

HETEROGENEITY OF HUMAN MAST CELLS

Two types of human mast cells have now been defined on the basis of distinct compositions of neutral proteases. TC mast cells contain tryptase together with chymase; T mast cells contain tryptase without chymase. These compositional differences have been demonstrated by immunohistochemistry with light[2] and electron[100] microscopy. The latter technique also showed that chymase and tryptase reside together in the same granules. The compositional differences between T and TC mast cells observed by microscopic techniques have been confirmed and quantified with dispersed preparations of predominantly T (lung) and TC (adult foreskin) mast cells. T mast cells contain about 10 pg of tryptase; TC mast cells contain about 35 pg of tryptase and 4.5 pg of chymase[18]. A recent observation that a carboxypeptidase is preferentially present in TC mast cells[98] further extends the compositional distinction between these two types of mast cells. It is of interest that distinct chymotryptic proteinases have been found in each type of rat mast cell[101].

Functional differences between types of human mast cells also have been observed. Compound 48/80, for example, causes histamine release from dispersed mast cells from skin[102] but not lung[103], presumably reflecting differences between corresponding TC and T types of mast cells. A similar difference in the response to compound 48/80 between rodent connective tissue and mucosal mast cells has been described[104].

The distribution and concentration of T and TC mast cells in normal skin, lung and intestine are shown in Table 4.4. TC mast cells predominate in skin and small bowel submucosa and T mast cells predominate in lung (particularly alveoli) and small bowel mucosa. TC mast cells are slightly larger than T mast cells, but cannot be distinguished on the basis of size alone[2]. Both types of mast cells are optimally-fixed in Carnoy's fluid. T and TC mast cells are both stained by basic dyes and cannot be distinguished on this basis. After formalin fixation, staining intensity with basic dyes is reduced, more so for T than TC mast cells. In addition, recognition of chymase by anti-

Table 4.4 Distribution of T (tryptase positive, chymase negative) and TC (tryptase positive, chymase positive) mast cells in human skin, bowel and lung

Tissue	%T	%TC	Mast cells/mm³
Skin (foreskin)	1	99	3000
Lung bronchi/bronchial			
epithelial	90	10	8500
subepithelial	77	23	18 000
alveoli	93	7	26 500
Small bowel			
mucosa	96	4	20 000
submucosa	12	88	8000
Large bowel			
mucosa	75	25	16 000
submucosa	8	92	10 000

chymase antibodies in formalin-fixed TC mast cells is lost, making it impossible to distinguish formalin-fixed T and TC types of mast cells from one another by current immunohistochemical techniques. It is possible that distinct proteoglycans, additional proteases or membrane surface markers may also be found which distinguish different types of mast cells, even after formalin fixation.

The identification of two types of human mast cells provides a situation analogous to that in rodents for consideration of mast cell lineage. In rodents the evidence indicates that different mast cell types originate from a common stem cell[105]. How they further differentiate into distinct mature types of mast cells is not certain. Assuming a common precursor for T and TC mast cells in humans, recent evidence indicates divergent rather than linear pathways of maturation. This is based primarily on an analysis of mast cell types in the intestine of human subjects with either congenital (combined immunodeficiency disease) or acquired (AIDS) disorders of T lymphocyte function. In both cases there occurs a selective deficiency of the T mast cell, with no significant change in the distribution or concentration of TC mast cells[106]. This indicates a role for the T lymphocyte in the maturation/proliferation of human T but not TC mast cells, somewhat analogous to the situation in rodents[53]. A linear pathway of differentiation whereby TC mast cells are derived from T mast cells seems unlikely, because a deficiency of T mast cells, as above, does not lead to a decrease in TC mast cells. Furthermore, derivation of T from TC mast cells seems unlikely without a known mechanism for the selective removal of chymase from the TC mast cell secretory granules.

The nomenclature for different types of mast cells varies among species and laboratories. It appears that mucosal, atypical, mouse E and human T mast cells are analogous types, as are connective tissue, typical, mouse H and human TC mast cells. The rodent bone marrow-derived P (persisting) or IL-3-dependent tissue culture mast cell appears phenotypically similar to the mucosal type. The mucosal/connective tissue terminology is confusing because the mucosal type of mast cell can be found in connective tissues, and the connective tissue type of mast cell can reside in mucosal tissues. Furthermore, the term mucosal or connective tissue has been used incorrectly to designate mast cell type by location alone rather than by phenotype. The designation typical/atypical implies something is wrong or unusual with the latter type of mast cells, which is not the case. The T/TC terminology (see above) appears adequate for human mast cell types, but does not extend to other species. The H (heparin)/E (chondroitin sulphate E) designation was developed for murine mast cells, but did not extend to rat mast cells where heparin and chondroitin sulphate di-B are the distinguishing types of proteoglycan. Thus, readers must be famililar with the various nomenclatures in use until a universally-accepted terminology is developed.

CONCLUSIONS

In conclusion, the preformed mediators of human mast cells distinguish mast cells from other cell types and different types of mast cells from one another. The ability of mast cell mediators to facilitate the influx of plasma into tissues (histamine, leukotriene C_4, platelet activating factor), prevent local thrombosis (prostaglandin D_2, histamine) and coagulation (heparin, tryptase), activate latent collagenase (tryptase) and the C3a anaphylatoxin (tryptase) indicate an important role in connective tissue repair and inflammation (homeostasis). The development of sensitive and specific assays for histamine and tryptase enable one to determine mast cell involvement in a variety of clinical situations. Such measurements will provide a better understanding of mast cell pathophysiology, provide diagnostic information and provide an objective test for monitoring the effect of therapy and the mechanism of drug action. Finally, the recognition of two types of human mast cells requires an understanding of their tissue distribution and concentration in different clinical conditions, of the differences, if any, in the stimulatory agents and pharmacologic regulation for each mast cell type and their common and unique biologic functions.

References

1. Craig, S. S., DeBlois, G. and Schwartz, L. B. (1986). Mast cells in human keloid, small intestine and lung by an immunoperoxidase technique using a murine monoclonal antibody against tryptase. *Am. J. Pathol.*, **124**, 427
2. Irani, A. A., Schechter, N. M., Craig, S., DeBlois, G. and Schwartz, L. B. (1986). Two human mast cell subsets with different neutral protease compositions. *Proc. Natl. Acad. Sci. (USA)*, **83**, 4464
3. Lewis, R. A., Holgate, S. T., Roberts, II, L. J., Maguire, J. F., Oates, J. A. and Austen, K. F. (1979). Effects of indomethacin on cyclic nucleotide levels and histamine release from rat serosal mast cells. *J. Immunol.*, **123**, 1663
4. Razin E., Lewis, R. A., Corey, E. J. and Austen, K. F. (1984). An analysis of the relationship between 5-lipoxygenase product generation and the secretion of preformed mediators from mouse bone marrow-derived mast cells. *J. Immunol.*, **133**, 938
5. Marqardt, D. L., Walker, L. L. and Wasserman, S. I. (1984). Adenosine receptors on mouse bone marrow-derived mast cells: functional significance and regulation by aminophylline. *J. Immunol.*, **133**, 932
6. Shaff, R. E. and Beaven, M. A. (1976). Increased sensitivity of the enzymatic isotopic assay of histamine: measurement of histamine in plasma and serum. *Anal. Biochem.*, **94**, 425–30
7. Shore, P. A. (1976). Fluorometric assay of histamine. In Williams, C. A. and Chase, M. W., *Methods in Immunology and Immunochemistry* V. pp. 129–31. (NY: Academic Press)
8. Rauls, D. O., Ting, S. and Lund, M. (1986). Analysis of plasma histamine: A modification of the enzymatic isotopic assay. *J. Allergy Clin. Immunol.*, **77**, 673–6
9. Brown, M. J., Ind, P. W., Barnes, P. J., Jenner, D. A. and Dollery C. T. (1980). A sensitive and specific radiometric method for the measurement of plasma histamine in normal individuals. *Anal. Biochem.*, **109**, 142–6
10. Allenmark, S., Bergstrom, S. and Ennerback, L. (1985). A selective post column O-phthalaldehyde-derivatization system for the determination of histamine in a biological material by high-performance liquid chromatography. *Anal. Biochem.*, **144**, 98–103
11. Benditt, E. P., Wong, R. L. and Arase, M. (1955). 5-Hydroxytryptamine in mast cells. *Proc. Soc. Exp. Biol. Med.*, **90**, 303–4
12. Jenkinson, D. M., Thompson, G. E., Kenny, J. D. R. and Pearson, J. M. (1970). Histochemical studies on mast cells in cattle skin. *Histochem. J.*, **2**, 419–24
13. Grzanna, R. and Schultz, L. D. (1982). The contribution of mast cells to the histamine content of the central nervous system: A regional analysis. *Life Sci.*, **30**, 1959–64

14. Soll, A. H., Lewin, K. J. and Beaven, M. A. (1981). Isolation of histamine-containing cells from rat gastric mucosa: biochemical and morphologic differences from rat mast cells. *Gastroenterology*, **80**, 717
15. Meggs, W. J., Atkins, F. M., Wright, R., Fishman, M., Kaliner, M. A. and Metcalfe D. D. (1985). Failure of sulfites to produce clinical responses in patients with systemic mastocytosis or recurrent anaphylaxis: Results of a single-blind study. *J. Allergy Clin. Immunol.*, **76**, 840–6
16. MacGlashan, D. W., Jr. and Lichtenstein, L. M. (1980). The purification of human basophils. *J. Immunol.*, **124**, 2519–21
17. Toll, J. B. C., Wikberg, J. E. S. and Anderson, R. G. G. (1981). Purification of human basophils by affinity chromatography on anti-IgE-Sepharose 6MB. *Allergy*, **36**, 411–17
18. Schwartz, L. B., Irani, A. A., Roller, K., Castells, M. C. and Schechter, N. M. (1987). Quantitation of histamine, tryptase and chymase in dispersed human T and TC mast cells. *J. Immunol.*, **138**, 2611
19. Lagunoff, D. and Rickard, A. (1983). Evidence for control of mast cell granule protease *in situ* by low pH. *Exp. Cell Res.*, **144**, 353
20. Uvnas, B., Aborg, C. H. and Bergendoff, A. (1970). Storage of mast cells. Evidence for an ionic binding of histamine to protein carboxyls in the granule heparin protein complex. *Acta Physiol. Scand. (Suppl.)*, **336**, 3
21. Smith, P. C., Kagey-Sabotka, A., Bleecker, E. R. (1980). Physiologic manifestations of human anaphylaxis. *J. Clin. Invest.*, **66**, 1072–80
22. Sheffer, A. L., Soter, N. A., McFadden, E. R., Jr. and Austen, K. F. (1983). Exercise-induced anaphylaxis: a distinct form of physical allergy. *J. Allergy Clin. Immunol.*, **71**, 331–6
23. Myers, G., Donlon, M. and Kaliner, M. (1981). Measurement of urinary histamine: Development of methodology and normal values. *J. Allergy Clin. Immunol.*, **67**, 305
24. Keyzer, J. J., Breukelman, H., Wolthers, B. G., Richardson, F. J. and De Monchy J. G. R. (1985). Measurement of N^t-methylhistamine concentrations in plasma and urine as a parameter for histamine release during anaphylactoid reactions. *Agents Actions*, **16**, 76
25. Keyzer, J. J., De-Monchy, J. G., Van Doormaal, J. J. and Van Voorst-Vlader, P. C. (1983). Improved diagnosis of mastocytosis by measurement of urinary histamine metabolites. *N. Engl. J. Med.*, **309**, 1603
26. Rosenbaum, R. C., Frieri, M. and Metcalfe, D. D. (1984). Patterns of skeletal scintography and their relationship to plasma and urinary histamine levels in systemic mastocytosis. *J. Nucl. Med.*, **25**, 859
27. Black, J. W., Duncan, W. A. M., Durant, C. J. *et al.* (1972). Definition and antagonism of histamine H2-receptors. *Nature*, **236**, 385
28. Robertson, I. and Greaves, M. W. (1978). Responses of human skin blood vessels to synthetic histamine analogues. *Br. J. Clin. Pharmacol.*, **5**, 319
29. Cochrane, C. G. (1958). Studies on the localization of circulating antigen–antibody complexes and other macromolecules in vessels II. Pathogenic and pharmacodynamic studies. *J. Exp. Med.*, **65**, 503
30. Kaliner, M., Shelhamer, J. H. and Ottesen, E. A. (1982). Effects of infused histamine: correlation of plasma histamine levels and symptoms. *J. Allergy Clin. Immunol.*, **69**, 283
31. Douglas, W. D. (1980). Histamine and 5-hydroxytryptamine (serotonin) and their antagonists. In Gilman, A. G., Goodman, L. S. and Gilman, A. (eds.) *The Pharmacologic Basic of Therapeutics*, Edn. 6. p. 609. (NY: MacMillan Publishing)
32. Holgate, S. T., Emanuel, M. B. and Howarth, P. H. (1985). Astemizole and other H_1-antihistaminic drug treatment of asthma. *J. Allergy Clin. Immunol.*, **76**, 375
33. Braude, S., Royston, D., Coe, C. and Barnes, P. J. (1984). Histamine increases lung permeability by an H_2-receptor mechanism. *Lancet*, **2**, 372
34. Melmon, K. L., Rocklin, R. E. and Rosenkranz, R. P. (1981). Autocoids as modulators of the inflammatory and immune response. *Am. J. Med.*, **71**, 100
35. Anwar, A. R. E. and Kay, A. B. (1978). Enhancement of human eosinophil complement receptors by pharmacologic mediators. *J. Immunol.*, **121**, 1425
36. Anwar, A. R. E., McKean, J. R., Smithers, S. R. and Kay, A. B. (1980). Human eosinophil- and neutrophil-mediated killing of schistosomula of *Schistosoma mansoni in vitro*. I. Enhancement of C'-dependent damage by mast cell-derived mediators and formyl methionyl peptides. *J. Immunol.*, **124**, 1122

37. Baeziger, N. L., Fogerty, F. J., Mertz, L. F. and Chernuta, L. F. (1981). Regulation of histamine-mediated prostacyclin synthesis in cultured human vascular endothelial cells. *Cell*, **24**, 915
38. Naclerio, R. M., Meier, H. L., Kagey-Sobotka, A., Adkinson, J. R. N. F., Meyeres, D. A., Norman, P. S. and Lichtenstein, L. M. (1983). Mediator release after nasal airway challenge with allergen. *Am. Rev. Resp. Dis.*, **128**, 597–602
39. Talbot, S. F., Atkins, P. C., Valenzano and Zweiman, B. (1984). Correlations of *in vivo* mediator release with late cutaneous allergic responses in humans. I. Kinetics of histamine release. *J. Allergy Clin. Immunol.*, **74**, 819
40. Metcalfe, D. D., Lewis, R. A., Silbert, J. E., Rosenberg, R. D., Wasserman, S. I. and Austen, K. F. (1979). Isolation and characterization of heparin from human lung. *J. Clin. Invest.*, **64**, 1537
41. Metcalfe, D. D., Soter, N. A., Wasserman, S. I. and Austen, K. F. (1980). Identification of sulphated mucopolysaccharides including heparin in the lesional skin of a patient with mastocytosis. *J. Invest. Dermatol.*, **74**, 210
42. Eliakim, R., Gilead, L., Ligumsky, M., Okon, E., Rachmilewitz, D. and Razin, E. (1986). Histamine and chondroitin sulphate E proteoglycan released by cultured human colonic mucosa: Indication for possible presence of E mast cells. *Proc. Natl. Acad. Sci. (USA)*, **83**, 461
43. Metcalfe, D. D., Smith, J. A., Austen, K. F. and Silbert, J. E. (1980). Poydispersity of rat mast cell heparin: implications for proteoglycan assembly. *J. Biol. Chem.*, **255**, 11753
44. Horner, H. H. (1971). Macromolecular heparin from rat skin. Isolation, characterization and depolymerization with ascorbate. *J. Biol. Chem.*, **246**, 231
45. Stevens, R. L., Otsu, K. and Austen, K. F. (1985). Purification and analysis of the core protein of the protease-resistant intracellular chondroitin sulfate E proteoglycan from the interleukin 3-dependent mouse mast cell. *J. Biol. Chem.*, **260**, 14194–200
46. Seldin, D. C., Austen, K. F. and Stevens, R. L. (1985). Purification and characterization of protease-resistant secretory granule proteoglycans containing chondroitin di-B and heparin-like glycosaminoglycans from rat basophil leukemia cells. *J. Biol. Chem.*, **260**, 11131–9
47. Razin, E., Stevens, R. L., Akiyama, F., Schmid, K. and Austen, K. F. (1982). Culture from mouse bone marrow of a subclass of mast cells possessing a distinct chondroitin sulfate proteoglycan with glycosaminoglycans rich in N-acetylgalactosamine-4, 6-disulfate. *J. Biol. Chem.*, **257**, 7229
48. Stevens, R. L., Otsu, K. and Austen, K. F. (1985). Purification and analysis of the protease-resistant intracellular chondroitin sulfate E proteoglycan from the interleukin 3-dependent mouse mast cell. *J. Biol. Chem.*, **260**, 14194
49. Seldin, D. C., Austen, K. F. and Stevens, R. L. (1985). Purification and characterization of protease-resistant secretory granule proteoglycans containing chondroitin sulfate di-B and heparin-like glycosaminoglycans from rat basophilic leukemia cells. *J. Biol. Chem.*, **260**, 11131
50. Stevens, R. L., Lee, T. D. G., Seldin, D. C., Austen, K. F., Befus, A. D. and Bienenstock, J. (1986). Intestinal mucosal mast cells from rats infected with *Nippostrongylus brasiliensis* contain protease-resistant chondroitin sulfate di-B proteoglycans. *J. Immunol.*, **137**, 291–5
51. Metcalfe, D. D., Bland, C. E. and Wasserman, S. I. (1984). Biochemical and functional characterization of proteoglycans isolated from basophils of patients with chronic myelogenous leukemia. *J. Immunol.*, **132**, 1943
52. Katz, H. R., Stevens, R. L. and Austen, K. F. (1985). Heterogeneity of mammalian mast cells differentiated *in vivo* and *in vitro*. *J. Allergy Clin. Immunol.*, **76**, 250
53. Barrett, K. E. and Metcalfe, D. D. (1984). Mast cell heterogeneity: evidence and implications. *J. Clin. Immunol.*, **4**, 253
54. Yurt, R. W., Leid, R. W., Austen, K. F. and Silbert, J. E. (1977). Native heparin from rat peritoneal mast cells. *J. Biol. Chem.*, **252**, 518
55. Stevens, R. L., Razin, E., Austen, K. F., Hein, A., Caulfield, J. P., Seno, N., Schmid, K. and Akiyama, F. (1983). Synthesis of chondroitin SO_4 E glycosaminoglycan onto *p*-nitrophenyl β-D xyloside and its localization to secretory granules of rat serosal mast cells and mucosal bone marrow-derived mast cells. *J. Biol. Chem.*, **258**, 5977

56. Metcalfe, D. D., Wasserman, S. I. and Austen, K. F. (1980). Isolation and characterization of sulphated mucopolysaccharides from rat leukemic (RBL-1) basophils. *Biochem. J.*, **185**, 367

57. Schwartz, L. B. and Bradford, T. M. (1986). Regulation of tryptase from human lung mast cells by heparin: Stabilization of the active tetramer. *J. Biol. Chem.*, **261**, 7372

58. Alter, S. C., Metcalfe, D. D. and Schwartz, L. B. (0000). Stabilization of human mast cell tryptase: Effect of enzyme concentration, ionic strength and the structure and negative charge density of polysaccharides. *Biochem. J.*, **248**, 821

59. Rosenberg, R. D. and Lam, L. (1979). Correlation between structure and function of heparin. *Proc. Natl. Acad. Sci. (USA)*, **76**, 1218

60. Scully, M. F., Ellis, V., Seno, N. and Kakkar, V. V. (1986). The anticoagulant properties of mast cell product, chondroitin sulphate E. *Biochem. Biophys. Res. Commun.*, **137**, 15–22

61. Kazatchkine, M. D., Fearon, D. T., Silbert, J. E. and Austen, K. F. (1979). Surface-associated heparin inhibits zymosan-induced activation of the human alternative complement pathway by augmenting the regulatory action of the control proteins on particle-bound C3b. *J. Exp. Med.*, **150**, 1201

62. Loos, M., Volanakis, J. E. and Stroud, R. M. (1976). Mode of interaction of different polyanions with the first (C1, C̄1), second (C2), and the fourth (C4) component of complement. III. Inhibition of C4 and C2 binding site(s) of C̄1s by polyanions. *Immunochemistry*, **13**, 789

63. Hojima, Y., Cochrane, C. G., Wiggins, R. C., Austen, K. F. and Stevens, R. L. (1984). *In vitro* activation of the contact (Hageman Factor) system of plasma by heparin and chondroitin sulfate E. *Blood*, **63**, 1453

64. Schechter, N. M., Fraki, J. E., Geesin, J. C. and Lazarus, G. S. (1983). Human skin chymotryptic protease. Isolation and relation to cathepsin G and rat mast cell proteinase I. *J. Biol. Chem.*, **258**, 2973

65. Schwartz, L. B., Lewis, R. A. and Austen, K. F. (1981). Tryptase from human pulmonary mast cells: Purification and characterization. *J. Biol. Chem.*, **256**, 11939

66. Smith, T. J., Hougland, M. W. and Johnson, D. A. (1984). Human lung tryptase, purification and characterization. *J. Biol. Chem.*, **259**, 11046

67. Schwartz, L. B. (1985). Monoclonal antibodies against human mast cell tryptase demonstrate shared antigenic sites on subunits of tryptase and selective localization of the enzyme to mast cells. *J. Immunol.*, **134**, 256

68. Castells, M., Irani, A. A. and Schwartz, L. B. (1987). Evaluation of human peripheral blood leukocytes for mast cell tryptase. *J. Immunol.*, **138**, 2184

69. Glenner, C. G. and Cohen, L. A. (1960). Histochemical demonstration of a species-specific trypsin-like enzyme in mast cells. *Nature (London)*, **185**, 846

70. Schwartz, L. B., Lewis, R. A., Seldin, D. and Austen, K. F. (1981). Acid hydrolases and tryptase from secretory granules of dispersed human lung mast cells. *J. Immunol.*, **126**, 1290

71. Wenzel, S., Irani, A. A., Sanders, J. M., Bradford, T. R. and Schwartz, L. B. (1986). Immunoassay of tryptase from human mast cells. *J. Immunol. Meth.*, **86**, 139

72. Schwartz, L. B., Atkins, P. C., Fleekopp, P. and Zweiman, B. (1986). Release of tryptase and histamine during cutaneous challenge with allergen. *J. Allergy Clin. Immunol.*, **77**, 246

73. Shalit, M., Schwartz, L., Atkins, P. and Zweiman, B. (1987). Mediator release during late onset cutaneous reactions induced by continuous antigen stimulation. *J. Allergy Clin. Immunol.* (Abstr.), **79**, 248

74. Schwartz, L. B., Metcalfe, D. D., Miller, J., Earl, H. and Sullivan, T. (1987). Tryptase levels as an indicator of mast cell activation in systemic anaphylaxis and mastocytosis. *N. Engl. J. Med.*, **316**, 1622

75. Tanaka, T., McRae, B. J., Cho, K., Cook, R., Fraki, J. E., Johnson, D. A. and Powers, J. C. (1983). Mammalian tissue trypsin-like enzymes: comparative reactivities of human skin tryptase, human lung tryptase and bovine trypsin with peptide 4-nitroanilide and thioester substrates. *J. Biol. Chem.*, **258**, 13552–7

76. Fraki, J. E., Schechter, N. M., Harvima, I. T. and Lazarus, G. S. (1985). Human skin tryptase. In Ogawa, H., Lazarus, G. S. and Hopsu-Havo, V. K. (eds.) *The Biological Role of Proteinases and Their Inhibitors in Skin*. pp. 127–37. (Tokyo: University of Tokyo Press)

77. Alter, S. C., Yates, P., Margolius, H. S. and Schwartz, L. B. (1987). Tryptase and kinin generation: Tryptase from human mast cells does not activate human urinary prokallikrein. *Int. Arch. Allergy Appl. Immunol.*, **83**, 321

78. DeWater, R., Williams, L. N. A., Van Muigen, G. N. P., Granken, C., Fransen, J. A. M., Dijkman, J. H. and Kramps, J. A. (1986). Ultrastructural localization of bronchial antileukoprotease in central and peripheral human airways by a gold-labeling technique using monoclonal antibodies. *Am. Rev. Resp. Dis.*, **133**, 882–90

79. Kramps, J. A. and Klasen, E. C. (1985). Characterization of a low molecular weight antielastase isolated from human bronchial secretions. *Exp. Lung Res.*, **9**, 151

80. Schwartz, L. B., Kawahara, M. S., Hugli, T. E., Vik, D., Fearon, D. T. and Austen, K. F. (1983). Generation of C3a anaphylatoxin from human C3 by human mast cell tryptase. *J. Immunol.*, **130**, 18991

81. Gruber, B. L., Schwartz, L. B., Ramamurthy, N. S., Irani, A. M. and Marchese, M. J. (1988). Activation of latent rheumatoid synovial collagenase by human mast cell tryptase. *J. Immunol.* (In press)

82. Crisp, A. J., Chapman, C. M., Kirkham, S. E., Schiller, A. L. and Krane, S. M. (1984). Articular mastocytosis in rheumatoid arthritis. *Arthr. Rheum.*, **27**, 845–51

83. Schwartz, L. B., Bradford, T. M., Littman, B. L. and Wintroub, B. U. (1985). The fibrinogenolytic activity of purified tryptase from human lung mast cells. *J. Immunol.*, **135**, 2762

84. Maier, M., Spragg, J. and Schwartz, L. B. (1983). Inactivation of human high molecular weight kininogen by human mast cell tryptase. *J. Immunol.*, **130**, 2352

85. Schwartz, L. B., Maier, M. and Spragg, J. (1986). Interaction of low molecular weight kininogen with human mast cell tryptase. *Adv. Exp. Med. Biol.*, **198A**, 105

86. Schwartz, L. B., Bradford, T. M. and Griffin, J. H. (1985). The effect of tryptase from human mast cells on human prekallikrein. *Biochem. Biophys. Res. Commun.*, **129**, 76

87. Proud, D., Togias, A., Naclerio, R. M., Crush, S. A., Norman, P. S. and Lichtenstein, L. M. (1983). Kinins are generated *in vivo* following nasal airway challenge of allergic individuals with allergen. *J. Clin. Invest.*, **72**, 1678

88. Chiu, H. and Lagunoff, D. (1972). Histochemical comparison of vertebrate mast cells. *Histochem. J.*, **4**, 135

89. Schechter, N. M., Choi, J. K., Slavin, D. A., Deresienski, D. T., Sayama, S., Dong, G., Lavker, R. M., Proud, D. and Lazarus, G. S. (1986). Identification of a chymotrypsin-like proteinase in human mast cells. *J. Immunol.*, **137**, 962

90. Huntley, J. F., Newlands, G. F. J., Gibson, S., Ferguson, A. and Miller, H. R. P. (1985). Histochemical demonstration of chymotrypsin-like serine esterases in mucosal mast cells in four species including man. *J. Clin. Pathol.*, **38**, 375

91. Wintroub, B. U., Schechter, N. B., Lazarus, G. S., Kaempfer, C. E. and Schwartz, L. B. (1984). Angiotension I conversion by human and rat chymotryptic proteinases. *J. Invest. Derm.*, **83**, 336

92. Reilly, C. F., Tewksbury, D. A., Schechter, N. M. and Travis, J. (1982). Rapid conversion of angiotensin I to angiotensin II by neutrophil and mast cell proteinases. *J. Biol. Chem.*, **257**, 8619

93. Wintroub, B. U., Daempfer, B. S., Schechter, N. M. and Proud, D. (1986). A human lung mast cell chymotrypsin-like proteinase: Identification and partial characterization. *J. Clin. Invest.*, **77**, 196

94. Briggaman, R. A., Schechter, N. M., Fraki, J. and Lazarus, G. S. (1984). Degradation of the epidermal–dermal junction by a proteolytic enzyme from human skin and human polymorphonuclear leukocytes. *J. Exp. Med.*, **160**, 1027

95. Meier, H. L., Kaplan, A. P., Lichtenstein, L. M., Revak, S. D., Cochrane, C. G. and Newball, H. (1983). Anaphylactic release of a prekallikrein activator from human lung *in vitro*. *J. Clin. Invest.*, **72**, 574

96. Proud, D., MacGlashan, Jr., J. W., Newball, H. H., Schulman, E. S. and Lichtenstein, L. M. (1985). IgE-mediated release of a kininogenase from purified human lung mast cells. *Am. Rev. Resp. Dis.*, **132**, 405

97. Meier, H. L., Heck, L. W., Schulman, E. S. and MacGlashan, Jr., D. W. (1985). Purified human mast cells and basophils release human elastase and cathepsin G by an IgE-mediated mechanism. *Int. Arch. Allergy Appl. Immunol.*, **77**, 179

146

98. Goldstein, S. M., Kaempfer, C., Proud, D., Schwartz, L. B., Irani, A. M. and Wintroub, B. U. (1987). Detection and partial characterization of a human mast cell carboxy-peptidase. *J. Immunol.*, **139**, 2724

99. Schwartz, L. B., Riedel, C., Schratz, J. J. and Austen, K. F. (1982). Localization of carboxypeptidase A to the macromolecular heparin proteoglycan–protein complex in secretory granules of rat serosal mast cells. *J. Immunol.*, **128**, 1128–33

100. Craig, S. S., Schechter, N. M. and Schwartz, L. B. (1988). Ultrastructural analysis of human T and TC mast cells identified by immunoelectron microscopy. *Lab. Invest.* (In press)

101. Gibson, S. and Miller, H. R. P. (1986). Mast cell subsets in the rat distinguished immuno-histochemically by their content of serine proteinases. *Immunology*, **58**, 101

102. Benyon, R. C., Lowman, M. A. and Church, M. K. (1987). Human skin mast cells: their dispersion, purification and secretory characterization. *J. Immunol.*, **138**, 861

103. Church, M. K., Pao, G. J.-K. and Holgate, S. T. (1982). Characterization of histamine secretion from dispersed human lung mast cells: effects of anti-IgE, calcium ionophore A23187, compound 48/80, and basic polypeptides. *J. Immunol.*, **129**, 2116

104. Lee, T. D. G., Swieter, M., Bienenstock, J. and Befus, A. D. (1985). Heterogeneity in mast cell populations. *Clin. Immunol. Rev.*, **4**, 143

105. Kobayeshi, T., Nakano, T., Nakahata, T., Asai, H., Yogi, Y., Tsuji, K., Komiyama, A., Akabane, T., Kojima, S. and Kitamura, Y. (1986). Formation of mast cell colonies in methylcellulose by mouse peritoneal cells and differentiation of these cloned cells in both the skin and the gastric mucosa of W/Wᵛ mice: Evidence that a common precursor can give rise to both 'connective tissue-type' and 'mucosal' mast cells. *J. Immunol.*, **136**, 1378

106. Irani, A. A., Schechter, N. M. and Schwartz, L. B. (1987). Deficiency of the tryptase positive, chymase negative mast cell type in gastrointestinal mucosa of patients with defective T lymphocyte function. *J. Immunol.*, **138**, 4381

5
Mast Cells and Newly-Generated Lipid Mediators

C. ROBINSON

INTRODUCTION

In addition to their ability to release preformed, granule-derived mediators, activated mast cells from all species so far studied have the capacity to synthesize and release mediators on a *de novo* basis. The purpose of this chapter is to review the generation of newly-synthesized lipid mediators of inflammation by activated mast cells.

Biosynthesis of prostaglandins and thromboxanes

Prostaglandins and thromboxanes are synthesized quickly when required from their polyunsaturated fatty acid precursors dihomo-γ-linolenic acid (20:3 ω6), arachidonic acid (20:4 ω6) and eicosapentaenoic acid (20:5 ω3). A prerequisite is their release from storage sites in membrane lipids. In Western populations the most important eicosanoid precursor is arachidonic acid, which gives rise to the 2 series or dienoic prostaglandins. Although the arachidonic acid content of most cells is high, little of this is in a freely available form, and consequently its release from neutral and phospholipids is the initial reaction in prostanoid formation[1]. As far as is known no oxidative metabolism of the fatty acid occurs while it is esterified in lipids. It is currently believed that phospholipase A_2, phospholipase C/diglyceride lipase and neutral lipid lipases are involved in the mobilization of arachidonic acid[2-4]. In mast cells and macrophages it has also been claimed that arachidonic acid is stored in the form of cytoplasmic lipid bodies, although the significance of these observations is unknown[5].

The transformations of arachidonic acid to yield prostaglandins and thromboxanes (Figure 5.1) begin with the enzyme complex fatty acid cyclooxygenase (E.C. 1.14.99.1.1). This is a cytochrome b-like haemprotein from which the haem moiety is readily removed[6,7], and which is found in the endoplasmic reticulum of most cells[7,8]. The haem group is essential for both

149

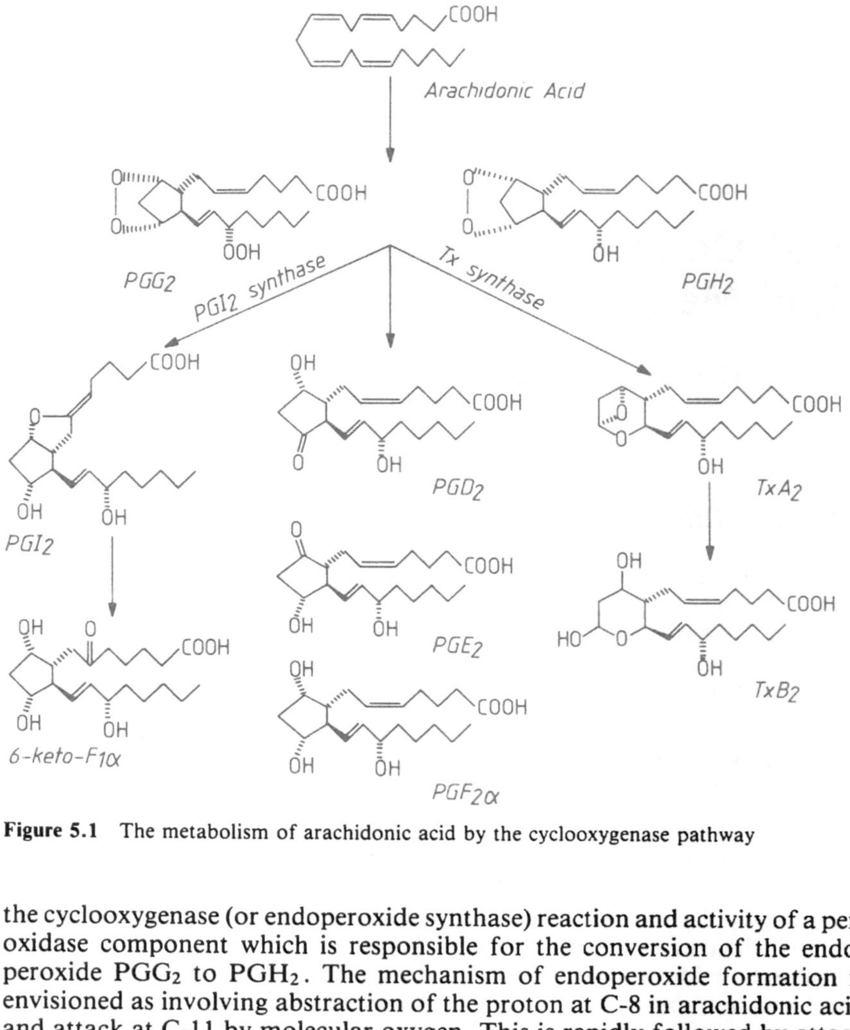

Figure 5.1 The metabolism of arachidonic acid by the cyclooxygenase pathway

the cyclooxygenase (or endoperoxide synthase) reaction and activity of a peroxidase component which is responsible for the conversion of the endoperoxide PGG_2 to PGH_2. The mechanism of endoperoxide formation is envisioned as involving abstraction of the proton at C-8 in arachidonic acid and attack at C-11 by molecular oxygen. This is rapidly followed by attack at C-9 by the 11-peroxy radical so generated, and subsequent cyclization and hydroperoxidation at C-15 to yield PGG_2[9]. The ability of the arachidonic acid molecule to fold facilitates these processes by enabling the appropriate groups to come into juxtaposition. The endoperoxide PGG_2 may then be converted by a C-15 peroxidase to produce PGH_2[9]. Both of these endoperoxides are relatively unstable (t½ ~ 5 min at pH 7.4) and they serve as key reactive intermediates in the formation of the primary 'classical' prostaglandins[10, 11], prostacyclin (PGI_2) and thromboxanes[12–15].

Formation of the classical prostaglandins may proceed enzymatically or by non-enzymatic reductive or disproportionate cleavage of the 9,11-endoperoxides. A protein catalysing the glutathione-dependent formation of

PGE$_2$ (prostaglandin endoperoxide E isomerase, E.C. 5.3.99.3.3) has been partially purified from bovine vesicular glands[16], and a series of glutathione-S-transferase dependent proteins promoting the formation of PGD$_2$ have been reported[17, 18]. PGD$_2$ may also be produced by simple aqueous decomposition of PG endoperoxides, particularly in the presence of albumin[19-21]. Some controversy exists over the formation of F series prostaglandins. Despite the fact that the capacity to synthesize PGF$_{2\alpha}$ is widely distributed, a specific enzyme catalysing the conversion of PGH$_2$ to PGF$_{2\alpha}$ has been reported only in guinea-pig uterus and bovine lung[22-24]. Later work with the partially purified bovine lung enzyme showed that the protein also catalysed the 11-ketoreduction of PGD$_2$ to 9α,11β-PGF$_2$[24].

Of the remaining primary prostaglandins PGA$_2$ is produced from PGE$_2$ under acidic dehydrating conditions. Under mildly basic conditions PGA$_2$ undergoes double bond migration to yield PGB$_2$ as the major product, with PGC$_2$ probably formed as a transient intermediate. Although PGA$_2$ and PGB$_2$ have been detected in biological samples it is hard to determine whether their formation is artefactual. Similarly, the PGC-isomerase enzyme described in the rabbit is of questionable specificity and relevance to human pathophysiology.

Thromboxane A$_2$ (TXA$_2$) is synthesized from PG endoperoxides in a reaction catalysed by a modified cytochrome P450 synthase enzyme[25]. 12-Hydroxyheptadecatrienoic acid (HHT) is co-produced from PGH$_2$ in this reaction, although it appears to arise independently and is not a metabolite of TXA$_2$[26]. Relatively little is known about the molecular properties of the enzyme, save that when subjected to immunoaffinity purification from porcine lung or human platelets the enzyme is a haemprotein of molecular weight 50 000–53 000 daltons (SDS gel) and that it can be readily and irreversibly deactivated by PGH$_2$ or 15-hydroperoxyeicosatetraenoic acid (15-HPETE)[27]. This catalytic inactivation may represent an important regulatory system for this enzyme. The mechanism of reaction leading to the formation of TXA$_2$ is envisaged as involving protonation and cleavage of the endoperoxides at C-9, cleavage at C-11/C-12 and the formation of two new C–O bonds[9].

Prostacyclin synthase is also a microsomal cytochrome P450 system of MW 49 000 and has been purified to homogeneity[28]. The mechanism of formation of prostacyclin is probably very similar to that of TXA$_2$, but protonation being initiated at C-11.

Biosynthesis of lipoxygenase products

In addition to reactions leading to prostaglandin and thromboxane formation, arachidonic acid and certain other polyunsaturated fatty acids can undergo lipoxygenation reactions to yield a wide variety of acyclic fatty acid metabolites (Figure 5.2), including the sulphidopeptide leukotrienes now known to comprise slow reacting substance of anaphylaxis (SRS-A) (for reviews see References 29–32). Unlike prostaglandin formation which requires liberation of arachidonic acid from phospholipid stores, there is some evidence that lipoxygenase product formation could occur by direct attack

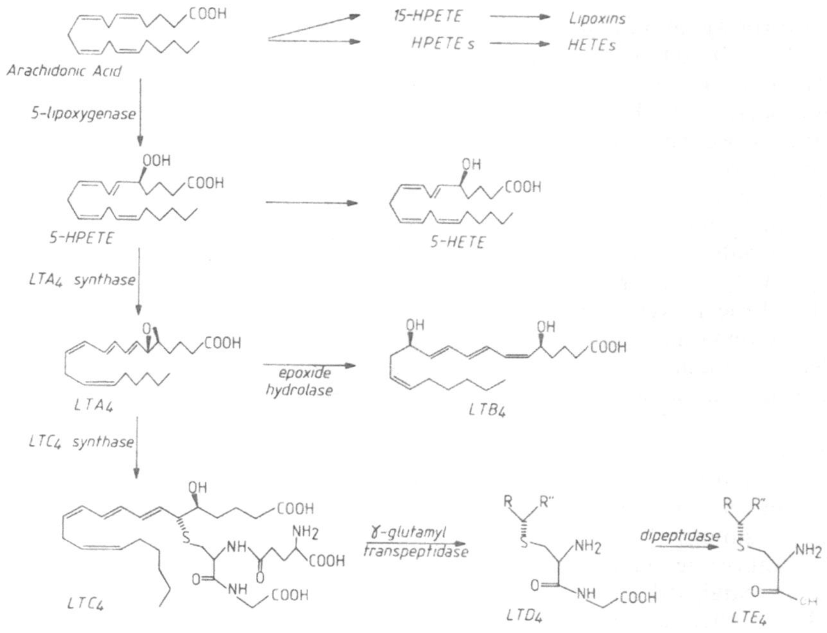

Figure 5.2 The metabolism of arachidonic acid by lipoxygenase pathways

of the enzyme on esterified arachidonic acid. Two partially purified lipoxy-genases, from soybean and rabbit reticulocytes respectively, can oxygenate with high positional and stereospecificity, the unsaturated fatty acids present in phosphoglycerides to yield the corresponding hydroperoxyphospho-glyceride[33]. Studies with $H_2{}^{18}O$-labelled buffers have shown that although this could occur in leukocytes, free arachidonic acid is still a preferred sub-strate for lipoxygenation[34].

Lipoxygenases (E.C. 1.13.11.12) are a family of iron-containing dioxy-genases which facilitate the hydroperoxidation of polyunsaturated fatty acids containing a penta-1,4-*cis*-diene system[35]. Thus, in the arachidonic acid molecule there are three possible pairs of carbon atoms at which lipoxy-genation may be initiated by the reaction of molecular oxygen with a fatty acid radical formed by hydrogen abstraction from position 3 of the penta-diene unit. The first mammalian lipoxygenase enzyme identified was in blood platelets in which the enzyme forms a 12(*S*)-hydroperoxy-(*Z,Z,E.Z*)-5,8,10,14-eicosatetraenoic product (12-HPETE)[36]. This hydroperoxy acid is converted by glutathione/glutathione peroxidase to the corresponding C-12 hydroxy acid (12-HETE). Since this observation, it has become recognized that other lipoxygenase enzymes with positional specificity for other points in the arachidonic acid molecule are widely distributed in a diverse range of cells known to subserve important roles in inflammation. The complexities of some of these pathways are only recently becoming realized. For example, the enzyme 15-lipoxygenase metabolizes arachidonic acid to 15-HPETE.

As well as giving rise to 15-HETE, in leukocytes 15-HPETE can also be metabolized to produce the fully conjugated tetraenes lipoxins A and B[37-39]. Although biologically active, little is known about the synthesis, fate and pathophysiological relevance of the lipoxins.

Unlike other lipoxygenase enzymes which read the substrate fatty acid from the terminal methyl group, the 5-lipoxygenase enzyme reads the molecule from the carboxyl end. In the case of the product of 5-lipoxygenation, 5(S)-hydroperoxy-(E,Z,Z,Z)-6,8,11,14-eicosatetraenoic acid, (5-HPETE), the molecule may undergo the usual two electron reduction of the hydroperoxide to produce 5-HETE. In addition, the same enzyme can also promote 5,6-epoxide formation to give rise to leukotriene A₄ (LTA₄)[40,41]. The cytosolic 5-lipoxygenase/LTA₄ synthase complex has been purified from human and porcine leukocytes, murine mastocytoma and RBL-1 cells[41-43], and is a Ca^{2+} and ATP-requiring enzyme of molecular weight 70 000–75 000. Being an allylic epoxide LTA₄ is a reactive molecule, and readily undergoes nucleophilic substitution under both enzymatic and non-enzymatic conditions. An LTA₄ hydrolase enzyme, present in human leukocytes, erythrocytes and plasma[44-46] catalyses the reaction of LTA₄ with water to produce 5(S),12(R)-dihydroxy-(Z,E,E,Z)-6,8,10,14-eicosatetraenoic acid (LTB₄), a molecule which is chemotactic for neutrophils and eosinophils, and which may play a considerable role in polymorphonuclear leukocyte-dependent inflammatory reactions. The cytosolic hydrolase enzyme has been purified to homogeneity from human leukocytes. It has a molecular weight of 70 000[44].

In addition to its reaction with water, LTA₄ also undergoes an important reaction with glutathione to form 5(S)-hydroxy-6(R)-S-glutathionyl-(E,E,Z,Z,)-7,9,11,14-eicosatetraenoic acid (LTC₄)[47]. This peptidolipid is the first member of a family now known to comprise slow reacting substances of anaphylaxis (SRS-A). The enzyme catalysing this reaction is a unique microsomal glutathione-S-transferase[48-50], now commonly referred to as LTC₄ synthase. LTC₄ may be converted to 5(S)-hydroxy-6(R)-S-cysteinyl-glycinyl-(E,E,Z,Z)-7,9,11,14-eicosatetraenoic acid (LTD₄) by γ-glutamyl-transpeptidase[51,52], and subsequently to 5(S)-hydroxy-6(R)-S-cysteinyl-(E,E,Z,Z)-7,9,11,14-eicosatetraenoic acid (LTE₄) by a dipeptidase[53]. At present, relatively little is known about the enzymology of these metabolic conversions of LTC₄, except that the dipeptidase enzyme has been found in the specific granules of leukocytes[53].

Biosynthesis of platelet activating factor (PAF-acether)

PAF-acether (1-O-alkyl-2-acetylglyceryl-3-phosphorylcholine) is a unique ether phospholipid which was originally considered to be a basophil derived mediator of anaphylaxis in the rabbit[54,55]. It is now realized that many other cell types have the capacity to synthesize PAF-acether, and this compound has attracted considerable attention as a putative mediator of inflammation. The biosynthesis of PAF-acether occurs in a concerted two-step process in which a phospholipase A₂ enzyme hydrolyses 1-O-alkyl-2-acyl-glyceryl-3-phosphorylcholine to yield the corresponding lyso derivative[56,57]. The lyso-PAF-acether is then converted to PAF-acether by an acetyltransferase

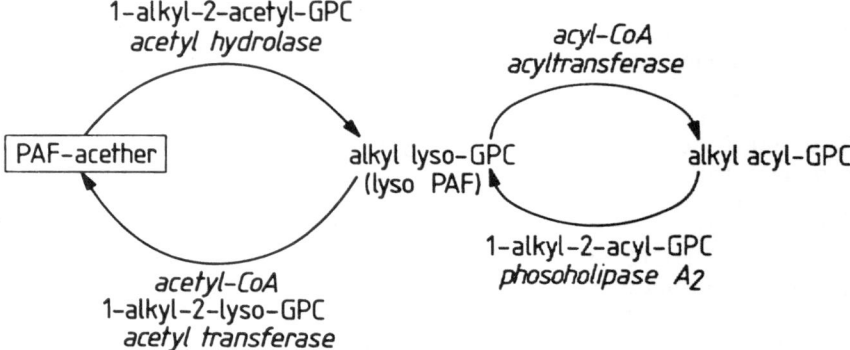

Figure 5.3 The biosynthesis of PAF-acether

enzyme (1-alkyl-2-lyso-*sn*-glycero-3-phosphocholine: acetyl-CoA acetyl-transferase) which has been described for a variety of cell types[58-62]. As well as being the precursor to PAF-acether, lyso-PAF is the degradation product of this mediator. The metabolic reaction is catalysed by a specific acetylhydrolase enzyme (1-alkyl-2-acetyl-*sn*-glycero-3-phosphocholine acetylhydrolase) (Figure 5.3). Lyso-PAF may be further degraded at *sn*-1 by an alkyl monooxygenase to yield a fatty alcohol and 3-phosphatidylcholine glycerol[63].

MAST CELLS AND NEWLY-GENERATED LIPID MEDIATORS

Traditionally, peritoneal mast cells from rodents have been used for the study of mediator release. Calcium-dependent activation of rat peritoneal mast cells with ionophore A23187 results in the liberation of PGD_2, together with smaller quantities of 6-keto-$PGF_{1\alpha}$, $PGF_{2\alpha}$ and TXB_2[64]. Lipoxygenase products identified as being released from these cells include 11-HETE, 12-HETE and LTB_4[64]. However, it has become increasingly apparent that there is heterogeneity of mast cells, not only between species but between different tissues of the same species[65-67]. In rodents these differences are relatively well demarcated, but in humans it appears that this heterogeneity is more subtle[68]. This realization has prompted detailed studies of mediator release from human mast cells. With this approach it is inevitable that the source of the mast cells may have a bearing on the results obtained as it is often necessary to rely on surgical specimens of diseased tissue from which to obtain the cells. This should be borne in mind in the following discussions.

To date, eicosanoid formation has been studied in populations of human mast cells of varying purity derived from lung parenchyma, airway epithelium, skin, colon and mastocytosis spleen[69-72]. With the exception of the lumenal mast cells of the respiratory tract, which are presumably derived from the epithelium, all of these systems require proteolytic digestion of the tissue in order to obtain suspensions of mast cells. Such suspensions may be enriched or depleted in mast cell content using a variety of strategies ranging from density gradient centrifugation to cell sorting and countercurrent centrifugal elutriation, or a combination of these.

Newly-generated lipid mediator release from human lung mast cells

The cellular complexity of lung tissue, together with the ability of all of the cells present to synthesize and release eicosanoids, creates tremendous problems when attempting to elucidate the cellular provenance of individual mediators. It may be somewhat surprising therefore, that connective tissue mast cells derived from human lung have been the most extensively characterized of human mast cells in the context of lipid mediator formation.

The most abundant cyclooxygenase product synthesized and released by the IgE-dependent activation of such cells is PGD_2[69, 73-75]. Maximal activation releases $50-100 \, ng/10^6$ mast cells, some 10-20 fold less than the amount of histamine released under the same conditions[74]. The release of PGD_2 is also observed in response to calcium-dependent activation with the ionophore A23187, although it is important to note that the amount of histamine released per unit amount of PGD_2 is approximately half the value seen with IgE-dependent activation[74]. These differences probably arise from the different activation–secretion processes triggered by the two secretagogues. In both cases, the release of PGD_2 from the mast cell is resistant to the inhibitory effects of corticosteroid drugs[75, 76], implying that these cells have a limited capacity for lipocortin synthesis. The release of PGD_2 in response to both secretagogues is also seen in protein-free media[77, 78]. This is an important observation because PGD synthase has yet to be characterized in human mast cells, and this prostanoid could theoretically arise by the albumin-catalysed decomposition of PG endoperoxides. Highly purified human pulmonary mast cells generate small quantities of TXB_2, 6-keto-$PGF_{1\alpha}$, PGE_2 and $PGF_{2\alpha}$[73, 79]. This is in contrast to rat peritoneal mast cells where 6-keto-$PGF_{1\alpha}$ and TXB_2 are more abundant than in human cells[64, 73].

IgE- or calcium-dependent stimulation of human lung fragments[69, 80, 81] or of unfractionated dispersed cells[78, 82] also triggers the release of the sulphidopeptide leukotrienes (LTC_4, LTD_4 and LTE_4) which comprise SRS-A. Early experiments suggested that an accessory cell type was needed for the optimum generation of leukotrienes from enriched populations of human lung mast cells in response to immunological activation[83, 84]. More recent work has refuted this hypothesis[85], although it should be borne in mind that other cell types present in human lung, particularly macrophages, have a substantial capacity for leukotriene biosynthesis[86]. The presence of IgE Fc receptors on macrophages and other inflammatory cells may result in their being activated for mediator release together with mast cells. It is also possible that these other inflammatory cells may be activated by mast cell-dependent products such as the oligopeptide prostaglandin generating factor of anaphylaxis[87, 88]. Cell–cell communication mechanisms may also exert their effects at other levels. For example, experiments in mouse peritoneal mast cells and

155

macrophages have shown that free radical mechanisms may serve as mechanisms which limit the formation of sulphidopeptide leukotrienes[89]. Such regulatory mechanisms undoubtedly deserve examination in human cells.

The issue of leukotriene formation in human lung has unquestionably been controversial, partly as a result of the relative instability of the leukotrienes and the difficulties associated with their measurement. A survey of the amounts of sulphidopeptide leukotrienes released from human lung mast cells reveals a wide discrepancy of values[31, 78, 79, 82, 85]; more recent analytical work indicating net release of LTC_4 in the range 5–30 ng/10^6 mast cells. Experiments with mast cells of 83–96% purity which had been labelled with octatritiated arachidonic acid have confirmed the immunological release of LTC_4 from these cells[79], an observation implying that the formation of LTD_4 and LTE_4 in human lung must occur outside the mast cell. Although mast cells of parenchymal origin do have the capacity to release leukotrienes, it is noteworthy that mast cells recovered by bronchoalveolar lavage release them in only small amounts[90]. Furthermore, compared to parenchymal mast cells these cells have markedly different characteristics of PGD_2 release when corrected for their release of histamine (Table 5.1).

The release of LTB_4, 5- and 12-HETE has been detected following A23187 challenge of rat peritoneal mast cells and mouse MC-9 or bone marrow-derived mast cells grown in culture[91, 92]. Although one study has reported the immunological release of LTB_4 from human lung mast cells[79] this has not yet been substantiated by other groups using similar techniques.

Recently, a technique has been described which permits the culture of mast cells from human lung[93]. Maintenance of the colony – the cells do not divide – is achieved by growing mast cells dispersed from human lung in the presence of skin fibroblasts from 3T3 mice. Such cells maintain their cellular histamine content, and electron microscopically they have the oval nucleus and scroll-like granule structure classically described for human lung mast cells. Immunological activation of cells passively sensitized with IgE results in degranulation and liberation of histamine[93]. Of interest is the observation that freshly dispersed cells release relatively little LTC_4 and LTB_4, but that after cell culture these amounts increase considerably together with an approximate three-fold increase in PGD_2 release[93]. At present the meaning of these results is not clear. It could be argued that the proteolytic digestion techniques employed in work of this type result in the switching off of 5-lipoxygenase activity and that such activity is restored after

Table 5.1 The relative release of PGD_2 and histamine from human mast cells activated by IgE cross-linkage or with A23187

Cell source	PGD_2 release (pg/ng histamine)	
	A23187	anti-IgE
Human bronchoalveolar	86	43
Human skin	52	144
Human lung parenchyma	32	77
Human mastocytosis spleen	6	13

several days in culture. Alternatively, the colony of fibroblasts upon which such cells are grown may be providing a micro-environmental factor(s) which promotes the expression of 5-lipoxygenase activity[90]. Clearly, further work is necessary to investigate these possibilities as they could ultimately have important bearings on our perception of the role of the mast cell as a source of many newly-generated mediators.

In contrast to the eicosanoids much less is known about the release of PAF-acether from mast cells. Although early experiments with rodent peritoneal cells suggested that the mast cell was a source of PAF-acether[94] this view was later dismissed on the basis that macrophages could account for all of the PAF-acether released[95]. However, it was subsequently observed that mouse mast cells cultured from bone marrow not only synthesized PAF-acether but also released it upon immunological activation by IgE cross-linkage[96]. To date few investigations have been performed with human mast cells. In a limited series of studies Schleimer and colleagues[97] demonstrated that in human lung mast cells of 97–99% purity activated by anti-IgE there was a rapid synthesis of PAF-acether which reached a maximum 2 min after challenge. However, none of this PAF-acether was released into the extracellular environment. This surprising observation is a more extreme manifestation of the situation in other cell types (neutrophils, monocytes, endothelial cells and eosinophils) where the amount of PAF-acether released is a small proportion of the amount actually generated by the cell[98]. Whether this cell-associated PAF-acether exerts any biological effects is not known at present. By analogy with certain eicosanoids[99] such an intracellular role may be possible although it may be hard to demonstrate. Interestingly, when incorporated into liposomes PAF-acether does exhibit biological activity, raising the possibility that one explanation for its intracellular retention may be to protect it from inactivation[98].

Newly-generated lipid mediator release from other human mast cells

Human mast cells from other tissue sources have been examined for their ability to synthesize and release lipid mediators following cell activation. As with human lung, this work is hindered by the difficulty in obtaining relatively pure populations of mast cells, which themselves may show considerable inhomogeneity with respect to size and density. Such studies have been performed on impure populations of mast cells obtained by proteolytic digestion of human intestinal mucosa[100]. These cells respond to IgE-dependent activation with the release of histamine, PGD_2 and sulphido-peptide leukotrienes. The ratio of PGD_2 to LTC_4 release was approximately 5 : 1 although subsequent analysis showed that the major leukotriene present was actually LTE_4[100]. Although not reported, it is likely that LTC_4 is converted to LTE_4 after release from mast cells, as is the case in human lung.

Recently, a technique has been developed which permits the isolation and enrichment of human dermal mast cells[101]. The pathways of arachidonic acid metabolism have now been mapped in these cells[71,102]. In cells of >80% purity IgE or A23187 dependent activation results in the synthesis of large amounts of PGD_2 together with the release of histamine. Under conditions of maximal activation with anti-IgE approximately 40 ng of PGD_2 are released per 10^6 mast cells. Radiochemical studies have shown that the sole leukotriene released by these cells is LTC_4, and at maximal activation release is 5–12 ng per 10^6 cells (Robinson, Benyon, Church and Holgate, unpublished observations). The amount of PGD_2 released per unit mass of histamine in these and other human mast cells is shown in Table 5.1.

BIOLOGICAL EFFECTS OF NEWLY-GENERATED LIPID MEDIATORS

Newly-generated lipid mediators exert a wide array of pathobiological effects on both vascular and non-vascular smooth muscle, together with effects on cell motility and activation state. In terms of potency, LTC_4 and LTD_4 are some of the most powerful bronchoconstrictor agents when given to man by inhalation (reviewed in References 103, 104). In man they are capable of producing significant reductions in airway calibre at concentrations between 0.75–8 μmol/l. In comparison, the mast cell-derived prostaglandin PGD_2 and its initial metabolite $9\alpha,11\beta$-PGF_2 exert similar effects in patients with mild asthma at concentrations of approximately 100 μmol/l[105, 106]. It is not currently known whether PGD_2 released from pulmonary mast cells is metabolized to $9\alpha,11\beta$-PGF_2 in human lung, but if this did occur then a component of the bronchoconstrictor action of PGD_2 may be mediated by its initial metabolite. When given by inhalation both prostanoids exert a component of their action by reflex bronchoconstriction, since the muscarinic cholinergic antagonist ipratropium bromide attenuates the response[107]. Other biological effects of PGD_2 are shown in Table 5.2. At the time of writing, relatively less is known of the bronchopulmonary effects of PAF-acether in man. When given by inhalation to normal volunteers it elicits bronchoconstriction and produces a mild degree of bronchial hyper-responsiveness[108]. Whether the bronchoconstriction is dependent on platelet activation, as in the guinea pig[109], is not known.

Table 5.2 Pharmacological effects of prostaglandin D_2

Action	References
Bronchoconstrictor	105–107
Cutaneous vasodilatation and augmented vasopermeability	119, 120, 174
Inhibits platelet aggregation	175, 176
Neutrophil chemokinesis	113
Tussive	105, 177
Enhances basophil histamine secretion	178
Potentiates airway cholinergic responsiveness	179
Pulmonary and coronary vasoconstrictor	117, 121, 180
Negatively inotropic in heart	180
Inhibition of lysozyme synthesis	181
Inhibition of NK cell activity	182
Decrease in eosinophil count	183
Antinociceptive (CNS)	184
Inhibits tumour cell growth	185–188

Vascular smooth muscle is a significant end organ target for newly-generated lipid mediators. Prostaglandins E_2 and I_2 and the sulphidopeptide leukotrienes all augment vascular permeability in venules when injected singly into guinea pig skin[110, 111], or when applied topically to the buccal mucosa of the hamster[112]. After intradermal injection in man, nanomolar concentrations of LTC_4, LTD_4 and LTE_4 evoke a local weal, together with a more persistent erythema[113, 114]. When mixtures of PGE_1 or PGE_2 and LTC_4 or LTD_4 are co-injected in guinea pig skin it is possible to observe a synergistic inflammatory response[111]. This may arise as a result of the vaso-dilator action of PGE_2 opposing the arteriolar constrictor action of LTC_4 and LTD_4. The latter has been observed photomicrographically following intravascular administration of fluorescein or by local blanching after intra-dermal injection in man[110, 112]. Sulphidopeptide leukotrienes are potent con-tractile agonists on coronary and pulmonary vascular smooth muscle, but *in vivo* their overall effects are dependent on their route of administration and the species studied[115]. TXA_2 is a powerful contractile agent in vascular smooth muscle[116] and, together with PGD_2 which has similar but weaker effects[117], it could assume some considerable importance in cardiac anaphylaxis[118]. In the cutaneous vasculature PGD_2, PGE_2 and PGI_2 have vasodilator effects which may be synergistic or additive with other pro-inflammatory mediators[119, 120]. It is interesting to contrast the dilator action of PGD_2 in the cutaneous vasculature with its spasmogenic action on coronary and pulmonary vascular smooth muscle[117, 119, 121].

Although LTB_4 is released only in small amounts from activated human mast cells, it is likely to be an important secondary mediator since it can amplify inflammatory responses by virtue of its chemotactic effect on neutrophils[122, 123]. It also promotes neutrophil margination by triggering endothelial cell adherence for neutrophils[124].

Although the release of PAF-acether was originally described in rabbit basophils activated by IgE cross-linkage there is considerable controversy as to whether human basophils generate this mediator[125, 126]. As we have already seen in mast cells, it may be that basophils do actually make PAF-acether but release very little of this. Thus, although this fascinating mediator may be synthesized by a wide variety of cells which participate in inflamma-tory reactions (e.g. neutrophils, eosinophils, monocytes and alveolar macro-phages) its precise significance is just as unclear as some of the more recently discovered eicosanoids. An examination of its pharmacological actions raises some tantalizing possibilities, and some of these are described below.

PAF-acether was originally named for its ability to initiate the calcium and energy-dependent aggregation of platelets following anaphylactic activation of rabbit basophils. However, it is now clear that many other cells have the biochemical machinery to synthesize PAF-acether and that it exerts pharma-cological actions well beyond the domain of the platelet. For instance, PAF-acether is chemotactic for eosinophils[127], and induces neutrophil chemotaxis, shape change, superoxide generation and aggregation[128–131]. Some of these effects are dependent on the synthesis and release of LTB_4[132]. In support of this there are qualitative similarities between the neutrophil infiltration, plasma extravasation and hyperalgesic effects of PAF-acether

159

and LTB$_4$ when injected into the skin[133,134]. Fluid extravasation is also a characteristic effect of PAF-acether in the pulmonary vascular bed, although this may be due to a combination of enhanced vascular permeability and pulmonary hypertension[135-138].

EVIDENCE FOR NEWLY-GENERATED MEDIATOR RELEASE *IN VIVO*

In order to incriminate a mediator in a pathophysiological process one of the criteria which must be fulfilled is to demonstrate its release *in vivo* during the reaction concerned. Lipid derived inflammatory mediators are some of the most difficult compounds to measure due to problems with chemical decomposition, metabolism and the low concentrations involved. Great care must be exercised when reviewing older reports of plasma concentrations of many of these mediators: in general there has been a significant downward trend in the reported normal plasma concentrations of eicosanoids[139]. It is now well established that the plasma concentrations of most parent prostanoids lie below 5 pg/ml. This obviously creates tremendous analytical problems. It is usually necessary to concentrate samples prior to analysis, and this can itself be a source of considerable error. Certain prostaglandins also suffer from problems of instability; this being particularly true for prostanoids with a hydroxycyclopentanone structure (e.g. D and E series prostaglandins). In view of the potential interest in PGD$_2$ as a possible marker of mast cell activation *in vivo* it is worthwhile to consider in a little more detail why it may be poorly suited to this role.

Mass spectrometric investigations with a stable isotope internal standard have demonstrated that the normal plasma concentrations of PGD$_2$ are in the range 1–5 pg/ml[140] and that the halflife of this prostanoid in the circulation is approximately 2 min[140]. In addition to rapid metabolic breakdown, PGD$_2$ also undergoes a series of facile isomerization and dehydration reactions which may compromise its use as a biochemical marker[141-144]. In the simplest of these reactions, the Δ^{13} double bond migrates to C-12 with concomitant abstraction of the C-12 proton to yield a mixture of *cis* and *trans* isomers of the α,β-unsaturated ketone Δ^{12}-PGD$_2$ (Figure 5.4). Although much less biologically active than PGD$_2$ itself these isomers may be a source of possible error in the quantitative analysis of PGD$_2$. However, a more important error may be caused by dehydration of the PGD$_2$ ring system to produce a variety of products, including 9-deoxy-11-keto-15(S)-hydroxy-$\Delta^{5,9,12}$-prostenoic acid, 15-deoxy-11-keto-9α-hydroxy-$\Delta^{5,12,14}$-prostenoic acid and 9,15-dideoxy-11-keto-$\Delta^{5,9,13,14}$-prostenoic acid as shown in Figure 5.4[142]. Although trapping experiments have failed to isolate 9-deoxy-11-keto-15(S)-hydroxy-$\Delta^{5,9,13}$-prostenoic acid (PGJ$_2$), this may be an intermediate in the decomposition of PGD$_2$. These simple dehydration processes occur effectively in the presence of serum albumin thus necessitating immediate work-up of samples of PGD$_2$ from plasma[142,144].

A more fruitful approach to the measurement of prostaglandins in complex biological matrices has been to use metabolites of the parent

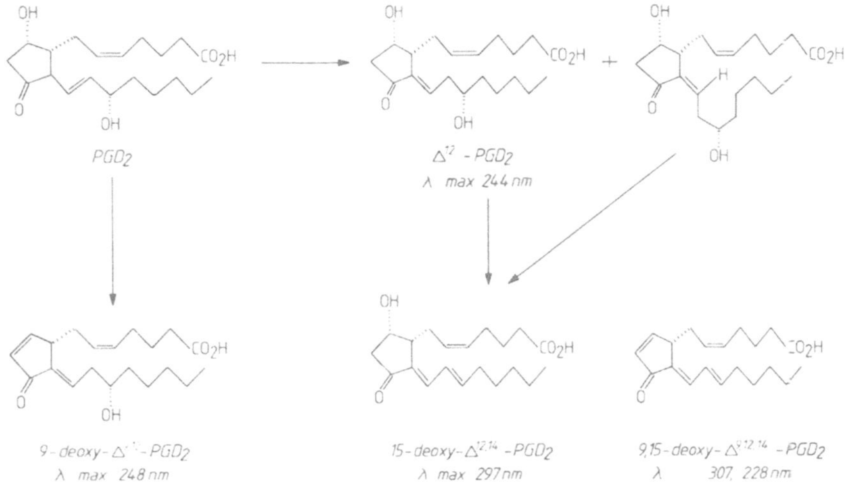

Figure 5.4 Possible events in the isomerization and decomposition of PGD₂

compound[139]. These are usually present in higher concentration than the parent compound and avoid the problem of artefactual generation upon sampling. However, this strategy can itself be of limited value due to the enzymatic redox interconversions of some cyclopentane ring systems. Unlike PGE and PGF series prostaglandins, PGD₂ is a poor substrate for the familiar combination of prostanoid metabolizing enzymes 15-hydroxy-prostaglandin dehydrogenase (15-PGDH, E.C. 1.1.1.141) and 15-keto-prostaglandin-Δ^{13}-reductase (Δ^{13}R)[145] (and Robinson and Hoult, unpublished experiments). Early reports demonstrated that in primates a significant proportion of PGD₂ may be metabolized by conversion to PGF ring compounds[146]. Although not tested directly it was assumed that these metabolites had the co-planar $9\alpha,11\alpha$-hydroxyl geometry of PGF$_{2\alpha}$ and its metabolites, and some support was presented for this hypothesis in man[147]. Had this been the case it is unlikely that such compounds could be used as indices of PGD₂ production in view of the impossibility of determining how much of each metabolite was derived from PGD₂. Fortunately, stereochemical analysis indicated that the PGD₂ metabolites actually had $9\alpha,11\beta$-hydroxyl geometry, and so the possibility that such metabolites of PGD₂ might be used to reflect the synthesis and release of PGD₂ is a real one.

Studies of PGD₂ metabolism in man following administration of a tritiated compound by either intravenous infusion or inhalation[148–150] and subsequent analysis of the metabolites present in the plasma or urine have indicated that the predominant reaction in the degradation of PGD₂ is the NADPH-dependent stereoselective reduction by a cytoplasmic 11-keto-reductase enzyme to yield $9\alpha,11\beta$-PGF$_2$[151–153]. This compound possesses an interesting spectrum of biological activities, including a contractile action on human airway smooth muscle *in vitro* and *in vivo*[106, 154]. This compound is then subjected to further metabolism by 15-PGDH/Δ^{13}R and subsequent

161

β- and ω-oxidation[148, 153]. It is likely that such metabolites of PGD_2 may prove to be suitable analytes. Relatively little metabolism of exogenous PGD_2 occurs in normal man by direct attack of 15-PGDH/Δ^{13}R, or by the formation of $PGF_{2\alpha}$ and its metabolites[148, 150]. However, it is likely that prostaglandins synthesized and released *in vivo* may be exposed to different profiles of metabolizing enzymes depending upon the tissues in which they are formed. Thus studies with exogenous tracers can only give a general overview of the likely fate of such compounds. Opportunities to perform detailed metabolic studies on endogenously formed compounds are rare, although one such study has been performed in a female patient suffering from systemic mastocytosis[155]. Interestingly, this patient had a larger proportion of urinary metabolites with PGD-rings than the healthy volunteer, studied by the same group, who received exogenous PGD_2.

Evidence for PGD₂ release in man

There are two principal reasons which make the measurement of PGD_2 or one of its metabolites an important goal. Firstly, it would provide an important opportunity to investigate the release of a newly-generated mast cell-derived mediator *in vivo*. Histamine has traditionally been used as a marker for mast cell activation, but there is no *a priori* reason to assume that the release of PGD_2, or any other newly-generated mediator, obeys the same characteristics. In fact recent evidence suggests that the release of PGD_2 and histamine may have different dose response characteristics[97], susceptibility to different secretagogues (Benyon, Robinson, Holgate and Church, unpublished observations) and a different susceptibility to antiallergic drugs[156]. The second reason for the measurement of PGD_2 is related to the lack of specificity of histamine as a marker of mast cell activation. As is well documented, basophils are a rich source of this amine and they may be activated by IgE-dependent mechanisms[157]. In contrast, PGD_2 is not made by human basophils[158], and thus offers the potential of being a more selective probe of mast cell activation.

A relatively small number of studies have been performed in which PGD_2 itself has been measured by radioimmunoassay or by GC/MS. These investigations have demonstrated parallel increases in the release of histamine and PGD_2 during local cutaneous anaphylaxis and following thermal challenge in patients with cold or heat urticaria[159-161]. Cold urticaria is characterized by an immediate weal and flare response associated with cutaneous mast cell degranulation and release of large amounts of histamine when the skin is cooled. Although the changes in PGD_2 concentration in blood draining the challenge site are convincing, it is interesting to note that there is little change in the concentration of PGD_2 in suction blister fluid harvested after cold challenge. The release of PGD_2 into human airways following acute antigen challenge has also been observed[162, 163]. In this study, bronchoalveolar lavage was performed in five patients with chronic stable asthma, before and up to 9 min after challenge with *Dermatophagoides pteronyssinus*. The concentration of PGD_2 in the lavage fluid in all five patients rose an average of 150-fold from < 8 to 322 ± 114 ng/ml following the antigen provocation procedure[162, 163].

A number of studies have also been made in the disease systemic mastocytosis, a condition in which there is a superabundance of mast cells and an overproduction of chemical mediators. In many of these investigations the urinary PGD_2 metabolite 9α-hydroxy-11,15-diketo-2,3,18,19-tetranorprost-5-ene-1,20-dioic acid has been quantified[164, 165]. The urinary excretion of this compound in normal subjects is approximately 250 ng/24 h, but in patients with systemic mastocytosis this excretion rate may be up to 150-fold higher even during remission. Further increases can occur during episodic exacerbations of the disease, and it is noteworthy that a reduction in PGD_2 production by aspirin therapy results in an alleviation of symptoms[165]. Supportive investigations have also been performed in which the urinary PGD_2 metabolite 9α-hydroxy-11,15-diketo-2,3,4,5-tetranor-prostane-1,20-dioic acid was measured[164, 165]. Investigations have also been made with $9\alpha,11\beta$-PGF_2 as the analyte, and here again there were marked elevations in the plasma and urinary concentrations of this compound which appeared to correlate with the disease activity[151]. To date, relatively little work has been published concerning the possible use of $9\alpha,11\beta$-PGF_2 and its metabolites as indices of PGD_2 production *in vivo*. It is known that several isomeric forms of $9\alpha,11\beta$-PGF_2 may exist. These probably arise by metabolism of PGD_2 isomers to yield *inter alia* 12-*epi*-$9\alpha,11\beta$-PGF_2, and analyses of PGD_2 metabolites should therefore take into account these isomeric structures.

Evidence for leukotriene release in man

The sulphidopeptide leukotrienes pose extreme analytical problems. Their biological potency suggests that they are unlikely to be present in biological fluids at high concentration. Unfortunately, they are not readily amenable to GC/MS analysis due to their low volatility and high polarity. In order to render them suitable for GC volatilization it is necessary to undertake chemical modification strategies, such as Birch reduction and thioether cleavage, to yield 5-hydroxyeicosanoic acid. Although some workers have attempted to measure leukotrienes in biological fluids using bioassay techniques it is now widely agreed that this assay technique provides an overestimate of the leukotriene content of complex matrices. For this reason a number of groups have attempted to measure the plasma concentrations of the sulphidopeptide leukotrienes using radioimmunoassay based techniques. The results from such studies are quite divergent; one study reporting resting concentrations of LTC_4 some 300-fold greater than those for the primary prostaglandins[166], whilst other estimates concluded that the plasma concentrations of LTC_4 and total sulphidopeptide leukotrienes must be below 30 pg/ml and 83 pg/ml, respectively[167, 168]. Given our experience with the analysis of prostaglandins it would seem reasonable that the maxim 'lowest is best' is equally applicable to the leukotrienes. It is interesting to note that in the same study in which significant elevations were detected in the concentration of PGD_2 in bronchoalveolar lavage fluid[162, 163] there was no detectable change in LTC_4 concentration after antigen challenge. The release of LTC_4, together with that of histamine, has been detected, however, in skin window fluid following epicutaneous challenge with specific antigen[169], and in tear fluid following immunological, but not chemical stimulation[170]. No immunological release of LTB_4 was detected in either of these studies. Further improvements in analytical strategies will be necessary in order to gain more meaningful information about the likely roles of sulphidopeptide leukotrienes in inflammatory disease.

Evidence for PAF-acether release in man

A number of analytical techniques have been applied to the measurement of PAF-acether in complex matrices: bioassay on platelets, high performance liquid chromatography and gas chromatography[171, 172]. All these methods have their attendant disadvantages – lack of specificity, lack of sensitivity or both. There is also a further problem in that PAF-acether is rapidly degraded to a substance which is also its precursor. We are currently at a very early stage in attempts to devise sensitive, specific and truly quantitative assay methods for PAF-acether, and even then the possibility that this mediator remains extensively cell-associated provides a difficult problem of interpretation. Some workers have provided indirect arguments for the systemic release of PAF-acether during experimental anaphylactic reactions in man[173]. In these experiments platelet factor 4 was measured with the unsupported rationale that this was dependent on PAF-acether release. Although an interesting approach, this cannot be viewed as formal evidence for PAF-acether release in human anaphylactic reactions.

CONCLUDING REMARKS

As has been seen there are a large number of newly-generated mediators which may participate in mast cell-dependent reactions. Whilst some of these compounds, such as PGD_2, have been conclusively identified as major products of the mast cell, the cellular provenance of many of the other compounds remains to be formally established. Great emphasis has been placed on the analytical methods for individual compounds since this is a key step in demonstrating the formation of such substances in human disease, and all too frequently also the Achilles heel of mediator pharmacology. In this context it will be of considerable interest to investigate whether the eicosanoid and PAF-acether antagonists and inhibitors currently being developed by the pharmaceutical industry are active in the mast cell-dependent reactions which present in the clinic.

References

1. Lands, W. E. M. and Samuelsson, B. (1968). Phospholipid precursor of prostaglandins. *Biochim. Biophys. Acta*, **164**, 426–9
2. Van den Bosch, H. (1980). Intracellular phospholipases A. *Biochim. Biophys. Acta*, **604**, 191–246

3. Prescott, S. M. and Majerus, P. W. (1983). Characterization of 1,2-diacylglycerol hydrolysis in human platelets. Demonstration of an arachidonyl monoacylglycerol intermediate. *J. Biol. Chem.*, **258**, 764–9

4. Bell, R. L., Kennerly, D. A., Stanford, N. and Majerus, P. W. (1979). Diglyceride lipase: a pathway for arachidonate release from human platelets. *Proc. Natl. Acad. Sci. USA*, **76**, 3238–41

5. Dvorak, A. M., Dvorak, H. F., Peters, S. P., Schulman, E. S., McGlashan, D. W., Pyne, K., Harvey, V. S., Galli, S. J. and Lichtenstein, L. M. (1983). Lipid bodies: cytoplasmic organelles important to arachidonate metabolism in macrophages and basophils. *J. Immunol.*, **131**, 2965–76

6. Van der Ouderaa, F. J., Buytenhek, M., Slikkerveer, F. J. and van Dorp, D. A. (1979). On the haemoprotein nature of prostaglandin endoperoxide synthetase. *Biochim. Biophys. Acta*, **572**, 29–42

7. Van Dorp, D. A. (1979). Isolation and characterization of enzymes involved in prostaglandin biosynthesis. In Roberts, S. M. and Scheinmann, F. (eds.) *Chemistry, Biochemistry and Pharmacological Activity of Prostanoids*, pp. 233–42. (Oxford: Pergamon Press)

8. Wlodawer, P. and Samuelsson, B. (1973). On the organization and mechanism of action of prostaglandin synthetase. *J. Biol. Chem.*, **248**, 5673–8

9. Hamberg, M., Svensson, J. and Samuelsson, B. (1976). Novel transformations of prostaglandin endoperoxides: formation of thromboxanes. In Samuelsson, B. and Paoletti, R. (eds.) *Advances in Prostaglandin and Thromboxane Research*, Vol. 1, pp. 19–27. (New York: Raven Press)

10. Hamberg, M. and Samuelsson, B. (1973). Detection and isolation of an endoperoxide intermediate in prostaglandin biosynthesis. *Proc. Natl. Acad. Sci. USA*, **70**, 899–903

11. Hamberg, M., Svensson, J. and Samuelsson, B. (1974). Prostaglandin endoperoxides: a new concept concerning the mode of action and release of prostaglandins. *Proc. Natl. Acad. Sci. USA*, **71**, 3824–8

12. Hamberg, M., Svensson, J. and Samuelsson, B. (1975). Thromboxanes a new group of biologically active compounds derived from prostaglandin endoperoxides. *Proc. Natl. Acad. Sci. USA*, **72**, 2994–8

13. Johnson, R. A., Morton, D. R., Kinner, J. H., Gorman, R. R., McGuire, J. C., Sun, F. F., Whittaker, N., Bunting, S., Salmon, J. A., Moncada, S. and Vane, J. R. (1976). The chemical structure of prostaglandin X (prostacyclin). *Prostaglandins*, **12**, 915–28

14. Moncada, S., Gryglewski, R. J., Bunting, S. and Vane, J. R. (1976). An enzyme isolated from arteries transforms prostaglandin endoperoxides to an unstable substance that inhibits platelet aggregation. *Nature*, **262**, 663–5

15. Hamberg, M., Svensson, J., Wakabayashi, T. and Samuelsson, B. (1974). Isolation and structure of two prostaglandin endoperoxides that cause platelet aggregation. *Proc. Natl. Acad. Sci. USA*, **71**, 345–9

16. Ogino, N., Miyamoto, T., Yamamoto, S. and Hayaishi, O. (1977). Prostaglandin endoperoxide E isomerase from bovine vesicular gland microsomes, a glutathione requiring enzyme. *J. Biol. Chem.*, **252**, 890–5

17. Urade, Y., Fujimoto, N., Ujihara, M. and Hayaishi, O. (1987). Biochemical and immunological characterization of rat spleen prostaglandin D_2 synthetase. *J. Biol. Chem.*, **262**, 3820–5

18. Christ Hazelhof, E. and Nugteren, D. H. (1979). Purification and characterization of prostaglandin endoperoxide D-isomerase, a cytoplasmic glutathione-requiring enzyme. *Biochim. Biophys. Acta*, **572**, 43–51

19. Nugteren, D. H. and Christ-Hazelhof, E. (1980). Chemical and enzymic conversion of prostaglandin endoperoxide PGH_2. In Samuelsson, B., Ramwell, P. W. and Paoletti, R. (eds.) *Advances In Prostaglandin and Thromboxane Research*, Vol. 6, pp. 129–37. (New York: Raven Press)

20. Hamberg, M. and Fredholm, B. B. (1976). Isomerization of PGH_2 into PGD_2 in the presence of serum albumin. *Biochim. Biophys. Acta*, **431**, 189–93

21. Christ Hazelhof, E., Nugteren, D. H. and van Dorp, D. A. (1976). Conversion of prostaglandin endoperoxides by glutathione-S-transferases and serum albumin. *Biochim. Biophys. Acta*, **450**, 450–61

165

22. Wlodawer, P., Kindahl, H., Hamberg, M. (1976). Biosynthesis of prostaglandin $F_{2\alpha}$ from arachidonic acid and prostaglandin endoperoxides in the uterus. *Biochim. Biophys. Acta*, **431**, 603–14

23. Burgess, J. R., Yang, H., Chang, M., Rao, M. K., Tu, C. P. D. and Reddy, C. C. (1987). Enzymic transformation of PGH_2 to $PGF_{2\alpha}$ catalyzed by glutathione-S-transferases. *Biochem. Biophys. Res. Commun.*, **142**, 441–7

24. Watanabe, K., Iguchi, Y., Iguchi, S., Arai, Y., Hayaishi, O. and Roberts, L. J. (1986). Stereospecific conversion of prostaglandin D_2 to (5Z,13E)-(15S)-9α,11β,15-trihydroxy-prosta-5,13-dien-1-oic acid (9α,11β-prostaglandin F_2) and of prostaglandin H_2 to prostaglandin $F_{2\alpha}$ by bovine lung prostaglandin F synthase. *Proc. Natl. Acad. Sci. USA*, **83**, 1583–7

25. Ullrich, V. and Haurand, M. (1980). Thromboxane as a cytochrome P_{450} enzyme. In Samuelsson, B., Ramwell, P. W. and Paoletti, R. (eds.) *Advances In Prostaglandin and Thromboxane Research*, Vol. 6, pp. 105–10. (New York: Raven Press)

26. Hall, E. R. and Tai, H. H. (1981). Purification of thromboxane synthetase and evidence for two distinct mechanisms for the formation of 12-L-hydroxy-5,8,10-heptadecatrienoic acid by porcine lung microsomes. *Biochim. Biophys. Acta*, **665**, 498–503

27. Shen, R. F. and Tai, H. H. (1986). Immunoaffinity purification and characterization of thromboxane synthase from porcine lung. *J. Biol. Chem.*, **261**, 11592–9

28. Graf, H., Ruf, H. H. and Ullrich, V. (1983). Prostacyclin synthetase, a cytochrome P_{450} enzyme. *Agnew. Chem. Int. Ed.*, **22**, 487–8

29. Samuelsson, B. (1981). Oxidative products of arachidonate: Leukotrienes, a new group of compounds, including slow-reacting substance of anaphylaxis (SRS-A). In Becker, E. L., Stolper Simon, A. and Austen, K. F. (eds.) *Biochemistry of the Acute Allergic Reactions*, pp. 1–11. (New York: Alan R. Liss)

30. Morris, H. R., Taylor, G. W. and Jones, C. M. (1981). Structure elucidation, biosynthesis and biodegradation of SRS-A from lung. In Piper, P. J. (ed.) *SRS-A and Leukotrienes*, pp. 19–44. (Chichester: John Wiley and Sons)

31. Lewis, R. A. and Austen, K. F. (1984). The biologically active leukotrienes. *J. Clin. Invest.*, **73**, 889–97

32. Parker, C. W. (1982). The chemical nature of slow reacting substances. In Weissmann, G. (ed.) *Advances in Inflammation Research*, Vol. 4, pp. 1–24. (New York: Raven Press)

33. Brash, A. R., Murray, J. J., Oates, J. A. (1985). The 5-lipoxygenase and 15-lipoxygenase of neutrophils and eosinophils. In Lefer, A. M. and Gee, M. H. (eds.) *Leukotrienes in Cardiovascular and Pulmonary Function*, pp. 143–52. (New York: Alan R. Liss)

34. Brash, A. R. and Ingram, C. D. (1986). Lipoxygenase metabolism of endogenous and exogenous arachidonate in leukocytes: GC/MS analyses of incubations in [^{18}O]-water buffers. *Prostaglandins Leukotrienes Med.*, **23**, 149–54

35. Taylor, G. W. and Morris, H. R. (1983). Lipoxygenase pathways. *Br. Med. Bull.*, **39**, 219–22

36. Nugteren, D. H. (1975). Arachidonate lipoxygenase in blood platelets. *Biochim. Biophys. Acta*, **380**, 299–307

37. Serhan, C. N., Hamberg, M. and Samuelsson, B. (1984). Lipoxins: Novel series of biologically active compound formed from arachidonic acid in human leukocytes. *Proc. Natl. Acad. Sci. USA*, **81**, 5335–9

38. Serhan, C. N., Hamberg, M. and Samuelsson, B. (1984). Trihydroxy-tetraenes: a novel series of compounds formed from arachidonic acid in human leukocytes. *Biochem. Biophys. Res. Commun.*, **118**, 943–9

39. Ramstedt, U., Serhan, C. N., Nicolaou, K. C., Webber, S. E., Wigzell, H. and Samuelsson, B. (1987). Lipoxin A-induced inhibition of human natural killer cell cytotoxicity: Studies on stereospecificity of inhibition and mode of action. *J. Immunol.*, **138**, 266–70

40. Shimizu, T., Rådmark, O. and Samuelsson, B. (1984). Enzyme with dual lipoxygenase activities catalyzes leukotriene A_4 synthesis from arachidonic acid. *Proc. Natl. Acad. Sci. USA*, **81**, 689–93

41. Shimizu, T., Izumi, T., Seyama, Y., Tadkoro, K., Radmark, O. and Samuelsson, B. (1986). Characterization of leukotriene A_4 synthase from murine mast cells: evidence for its identity to arachidonate 5-lipoxygenase. *Proc. Natl. Acad. Sci. USA*, **83**, 4175–9

42. Rouzer, C. A., Matsumoto, M. and Samuelsson, B. (1986). Single protein from human leucocytes possess 5-lipoxygenase and leukotriene A₄ synthase activities. *Proc. Nat!. Acad. Sci. USA*, **83**, 857–61

43. Goetze, A. M., Fayer, L., Bouska, J., Bornemeier, D. and Carter, G. W. (1985). Purification of a mammalian 5-lipoxygenase from rat basophilic leukemia cells. *Prostaglandins*, **29**, 689–701

44. Rådmark, O., Shimizu, T., Jornvall, M. and Samuelsson, B. (1984). Leukotriene A₄ hydrolase in human leukocytes. Purification and properties. *J. Biol. Chem.*, **259**, 12339–45

45. Fitzpatrick, F. A., Morton, D. R. and Wynalda, M. A. (1982). Albumin stabilizes leukotriene A₄. *J. Biol. Chem.*, **257**, 4680–3

46. Fitzpatrick, F. A., Haeggstrom, J., Granstrom, E. and Samuelsson, B. (1983). Metabolism of leukotriene A₄ by an enzyme in blood plasma: a possible leukotactic mechanism. *Proc. Natl. Acad. Sci. USA*, **80**, 5425–9

47. Hammarström, S. (1983). Leukotrienes. *Ann. Rev. Biochem.*, **52**, 355–77

48. Bach, M. K. and Brashler, J. R. (1985). A comparison of the leukotriene synthesizing ability of subfractions of rat liver glutathione-S-transferases. *Prostaglandins Leukotrienes Med.*, **17**, 125–36

49. Bach, M. K., Brashler, J. R. and Murphy, R. C. (1984). Solubilization and characterization of the leukotriene C₄ synthetase of rat basophil leukemic cells: a novel, particulate glutathione-S-transferase. *Arch. Biochem. Biophys.*, **230**, 455–65

50. Jakschik, B. A., Harper, T. and Murphy, R. C. (1982). Leukotriene C₄ and D₄ formation by particulate enzymes. *J. Biol. Chem.*, **257**, 5342–9

51. Hammarström, S., Samuelsson, B., Clark, D. A., Goto, G., Marfat, A., Miowskowski, C. and Corey, E. J. (1980). Stereochemistry of leukotriene C-1. *Biochem. Biophys. Res. Commun.*, **92**, 946–53

52. Orning, L., Hammarström, S. and Samuelsson, B. (1980). Leukotriene D: A slow reacting substance from rat basophilic leukemia cells. *Proc. Natl. Acad. Sci. USA*, **77**, 2014–17

53. Lee, C. W., Lewis, R. A., Corey, E. J. and Austen, K. F. (1983). Conversion of leukotriene D₄ to E₄ by a dipeptidase released from the specific granule of human polymorphcnuclear leukocytes. *Immunology*, **48**, 27–35

54. Pinckard, R. N., McManus, L. M. and Hanahan, D. J. (1982). Chemistry and biology of acetyl glyceryl ether phosphorylcholine (platelet-activating factor). In Weissman, G. (ed.) *Advances in Inflammation*, Vol. 4, pp. 147–80. (New York: Raven Press)

55. Lynch, J. M., Worthen, G. S. and Henson, P. M. (1984). Platelet-activating factor. In Buckle, D. R., Smith, H. (eds.) *Development of Anti-asthmatic Drugs*, pp. 73–88. (London: Butterworth)

56. Mencia-Huerta, J. M., Ninio, E., Roubin, R. and Benveniste, J. (1981). Is platelet-activating factor (PAF-acether) synthesis by murine peritoneal cells (PC) a two step process. *Agents Actions*, **11**, 556–8

57. Benveniste, J., Chignard, M., LeCouedic, J. P. and Vargaftig, B. B. (1982). Biosynthesis of platelet-activating factor. II. Involvement of phospholipase A₂ in the formation of PAF-acether and lyso-PAF-acether from rabbit platelets. *Thromb. Res.*, **25**, 375–85

58. Wykle, R. L., Malone, B. and Snyder, F. (1980). Enzymatic synthesis of 1-alkyl-2-acetyl-sn-glycero-3-phosphocholine, a hypotensive and platelet aggregating lipid. *J. Biol. Chem.*, **255**, 10256–60

59. Lee, T. C., Malone, B., Wasserman, S. I., Fitzgerald, V. and Snyder, F. (1982). Activities of enzymes that metabolize platelet-activating factor (1-alkyl-2-acetyl-sn-glycero-3-phosphocholine) in neutrophils and eosinophils from humans and the effect of a calcium ionophore. *Biochem. Biophys. Res. Commun.*, **105**, 1303–8

60. Ninio, E., Mencia-Huerta, J. M., Heymans, F. and Benveniste, J. (1982). Biosynthesis of platelet activating factor. I. Evidence for an acetyltransferase activity in murine macrophages. *Biochim. Biophys. Acta*, **710**, 23–31

61. Mencia-Huerta, J. M., Roubin, R., Morgat, J. L. and Benveniste, J. (1982). Biosynthesis of platelet activating factor (PAF acether). III. Formation of PAF-acether from synthetic substrates by stimulated murine macrophages. *J. Immunol.*, **129**, 804–8

62. Roubin, R., Mencia-Huerta, J. M., Landes, A. and Benveniste, J. (1982). Biosynthesis of platelet activating factor (PAF-acether). IV. Impairment of acetyltransferase activity in thioglycollate-elicited mouse macrophages. *J. Immunol*, **129**, 809–13

63. Lee, T. C., Blank, M. L., Fitzgerald, V. and Snyder, F. (1981). Substrate specificity in the biocleavage of the O-alkyl bond: 1-alkyl-2-acetyl-sn-glycero-3-phosphocholine (a hypotensive and platelet activating lipid) and its metabolites. *Arch. Biochem. Biophys.*, **208**, 353–7

64. Roberts, L. J., Lewis, R. A., Oates, J. A. and Austen, K. F. (1979). Prostaglandin, thromboxane and 12-hydroxy-5,8,10,14-eicosatetraenoic acid production by ionophore-stimulated rat serosal mast cells. *Biochim. Biophys. Acta*, **575**, 185–92

65. Metcalfe, D. D. (1983). Effector cell heterogeneity in immediate hypersensitivity reactions. *Clin. Rev. Allergy*, **1**, 311–25

66. Enerback, L. (1986). Mast cell heterogeneity: The evolution of the concept of a specific mucosal mast cell. In Befus, A. D., Bienenstock, J. and Denburg, J. A. (eds.) *Mast Cell Differentiation and Heterogeneity*, pp. 1–26. (New York: Raven Press)

67. Lee, T. D. G., Swieter, M., Bienenstock, J. and Befus, A. D. (1985). Heterogeneity in mast cell populations. *Clin. Immunol. Rev.*, **4**, 143–99

68. Irani, A. A., Schechter, N. M., Craig, S., DeBlois, G. and Schwartz, L. B. (1986). Two types of human mast cells that have distinct neutral protease compositions. *Proc. Natl. Acad. Sci. USA*, **83**, 4464–8

69. Robinson, C., Holgate, S. T. (1986). The synthesis, release and effects of prostaglandins in the lung. In Kay, A. B. (ed.) *Asthma: Clinical Pharmacology and Therapeutic Progress*, pp. 213–25. (Oxford: Blackwell Scientific Publications)

70. Agius, R. M., Robinson, C., Church, M. K. and Holgate, S. T. (1988). Prostaglandin (PG) D_2 synthesis by human bronchoalveolar mast cells. (Abstr.). *Br. J. Pharmacol.* (In press)

71. Benyon, R. C., Robinson, C., Holgate, S. T. and Church, M. K. (1987). Prostaglandin D_2 release from human skin mast cells in response to ionophore A23187. *Br. J. Pharmacol.*, **92**, 635–8

72. Robinson, C., Benyon, C., Agius, R. M., Jones, D. B., Wright, D. H. and Holgate, S. T. (1988). The immunological- and calcium-dependent release of histamine and eicosanoids from human dispersed mastocytosis spleen cells. *J. Invest. Dermatol.* (In press)

73. Lewis, R. A., Soter, N. A., Diamond, P. T., Austen, K. F., Oates, J. A. and Roberts, L. J. (1982). Prostaglandin D_2 generation after activation of rat and human mast cells with anti-IgE. *J. Immunol.*, **129**, 1627–31

74. Holgate, S. T., Burns, G. B., Robinson, C. and Church, M. K. (1984). Anaphylactic and calcium dependent generation of prostaglandin D_2 (PGD$_2$), thromboxane B$_2$ and other cyclooxygenase products of arachidonic acid by dispersed human lung cells and relationship to histamine release. *J. Immunol.*, **133**, 2138–44

75. Schleimer, R. P., Schulman, E. S., MacGlashan, D. W., Peters, S. P., Hayes, E. C., Adams, G. K., Lichtenstein, L. M. and Adkinson, N. F. (1983). Effects of dexamethasone on mediator release from human lung fragments and purified human lung mast cells. *J. Clin. Invest.*, **71**, 1830–5

76. Schleimer, R. P., Davidson, D. A., Lichtenstein, L. M. and Adkinson, N. F. (1986). Selective inhibition of arachidonic acid metabolite release from human lung tissue by anti-inflammatory steroids. *J. Immunol.*, **136**, 3006–11

77. Holgate, S. T. and Robinson, C. (1984). 6,9-Deepoxy-6,9-(phenylimino)-$\Delta^{6,8}$-prostaglandin I_1 (U-60,257) stimulates prostaglandin D_2 and inhibits thromboxane B$_2$ release from ionophore challenged human dispersed lung cells. *Br. J. Pharmacol.*, **83**, 603–5

78. Robinson, C. and Holgate, S. T. (1986). Ionophore-dependent generation of eicosanoids in human dispersed lung cells: modulation by 6,9-Deepoxy-6,9-(phenylimino)-$\Delta^{6,8}$-prostaglandin I_1 (U-60, 257). *Biochem. Pharmacol.*, **35**, 1903–8

79. Peters, S. P., MacGlashan, D. W., Schulman, E. S., Schleimer, R. P., Hayes, E. C., Rokach, J., Adkinson, N. F. and Lichtenstein, L. M. (1984). Arachidonic acid metabolism in purified human lung mast cells. *J. Immunol.*, **132**, 1972–9

80. Dahlén, S. E., Hansson, G., Hedqvist, P., Bjorck, T., Granstrom, E. and Dahlen, B. (1983). Allergen challenge of lung tissue from asthmatics elicits bronchial contraction that correlates with the release of leukotrienes C$_4$, D$_4$, and E$_4$. *Proc. Natl. Acad. Sci. USA*, **80**, 1712–6

81. Sautebin, L., Vigano, T., Grassi, E., Crivellari, M. T., Galli, G., Berti, F., Mezzetti, M. and Folco, G. (1985). Release of leukotrienes, induced by the Ca^{++} ionophore A23187, from human lung parenchyma *in vitro*. *J. Pharmacol. Exp. Ther.*, **234**, 217–21

82. Harvey, J., Holgate, S. T., Peters, B. J., Robinson, C. and Walker, J. R. (1985). Oxidative transformations of arachidonic acid in human dispersed lung cells: disparity between utilization of endogenous and exogenous substrate. *Br. J. Pharmacol.*, **86**, 417–26

83. Paterson, N. A. M., Wasserman, S. I., Said, J. W. and Austen, K. F. (1976). Release of chemical mediators from partially purified human lung mast cells. *J. Immuncl.*, **117**, 1356–62

84. Lewis, R. A., Drazen, J. M., Corey, E. J. and Austen, K. F. (1981). Structural and functional characteristics of the leukotriene components of slow reacting substance of anaphylaxis. In Piper, P. J. (ed.) *SRS A and Leukotrienes*, pp. 101–17. (Chichester: Wiley) .

85. MacGlashan, D. W., Schleimer, R. P., Peters, S. P., Schulman, E. S., Adams, G. K., Newball, H. H. and Lichtenstein, L. M. (1982). Generation of leukotrienes by purified human lung mast cells. *J. Clin. Invest.*, **70**, 747–51

86. Damon, M., Chavis, C., Godard, P. H., Michel, F. B. and Crastes de Paulet, A. (1983). Purification and mass spectrometry identification of leukotriene D_4 synthesized by human alveolar macrophages. *Biochem. Biophys. Res. Commun.*, **111**, 518–24

87. Steel, L. K. and Kaliner, M. A. (1981). Prostaglandin generating factor of anaphylaxis. Identification and isolation. *J. Biol. Chem.*, **256**, 12692–8

88. Marom, Z., Shelhamer, J. H., Steel, L., Goetzl, E. J. and Kaliner, M. (1984). Prostaglandin generating factor of anaphylaxis induces mucus glycoprotein release and the formation of lipoxygenase products of arachidonate from human airways. *Prostaglandins*, **28**, 79–91

89. Wei, Y., Heghinian, K., Bell, R. L. and Jakschik, B. A. (1986). Contribution of macrophages to immediate hypersensitivity reaction. *J. Immunol.*, **137**, 1993–2000

90. Flint, K. C., Hudspith, B. N., Leung, K. B. P., Pearce, F. L., Seiger, K., Hammond, M. D. H., Brostoff, J. and Johnson, N. McI. (1985). IgE-dependent release of leukotriene C_4 and prostaglandin D_2 from human bronchoalveolar cells. (Abstr.). *Thorax*, **40**, 716

91. Musch, M. W., Bryant, R. W., Coscolluella, C., Myers, R. F. and Siegel, M. I. (1985). Ionophore-stimulated lipoxygenase activity and histamine release in a cloned murine mast cell, MC9. *Prostaglandins*, **29**, 405–30

92. Mencia-Huerta, J. M., Lewis, R. A., Razin, E. and Austen, K. F. (1983). Antigen-initiated release of platelet-activating factor (PAF-acether) from mouse bone marrow-derived mast cells sensitized with monoclonal IgE. *J. Immunol.*, **131**, 2958–64

93. Levi-Schaffer, F., Austen, K. F., Caulfield, J. P., Hein, A., Gravallese, P. M. and Stevens, R. L. (1987). Coculture of human lung-derived mast cells with mouse 3T3 fibroblasts: morphology and IgE-mediated release of histamine, prostaglandin D_2 and leukotrienes. *J. Immunol.*, **139**, 494–500

94. Camussi, G., Mencia-Huerta, J. M., Benveniste, J. (1977). Release of platelet-activating factor and histamine. II. Effect of immune complexes, complement and neutrophils on human and rabbit mastocytes and basophils. *Immunology*, **33**, 523–34

95. Mencia-Huerta, J. M. and Benveniste, J. (1979). Platelet-activating factor (PAF) and macrophages. I. Evidence for the release from rat and mouse peritoneal macrophages and not from mastocytes. *Eur. J. Immunol.*, **9**, 409–15

96. Mencia-Huerta, J. M. and Benhamou, M. (1986). PAF-acether (platelet activating factor): an update. In Kay, A. B. (ed.) *Asthma: Clinical Pharmacology and Therapeutic Progress*, pp. 237–50. (Oxford: Blackwell Scientific Publications)

97. Schleimer, R. P., MacGlashan, D. W., Peters, S. P., Pinckard, R. N., Adkinson, N. F. and Lichtenstein, L. M. (1986). Characterization of inflammatory mediator release from purified human lung mast cells. *Am. Rev. Resp. Dis.*, **133**, 614–17

98. Lynch, J. M. and Henson, P. M. (1986). The intracellular retention of newly synthesized platelet-activating factor. *J. Immunol.*, **137**, 2653–61

99. Dubose, D. A., Shapro, D. and Hechtman, H. B. (1987). Correlation among endothelial cell shape, F-actin arrangement and prostacyclin synthesis. *Life Sci.*, **40**, 447–53

100. Fox, C. C., Dvorak, A. M., Peters, S. P., Kagey-Sobotka, A. and Lichtenstein, L. M. (1985). Isolation and characterization of human intestinal mucosal mast cells. *J. Immunol.*, **135**, 483–91

101. Benyon, R. C., Lowman, M. A. and Church, M. K. (1987). Human skin mast cells: their dispersion, purification and secretory characterization. *J. Immunol.*, **138**, 861–7

102. Robinson, C., Benyon, R. C., Holgate, S. T. and Church, M. K. (1987). The calcium- and IgE-dependent release of eicosanoids from human cutaneous mast cells. (Abstr.) *Br. J. Pharmacol.*, **92**, 516 p.
103. Drazen, J. M. (1986). Inhalation challenge with sulphidopeptide leukotrienes in human subjects. *Chest*, **89**, 414–18
104. Robinson, C. (1988). Current concepts on the role of eicosanoids in the pathogenesis of asthma. In Church, M. K. and Robinson, C. (eds.) *The Role of Eicosanoids in Diseases of the Lung, Skin and Joints.* (Lancaster: MTP Press) (In press)
105. Hardy, C. C., Robinson, C., Tattersfield, A. E. and Holgate, S. T. (1984). The bronchoconstrictor effect of inhaled prostaglandin D_2 in normal and asthmatic men. *N. Engl. J. Med.*, **311**, 209–13
106. Beasley, C. R. W., Robinson, C., Featherstone, R. L., Varley, J. G., Hardy, C. C., Church, M. K. and Holgate, S. T. (1987). 9-α,11β-Prostaglandin F_2, a novel metabolite of prostaglandin D_2, is a potent contractile agonist of human and guinea pig airways. *J. Clin. Invest.*, **79**, 978–83
107. Beasley, R., Varley, J., Robinson, C. and Holgate, S. T. (1987). Cholinergic-mediated bronchoconstriction induced by prostaglandin D_2, its initial metabolite 9α,11β-PGF_2 and PGF_2 in asthma. *Am. Rev. Resp. Dis.*, **136**, 1140–4
108. Cuss, F. M., Dixon, C. M. S. and Barnes, P. J. (1986). Effects of inhaled platelet activating factor on pulmonary function and bronchial responsiveness in man. *Lancet*, **2**, 189–92
109. Page, C. P., Paul, W. and Morley, J. (1984). Platelets and bronchospasm. *Int. Arch. Allergy Appl. Immunol.*, **74**, 347–50
110. Drazen, J. M., Austen, K. F., Lewis, R. A., Clark, D. A., Goto, G., Marfat, A. and Corey, E. J. (1980). Comparative airway and vascular activities of leukotrienes C-1 and D *in vivo* and *in vitro. Proc. Natl. Acad. Sci. USA*, **77**, 4354–8
111. Peck, M. J., Piper, P. J. and Williams, T. J. (1981). The effect of leukotrienes C_4 and D_4 on the microvasculature of guinea-pig skin. *Prostaglandins*, **21**, 315–21
112. Dahlén, S. E., Bjork, J., Hedqvist, P., Arfors, K.-E., Hammarstrom, S., Lindgren, N.-A. and Samuelsson, B. (1983). Leukotrienes promote plasma leakage and leukocyte adhesion and postcapillary vasodilatation: *In vitro* effects with relevance to the acute inflammatory reaction. *Proc. Natl. Acad. Sci. USA*, **78**, 3887–91
113. Soter, N. A., Lewis, R. A., Corey, E. J. and Austen, K. F. (1983). Local effects of synthetic leukotrienes (LTC_4, LTD_4, LTE_4 and LTB_4) in human skin. *J. Invest. Dermatol.*, **80**, 115–19
114. Bisgaard, H. (1987). Vascular effects of leukotriene D_4 in human skin. *J. Invest. Dermatol.*, **88**, 109–14
115. Piper, P. J. (1983). Pharmacology of leukotrienes. *Br. Med. Bull.*, **39**, 255–9
116. Moncada, S., Vane, J. R. (1978). Pharmacology and endogenous roles of prostaglandin endoperoxides, thromboxane A_2 and prostacyclin. *Pharmacol. Rev.*, **30**, 293–331
117. Schrör, K. (1978). Prostaglandin D_2 (PGD_2) – a potent coronary vasoconstrictor agent in the guinea pig isolated heart. *Naunyn Schmeideberg's Arch. Pharmacol.*, **302**, 61–2
118. Allan, G. and Levi, R. (1981). Thromboxane and prostacyclin release during cardiac immediate hypersensitivity reactions *in vitro. J. Pharmacol. Exp. Ther.*, **217**, 157–61
119. Beasley, C. R. W., Hovell, C. J., Mani, R., Robinson, C. and Holgate, S. T. (1987). The comparative vascular effects of histamine, prostaglandin D_2 and its metabolite 9α,11β-PGF_2 in human skin. *Br. J. Clin. Pharmacol.*, **42**, 605–6P
120. Flower, R. J., Harvey, E. A., Kingston, W. P. (1976). Inflammatory effects of prostaglandin D_2 in rat and human skin. *Br. J. Pharmacol.*, **56**, 229–33
121. Gruetter, C., McNamara, D., Hyman, A. and Kadowitz, P. (1978). Contractile effects of a PGH_2 analog and PGD_2 on intrapulmonary vessels. *Am. J. Physiol.*, **234**, H139–45
122. Ford-Hutchinson, A. W., Bray, M. A., Doig, M. V., Shipley, M. E. and Smith, M. J. H. (1980). Leukotriene B_4, a potent chemotactic and aggregating substance released from polymorphonuclear leucocytes. *Nature*, **286**, 264–5
123. Haines, K. A., Giedd, K. N., Rich, A. M., Reibman, J., Korchak, H. M. and Weissman, G. (1987). Leukotriene B_4 paradox: Neutrophils can, but will not, respond to ligand-receptor interactions by forming leukotriene B_4 or its ω metabolites. In Samuelsson, B., Paoletti, R. and Ramwell, P. W. (eds.) *Advances in Prostaglandin, Thromboxane and Leukotriene Research*, Vol. 17B, pp. 890–99. (New York: Raven Press)

124. Hoover, R. L., Karnovsky, M. J., Austen, K. F., Corey, E. J. and Lewis, R. A. (1984). Leukotriene B₄ action on endothelium mediates augmented neutrophil/endothelial adhesion. *Proc. Natl. Acad. Sci. USA*, **81**, 2191–3

125. Pinckard, R. N., Farr, R. S. and Hanahan, D. J. (1979). Physicochemical and functional identity of rabbit platelet-activating factor (PAF) released *in vivo* during IgE anaphylaxis with PAF released *in vitro* from IgE sensitized basophils. *J. Immunol.*, **123**, 1847–57

126. Betz, S. J., Lotner, G. Z. and Henson, P. M. (1980). Generation and release of platelet-activating factor (PAF) from enriched preparations of rabbit basophils; failure of human basophils to release PAF. *J. Immunol.*, **125**, 2749–55

127. Wardlaw, A., Moqbel, R., Cromwell, O. and Kay, A. B. (1986). Platelet-activating factor: A potent chemotactic and chemokinetic factor for eosinophils. *J. Clin. Invest.*, **78**, 1701–6

128. Czarnetzki, B. M. and Benveniste, J. (1981). 1-O-octadecyl-2-O-acetyl-sn-glycero-3-phosphocholine (PAF-acether) on leukocytes. I. Analysis of the *in vitro* migration of human neutrophils. *Chem. Phys. Lipids*, **29**, 317–26

129. Camussi, G., Tetta, C., Bussolino, F., Caligaris Cappio, F., Coda, R. Masera, C. and Segolini, G. (1981). Mediators of immune-complex-induced aggregation of polymor-phonuclear neutrophils. II. Platelet activating factor as the effector substance of immune-induced aggregation. *Int. Arch. Allergy Appl. Immunol.*, **64**, 25–41

130. O'Flaherty, J. T., Miller, C. H., Lewis, J. C., Wykle, R. L., Bass, D. A., McCall, C. E., Waite, M. and DeChatelet, L. R. (1981). Neutrophil responses to platelet-activating factor. *Inflammation*, **5**, 193–201

131. O'Flaherty, J. T., Wykle, R. L., Lees, C. J., Shewmake, T., McCall, C. E. and Thomas, M. J. (1981). Neutrophil-degranulating action of 5,12-dihydro-6,8,10,14-eicosatetraenoic acid and 1-O-alkyl-2-O-acetyl-sn-glycero-3-phosphocholine. *Am. J. Pathol.*, **105**, 264–9

132. Lin, A. H., Morton, D. R. and Gorman, R. R. (1982). Acetylglycerylether-phosphoryl-choline stimulates leukotriene B₄ synthesis in human polymorphonuclear leukocytes. *J. Clin. Invest.*, **70**, 1058–65

133. Pinckard, R. N., Kniker, W. T., Lee, L., Hanahan, D. J., McManus, L. M. (1980). Vasoactive effects of 1-O-alkyl-2-acetyl-sn-glyceryl-3-phosphorylcholine (AcGEPC) in human skin. (Abstr.) *J. Allergy Clin. Immunol.*, **65**, 196

134. Stimler, N. P., Bloor, C. M., Hugli, T. E., Wykle, R. L., McCall, C. E. and O'Flaherty, J. T. (1981). Anaphylactic actions of platelet-activating factor. *Am. J. Pathol.*, **105**, 64–9

135. Heffner, J. E., Shoemaker, S. A., Canham, E. M., Patel, M., McMurtry, I. F., Morris, H. G. and Repine, J. E. (1983). Acetylglyceryletherphosphorylcholine-stimulated human platelets cause pulmonary hypertension and edema in isolated rabbit lungs. Role of thromboxane A₂. *J. Clin. Invest.*, **71**, 351–7

136. Hamasaki, Y., Mojarad, M., Saga, T., Tai, H.-H. and Said, S. I. (1984). Platelet-activating factor raises airway and vascular pressures and induces edema in lungs perfused with platelet-free solution. *Am. Rev. Respir. Dis.*, **129**, 742–6

137. Mojorad, M. and Said, S. I. (1982). Platelet activating factor increases pulmonary microvascular permeablity (Abstr.) *Am. Rev. Resp. Dis.*, **125** (Suppl.), 278

138. Worthen, G. S., Goins, A. I., Mitchell, B. C., Larsen, G. L., Reeves, J. R. and Henson, P. M. (1983). Platelet activating factor causes neutrophil accumulation and edema in rabbit lungs. *Chest*, **83** (Suppl.), 13S–15S

139. Granstrom, E. and Kindahl, H. (1978). Radioimmunoassay of prostaglandins and thromboxanes. In Frolich, J. C. (ed.) *Advances in Prostaglandin and Thromboxane Research*, Volume 5, pp. 119–210. (New York: Raven Press)

140. Heavey, D. J., Lumley, P., Barrow, S. E., Murphy, M. B., Humphrey, P. P. A. and Dollery, C. T. (1984). Effects of intravenous infusions of prostaglandin D₂ in man. *Prostaglandins*, **28**, 755–67

141. Bundy, G. L., Morton, D. R., Peterson, D. C., Nishizawa, E. E. and Miller, W. L. (1983). Synthesis and platelet aggregation inhibiting activity of prostaglandin D analogues. *J. Med. Chem.*, **26**, 790

142. Fitzpatrick, F. A. and Wynalda, M. A. (1983). Albumin-catalysed metabolism of prostaglandin D₂: identification of products formed *in vitro*. *J. Biol. Chem.*, **258**, 11713–18

143. Kikawa, Y., Narumiya, S., Fukushima, M., Wakatsuka, H. and Hayaishi, O. (1984). 9-deoxy-$\Delta^{9,12}$-13,14-dihydroprostaglandin D_2, a metabolite of prostaglandin D_2 formed in human plasma. *Proc. Natl. Acad. Sci. USA*, **81**, 1317–21
144. Fitzpatrick, F. A. and Wynalda, M. A. (1981). Albumin–lipid interactions: prostaglandin stability as a probe for characterizing binding sites on vertebrate albumins. *Biochemistry*, **20**, 6129–34
145. Sun, F. F., Armour, S. B., Bockstanz, V. R. and McGuire, J. C. (1976). Studies on 15-hydroxyprostaglandin dehydrogenase from monkey lung. In Samuelsson, B. and Paoletti, R. (eds.) *Advances in Prostaglandin Research*, Vol. 1, pp. 163–9. (New York: Raven Press)
146. Ellis, C. K., Smigel, M. D., Oates, J. A., Oelz, O. and Sweetman, B. J. (1979). Metabolism of prostaglandin D_2 in the monkey. *J. Biol. Chem.*, **254**, 4152–63
147. Barrow, S. E., Heavey, D. J., Ennis, M., Chappell, C. G., Blair, I. A. and Dollery, C. T. (1984). Measurement of prostaglandin D_2 and identification of metabolites in human plasma during intravenous infusion. *Prostaglandins*, **28**, 743–54
148. Liston, T. E. and Roberts, L. J. (1985). Metabolic fate of radiolabelled prostaglandin D_2 in a normal human male volunteer. *J. Biol. Chem.*, **260**, 13172–80
149. Robinson, C., Wendelborn, D. F., Roberts, L. J. and Holgate, S. T. (1987). Prostaglandin D_2 plasma metabolites after inhalation in normal men. (Abstr.) *Fed. Proc.*, **46**, 873
150. Robinson, C., Hardy, C. C. and Holgate, S. T. (1988). Formation of plasma metabolites of prostaglandin D_2 in man following administration by inhalation and intravenous infusion. *Br. J. Pharmacol.* (Submitted)
151. Liston, T. E. and Roberts, L. J. (1985). Transformation of prostaglandin D_2 to $9\alpha,11\beta$-(15S)-trihydroxy-prosta-(5Z,13E)-dien-1-oic acid ($9\alpha,11\beta$-prostaglandin F_2): a unique biologically active prostaglandin produced enzymatically *in vivo* in humans. *Proc. Natl. Acad. Sci. USA*, **82**, 6030–4
152. Pugliese, G., Spokas, E. G., Marcinkiewicz, E. and Wong, P. Y. K. (1985). Hepatic transformation of prostaglandin D_2 to a new prostanoid, $9\alpha,11\beta$-prostaglandin F_2, that inhibits platelet aggregation and constricts blood vessels. *J. Biol. Chem.*, **260**, 14621–5
153. Bacon, K. B., Hoult, J. R. S., Osborne, D. J. and Robinson, C. (1987). Metabolism of prostaglandin D_2 to $9\alpha,11\beta$-PGF$_2$ and subsequent transformation in rat, rabbit and guinea-pig. *Br. J. Pharmacol.*, **91**, 322 p.
154. Seibert, K., Sheller, J. R. and Roberts, L. J. (1987). (5Z,13E)-(15S)-9α,11β-15-trihydroxy-prosta-5,13-dienoic-1-oic acid ($9\alpha,11\beta$-prostaglandin F_2): formation and metabolism by human lung and contractile effects on human bronchial smooth muscle. *Proc. Natl. Acad. Sci. USA*, **84**, 256–60
155. Roberts, L. J. and Sweetman, B. J. (1985). Metabolic fate of endogenously synthesised prostaglandin D_2 in a human female with mastocytosis. *Prostaglandins*, **30**, 383–401
156. Church, M. K. and Hiroi, J. (1987). Inhibition of IgE-dependent histamine release from human lung mast cells by anti-allergic drugs and salbutamol. *Br. J. Pharmacol.*, **90**, 421–9
157. Church, M. K. and Holgate, S. T. (1980). The basophil leucocyte: Morphological, immunological and biochemical considerations. In Roath, S. (ed.) *Topical Reviews in Haematology*, Vol. 1, pp. 65–86. (Bristol: Wright)
158. MacGlashan, D. W., Schleimer, R. P., Peters, S. P., Schulman, E. S., Adams, G. K., Kagey-Sobotka, A., Newball, H. H. and Lichtenstein, L. M. (1983). Comparative studies of human basophils and mast cells. *Fed. Proc.*, **42**, 2504–9
159. Barr, R. M., Black, A. K., Francis, D. M., Koro, O., Numata, T. and Greaves, M. W. (1986). Release of prostaglandin D_2 (PGD$_2$) from human skin *in vivo* during cutaneous anaphylaxis (Abstr.) *Br. J. Pharmacol.*, **88** (Proceedings Suppl.), 394 p.
160. Heavey, D. J., Kobza-Black, A., Barrow, S. E., Chappell, C. G., Greaves, M. W. and Dollery, C. T. (1986). Prostaglandin D_2 and histamine release in cold urticaria. *J. Allergy Clin. Immunol.*, **78**, 458–61
161. Koro, O., Dover, J. S., Francis, D. M., Kobza-Black, A., Kelly, R. W., Barr, R. M. and Greaves, M. W. (1986). Release of prostaglandin D_2 and histamine in a case of localized heat urticaria and effects of treatments. *Br. J. Dermatol.*, **115**, 721–8
162. Murray, J. J., Tonel, A. B., Brash, A. R., Roberts, L. J., Gosset, P., Workman, R., Capron, A. and Oates, J. A. (1985). Prostaglandin D_2 is released during acute allergic bronchospasm in man. *Trans. Assoc. Am. Physicians.*, **98**, 275–80

163. Murray, J. J., Tonel, A. B., Brash, A. R., Roberts, L. J., Gosset, P., Workman, R., Capron, A. and Oates, J. A. (1986). Release of prostaglandin D_2 into human airways during acute antigen challenge. *N. Engl. J. Med.*, **315**, 800–4

164. Roberts, L. J., Sweetman, B. J., Lewis, R. A., Austen, K. F. and Oates, J. A. (1980). Increased production of prostaglandin D_2 in patients with systemic mastocytosis. *N. Engl. J. Med.*, **303**, 1400–4

165. Oates, J. A., Sweetman, B. J. and Roberts, L. J. (1984). The release of mediators of the human mast cell: investigations in mastocytosis. In Kay, A. B., Austen, K. F. and Lichtenstein, L. M. (eds.) *Asthma: Physiology, Immunopharmacology and Treatment, Third International Symposium*, pp. 55–62. (London: Academic Press)

166. Schwartzberg, S. R., Shelov, S. P. and Van Praag, D. (1987). Blood leukotriene levels during acute asthma attack in children. *Prostaglandins Leukotrienes Med.*, **26**, 143–55

167. Heavey, D. J., Richmond, R., Turner, N. C., Kobza-Black, A., Taylor, G. W., Chappell, C. G., Barrow, S. E. and Dollery, C. T. (1986). Measurement of leukotrienes C_4 and D_4 in inflammatory fluids. In Piper, P. J. (ed.) *The Leukotrienes – Their Biological Significance*, pp. 185–98. (New York: Raven Press)

168. Heavey, D. J., Soberman, R. J., Lewis, R. A., Spur, B. and Austen, K. F. (1987). Critical considerations in the development of an assay for sulfidopeptide leukotrienes in plasma. *Prostaglandins*, **33**, 693–708

169. Talbot, S. F., Atkins, P. C., Goetzl, E. J. and Zweiman, B. (1985). Accumulation of leukotriene C_4 and histamine in human allergic skin reactions. *J. Clin. Invest.*, **76**, 650–6

170. Bisgaard, H., Ford-Hutchinson, A. W., Charleson, S. and Taudorf, E. (1985). Production of leukotrienes in human skin and conjunctival mucosa after specific allergen challenge. *Allergy*, **40**, 417–23

171. Mallet, A. I., Cunningham, F. M. and Daniel, R. (1984). Rapid isocratic high performance liquid chromatographic purification of platelet activating factor (PAF) and lyso-PAF in human skin. *J. Chromatog.*, **309**, 160–4

172. Hanahan, D. J. and Weintraub, S. T. (1985). Platelet-activating factor isolation, identification, and assay. *Meth. Biochem. Anal.*, **31**, 195–219

173. Knauer, K. A., Lichtenstein, L. M., Adkinson, N. F. and Fish, J. E. (1981). Platelet activation during antigen-induced airway reactions in asthmatic subjects. *N. Engl. J. Med.*, **304**, 1404–7

174. Barnes, V. F. and Heavey, D. J. (1986). Effect of prostaglandin D_2 on histamine induced weals in human skin. *Br. J. Pharmacol.*, **87**, 357–60

175. Whittle, B. J. R., Moncada, S. and Vane, J. R. (1978). Comparison of the effects of prostacyclin (PGI_2), prostaglandin E_1 and D_2 on platelet aggregation in different species. *Prostaglandins*, **16**, 373–88

176. Mills, D. C. and MacFarlane, D. E. (1974). Stimulation of human platelet adenylate cyclase by prostaglandin D_2. *Thromb. Res.*, **5**, 401–12

177. Gardiner, P. J. and Browne, J. L. (1984). Tussive activity of inhaled PGD_2 in the rat and characterization of the receptors involved. *Prostaglandins Leukotrienes Med.*, **14**, 153–9

178. Peters, S. P., Kagey-Sobotka, A., MacGlashan, D. W. and Lichtenstein, L. M. (1984). Effect of prostaglandin D_2 in modulating histamine release from human basophils. *J. Pharmacol. Exp. Ther.*, **228**, 400–6

179. Omini, C., Brunelli, G., Daffonchio, L., Mapp, C., Fabbri, L. and Berti, F. (1986). Prostaglandin D_2 (PGD_2) potentiates cholinergic responsiveness in guinea-pig trachea. *J. Autonom. Pharmacol.*, **6**, 181–6

180. Hattori, Y. and Levi, R. (1986). Effect of PGD_2 on cardiac contractility: a negative inotropism secondary to coronary vasoconstriction conceals a primary positive inotropic action. *J. Pharmacol. Exp. Ther.*, **237**, 719–24

181. Kasukabe, T., Honma, Y. and Hozumi, M. (1985). Specific inhibition by prostaglandin D_2 and its metabolites of lysozyme synthesis in mouse macrophage-like cell line Mm-1. *Biochim. Biophys. Acta*, **844**, 330–6

182. Hall, T. J. and Brostoff, J. (1983). Inhibition of human natural killer cell activity by prostaglandin D_2. *Immunol. Lett.*, **7**, 141–4

183. Marsden, K. A., Rao, P. S., Papineni, S., Cavanagh, D. and Spaziani, E. (1984). The effect of prostaglandin D_2 (PGD_2) on circulating eosinophils. *Prostaglandins Leukotrienes Med.*, **15**, 387–97

184. Bhattacharya, S. K. (1986). The antinociceptive effect of intracerebroventricularly administered prostaglandin D₂ in the rat. *Psychopharmacology*, **89**, 121–4

185. Todo, S., Hashida, T., Shimizu, Y., Imashuku, S., Takamatsu, T. and Fujita, S. (1986). Cell kinetic studies of PGD₂ cytotoxicity on the *in vitro* growth of human neuroblastoma. *Prostaglandins Leukotrienes Med.*, **23**, 55–65

186. Todo, S., Shimizu, Y., Hashida, T., Imashuku, S. and Takamatsu, T. (1985). Antineoplastic effect of prostaglandin D₂ on cultured human neuroblastoma – effect on cell motion. *Oncologia*, **15**, 140–3

187. Kawamura, M. and Koshihara, Y. (1983). Prostaglandin D₂ strongly inhibits growth of murine mastocytoma cells. *Prostaglandins Leukotrienes Med.*, **12**, 85–93

188. Narumiya, S. and Fukushima, M. (1985). Δ^{12}-Prostaglandin J₂, an ultimate metabolite of prostaglandin D₂ exerting cell growth inhibition. *Biochem. Biophys. Res. Commun.*, **127**, 739–45

6
Mast Cell Heterogeneity

F. L. PEARCE

INTRODUCTION

Most allergic disorders are now recognized to be complex inflammatory processes involving the participation of a number of different cell types. Of these, the mast cell has assumed a pre-eminent position both because of its ability to release a diversity of spasmogenic, chemotactic and inflammatory mediators, and in view of its strategic location at the portals of entry into the body of foreign substances. Thus, while the mast cell is widely distributed throughout the human body, it is found in the largest numbers in the loose connective tissues of the bronchi, conjunctiva, gut, ear, nose, throat and skin. The mast cell is then uniquely placed to participate in allergic responses and, as such, has been incriminated in the aetiology and pathogenesis of asthma, rhinitis, conjunctivitis and inflammatory disorders of the gut and skin. Given the diversity and widespread occurrence of these conditions, it is essential to our understanding of the origins and management of allergic disorders to appreciate that mast cells from different locations may exhibit marked variations in their functional properties.

Much of our knowledge of the detailed biochemical events involved in the release from mast cells of inflammatory mediators, typified by the autacoid histamine and products of the oxidative metabolism of arachidonic acid such as thromboxanes, prostaglandins and leukotrienes, has come from studies on the serosal mast cells of rodents. These cells are simply obtained by direct lavage and are readily purified to homogeneity. However, more recently, methods have been developed for the enzymic dissociation of mast cells from a number of target tissues of experimental animals and man, including the adenoids[1], heart[2], intestine[3,4], lung[5-7], mesentery[8], skin[9,10] and tonsils[11]. Comparative studies on these preparations together with human basophil leukocytes and tissue cultures of mast cells and basophiloid cells have shown that histaminocytes from different locations exhibit marked heterogeneity in their morphological, histochemical and functional properties. In the latter respect, they may vary in their responses to given secretory stimuli and to particular mast cell stabilizing drugs. This chapter will provide examples of this heterogeneity and consider its clinical implications.

175

THE 'MUCOSAL' MAST CELL

The concept of mast cell heterogeneity was widely recognized by early pharmacologists, but current interest in the topic was undoubtedly stimulated by the pioneering work of Enerbäck[12] and his colleagues on the distribution and properties of mast cells in the gastrointestinal tract of the rat. Two distinct types of mast cell may be identified and provide probably the best example of mast cell heterogeneity within a single species. The mast cells in the lower layer of the intestinal wall resemble those found in other connective tissues and the serosal cavity, whereas the cells in the mucosa show very different properties. They are smaller in size and more variable in shape than the connective tissue cells, have a lower content of histamine and 5-hydroxytryptamine and possess fewer granules. The latter contain the less highly sulphated glycosaminoglycan chondroitin sulphate rather than heparin. These properties require that special conditions of fixation and staining be used to reveal this cell type. A characteristic feature of the mast cell is its ability to stain metachromatically with certain cationic dyes such as toluidine blue. This metachromasia arises from a shift in the colour spectrum of the dye following its interaction with the anionic proteoglycan granular matrix. Most importantly, the granules of the rat mucosal mast cell may become resistant to metachromatic staining after routine processing in common, formalin-based fixatives. The cells may also be distinguished by sequential staining with combinations of dyes such as alcian blue and safranin. The mature rat connective tissue cell stains metachromatically with safranin whereas the intestinal mucosal cell stains orthochromatically with alcian blue, consistent with the lower degree of sulphation of its proteoglycan matrix. Similarly, the cationic fluorescent dye berberine stains only the connective tissue cell. The mucosal cells have a shorter life-span than those in the connective tissues and proliferate in thymus-dependent fashion in response to certain parasitic infections. They also contain an antigenically distinct serine protease, the rat mast cell protease II, which has been used as a marker in studies of their oncogenesis.

Rat mucosal mast cells are additionally functionally quite distinct from those cells in the connective tissues and serosa. Thus, they do not release histamine in response to classical polyamine mast cell degranulating agents, such as compound 48/80 and peptide 401 from bee venom, and indeed proliferate on administration of the former agent *in vivo*, and are refractory to the action of the prototype anti-allergic drug disodium cromoglycate[3, 13]. These properties are summarized in Table 6.1 and are discussed further below.

While the above studies have undoubtedly served to focus attention on the problem of mast cell heterogeneity they have, rather unfortunately, polarized the issue and tended simply to divide mast cells into two extreme types, namely connective tissue or mucosal cells. Almost by definition, the latter cell has become one which is sensitive to routine formalin fixation, stains with alcian blue but does not counterstain with safranin, and is insensitive to compound 48/80 and disodium cromoglycate. This approach fails to recognize the full extent of mast cell heterogeneity and, as discussed below, both compound 48/80 and cromoglycate show a striking specificity in their action, and

Table 6.1 Some properties of mucosal and connective tissue mast cells from the gastrointestinal tract of the rat

Mucosal mast cells	*Connective tissue mast cells*
Small, variable shape, sparsely granulated	large, uniform, densely granulated
Soluble granular proteoglycan matrix	less soluble proteoglycan matrix
Chondroitin sulphate	Heparin
Low content of histamine and 5-hydroxytryptamine	high monoamine content
Proliferative, non-secretory polyamine response	secretory polyamine response
Short life span	long life span
Proliferative response to nematode infections	no proliferative response
IgE in cytosol	no IgE in cytosol
Berberine negative	berberine positive
Do not counterstain with safranin	counterstain with safranin
Contain rat mast cell protease II	contain rat mast cell protease I
Cromoglycate insensitive	cromoglycate sensitive

Modified from Enerbäck[12]. For further details and explanation, see text

affect, to varying extents, connective tissue mast cells from certain locations but not others. Moreover, it must be emphasized that the above histochemical criteria for distinguishing between subpopulations of mast cells have been developed exclusively for the gastrointestinal tract of the rat. The extent to which these findings may be extrapolated to other species, and especially to man, is by no means clear. It would currently appear that there may be two types of mast cell in the nose[14] and intestine[15–17] of man, and that these may respectively bear some structural and histochemical similarity to the connective tissue and mucosal mast cells of the rat. However, the distinction between the cell types is considerably more subtle and less obvious than in the gastrointestinal tract of the rodent[17]. Moreover, the subpopulations are no longer confined to particular anatomical areas of the target organ. Thus, the 'mucosal' mast cell of the human intestine, as defined by its histochemical characteristics, is not restricted to the laminar propria but is seen in densities as great or greater than the other population in the submucosa and muscle[16]. Furthermore, sequential staining with alcian blue and safranin has failed to reveal any convincing evidence of mast cell heterogeneity in human lung, and essentially all of the cells stain orthochromatically with the former dyestuff irrespective of whether they are located deep in the airways, in the alveoli or adjacent to the pleural surface[17, 18]. Under these conditions, the terms 'mucosal' and 'connective tissue' mast cells, which should be used strictly to define the topographical location of the cell type, must be applied with extreme caution[19]. The extent of functional mast cell heterogeneity in man is discussed further below.

DIFFERENCES IN MAST CELL MEDIATORS

Mast cell mediators are either preformed and stored in association with the secretory granules are synthesized *de novo* following cell activation. The preformed mediators include vasoactive and spasmogenic amines, hydrolytic

177

enzymes and chemotactic factors. The newly generated mediators consist of the products of the oxidative metabolism of arachidonic acid, which is liberated following cleavage of membrane phospholipids by phospholipases. Two major pathways for the oxidation of arachidonate have been delineated, the cyclooxygenase pathway which leads to the generation of prostaglandins (PGs) and thromboxanes (TXs), and the 5-lipoxygenase pathway which produces hydroxyeicosatetraenoeic acids (HETEs) and leukotrienes (LTs).

The matrix of the mast cell granule is largely comprised of heparin or a related glycosaminoglycan and associated cationic polypeptides. Some preformed mediators, such as histamine, are electrostatically bound to the granule and are sequentially eluted by an ion-exchange mechanism upon exposure to the external environment while others form a more integral part of the matrix. The exact constituents of the mast cell granule vary according to the species and have probably been most closely compared for rat peritoneal and human lung mast cells (Table 6.2). Both cell types contain histamine, but only the rodent cell possesses 5-hydroxytryptamine. The cells contain a variety of exoglycosidases of somewhat different specificities. The major neutral protease in the human cell is a trypsin-like enzyme (tryptase, MW 130 000) whereas the rat cells contain a chymotrypsin-like enzyme (chymase, MW 25 000). Both cells contain superoxide dismutase and peroxidase, carboxypeptidases of different specificities, and chemotactic factors for neutrophils and eosinophils of differing molecular size. The human cells also contain elastase and cathepsin. In addition, the heparin proteoglycan of the human lung mast cell is of considerably lower molecular weight than that of the rat.

Table 6.2 Preformed mediators of rat peritoneal and human lung mast cells

	Rat peritoneal mast cell	*Human lung mast cell*
Amines	histamine 5-hydroxytryptamine	histamine
Exoglycosidases	arylsulphatase A β-hexosaminidase A β-glucuronidase β-galactosidase	arylsulphatase B β-hexosaminidase B β-glucuronidase β-galactosidase
Proteases	chymase carboxypeptidase A	tryptase carboxypeptidase B elastase cathepsin G
Chemotactic factors (CF)	eosinophil CF oligopeptides and tetrapeptides neutrophil CF oligopeptides	eosinophil CF oligopeptides neutrophil CF, high MW
Other enzymes	superoxide dismutase peroxidase	superoxide dismutase peroxidase
Proteoglycan	heparin (MW 750 000)	heparin (MW 60 000)

Taken from Agius *et al.*[18] and reproduced with the permission of Blackwell Scientific Publications, Oxford

Table 6.3 Ability of human basophils and various mast cells (MC) to produce eicosanoids upon immunological stimulation

Cell type	*Eicosanoid* (ng/10^6 histaminocytes)	
	LTC$_4$	*PGD$_2$*
Human intestinal MC	31	21
Human lung MC	50	60
Human basophil	80	—
Murine bone marrow MC	90	6
Rat peritoneal MC	< 1	50

Taken from the data of Schulman *et al.*[22] and Fox *et al.*[25]

Mast cells also differ in the newly synthesized mediators of anaphylaxis that they produce by the oxidative metabolism of arachidonic acid. Rat peritoneal mast cells process arachidonate almost exclusively through the cyclooxygenase pathway to form PGD_2 with little or no generation of LTs[20]. In sharp contrast, cultures of bone marrow-derived mouse mast cells, which show some of the characteristics of 'mucosal' mast cells, preferentially synthesize LTC_4[21]. The situation in the human lung parenchymal cell has been the subject of conflicting reports, but it would appear [22-24] that this cell is capable of producing both PGD_2 and LTC_4 (see also below). The human intestinal mast cell similarly produces both eicosanoids although, unlike the situation in the lung, the leukotriene is primarily recovered as the degradation product LTE_4. It was originally reported that human basophils release only very small amounts of arachidonic acid metabolites of any type[22], but more recent work[24] has shown that the cell can produce significant amounts of LTC_4. Whether the basophil generates any cyclooxygenase products remains unclear. Attempts by radioimmunoassay have failed to identify PGD_2 or any other prostanoid, but recent studies by high performance liquid chromatography, in which cells were preincubated with exogenous radiolabelled arachidonic acid, have revealed a product moving in the prostaglandin area. The abilities of various mast cells to produce eicosanoids are summarized in Table 6.3.

An additional lipid-derived inflammatory mediator which is currently receiving great attention is platelet aggregating factor (PAF-acether, 1-*O*-alkyl-2-acetyl-*sn*-glyceryl-3-phosphoryl-choline)[26, 27]. In addition to its effects on platelets, PAF causes successive accumulation and activation of neutrophils, eosinophils and mononuclear cells. The molecule is a potent bronchoconstrictor and increases airway resistance in man and also induces a sustained inflammation and hyperreactivity of the airways. PAF additionally increases vascular permeability with resulting pulmonary oedema, and evokes both immediate and late reactions in lung and skin. A variety of inflammatory cells are able to produce PAF, including eosinophils, macrophages, monocytes, neutrophils and platelets, but mast cells and basophils vary considerably in their ability to generate the factor. Thus, the IgE-dependent activation of basophil leukocytes from the rabbit[26] but not of man[24] leads to the release of the molecule. Stimulation of isolated human lung mast cells leads to the rapid generation of several varieties of PAF

179

which differ in the length of the carbon chain in position one[26]. Interestingly, most of the PAF produced by this cell is not released. The significance of this observation, and whether the same situation pertains *in vivo*, remains as yet unclear. In contrast, tissue culture preparations of mouse bone marrow-derived mast cells release significant quantities of PAF following sensitization with monoclonal IgE and activation with specific antigen[26]. Whether other mast cell subpopulations release the factor under appropriate conditions *in vivo* or *in vitro* is obviously of great interest.

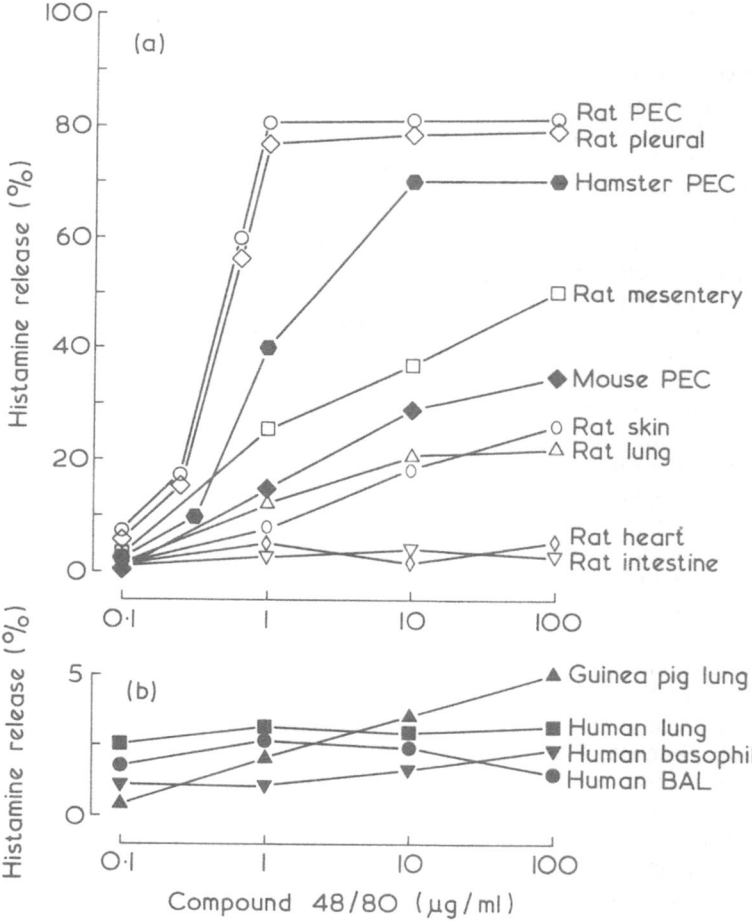

Figure 6.1 Histamine release induced by compound 48/80 from isolated mast cells from various sources. Results are based on at least four experiments and error bars are omitted for clarity. Mast cells were obtained by enzymic dissociation of the named tissues or by direct lavage. PEC denotes peritoneal exudate cells, and BAL indicates those cells obtained by broncho-alveolar lavage. Basophils were isolated by conventional techniques. Taken from Pearce[29] and reproduced with the permission of Raven Press, New York

FUNCTIONAL DIFFERENCES BETWEEN MAST CELLS

Responsiveness towards secretory stimuli

The pathophysiological stimulus for the release of histamine from the mast cell is provided by the combination of specific antigen with reaginic antibodies fixed to the cell surface. In addition, secretion may be induced by a variety of pharmacological agents which act independently of the immunological mechanism. In total, several hundred such histamine liberators have been characterized. Some of these exhibit a broad spectrum of activity, whereas others are extremely selective in their action. This topic has been previously reviewed in detail by the present author[19, 28-30], and representative examples only will be briefly discussed here.

The synthetic polyamine compound 48/80 is probably the best studied and most widely used chemical histamine liberator, and has been employed in several hundred investigations. It is often described as the 'classical mast cell degranulating agent' but is, in fact, highly specific in its action. As is well known, the compound is a remarkably potent releaser of histamine from rat peritoneal and pleural mast cells (Figure 6.1). Enzymically dispersed tissue mast cells of the rat show a continuous gradation in response to the polyamine with the mesenteric and, to a lesser extent, the skin and lung cells showing significant reactivity, while the cardiac and intestinal cells of this species are totally unresponsive. Peritoneal mast cells of the hamster, and particularly of the mouse, are less reactive than those of the rat, and tissue mast cells of the guinea pig and man are generally refractory to the compound. Additional examples of the differential reactivity of various histaminocytes to compound 48/80 have recently been reviewed[29] and will be further discussed here, along with other secretagogues, only in so far as they relate to serosal and intestinal mast cells of the rat and man and to the human basophil leukocyte. The responsiveness of these cells to various stimuli is summarized in Table 6.4.

Peptide 401, the mast cell degranulating (MCD) peptide from bee venom closely resembles compound 48/80 in its mode of action in that it is a potent histamine releaser from rat peritoneal but not intestinal mast cells, and is similarly without effect on the human basophil and on mast cells from human lung and intestine. Where tested, polylysine exhibits a similar spectrum of activity, but additionally activates the human basophil. The polysaccharide dextran is again extremely selective for rat serosal cells.

Three bioactive peptides, F-met-leu-phe (F-met peptide), the split complement component C5a and substance P, are of special interest. The former two agents are potent histamine releasers from the human basophil, while the F-met peptide is completely inactive against all of the mast cells tested, and C5a shows limited reactivity only towards the rat peritoneal cell. In sharp contrast, substance P is stongly active against the rat peritoneal cell, affects the rat intestinal cell only at relatively high concentrations and is ineffective against the human lung mast cell and basophil.

The tissue mast cells are generally hyporesponsive to the ionophore A23187, and the lipid phosphatidylserine is unique in potentiating IgE-mediated histamine secretion only from the rat serosal mast cell.

Table 6.4 Effect of various secretagogues on human basophils and mast cells (MC) from different sources

Secretagogue	Rat peritoneal MC	Rat intestinal MC	Human lung MC	Human intestinal MC	Human basophil
Compound 48/80	+ + +	—	—	—	—
Peptide 401	+ + +	—	—	—	—
Polylysine	+ + +	?	—	?	+ +
Dextran	+ + +	—	—	?	—
F–met peptide	—	?	—	—	+ + +
C5a	+	?	—	—	+ + +
Substance P	+ + +	+	—	?	—
Ionophore A23187	+ + +	+	+	+	+ + +
Phosphatidylserine	+ + +	—	—	?	—

The ability of various secretagogues to induce non-cytotoxic histamine release from various mast cells and basophils is subjectively graded. For discussion and explanation of abbreviations, see text. Taken from the data of Befus et al.[3, 31], Fox et al.[4, 25], Lichtenstein et al.[24], Ali et al.[32], Pearce et al.[28, 30, 33] and unpublished work

The above data, summarized in Table 6.4, then clearly illustrate the marked functional differences between rat connective tissue and intestinal mucosal mast cells, while the human lung and gut cells appear to behave identically in response to all of the stimuli so far tested. In contrast, there are striking differences between the human mast cells and basophils. These data then obviously raise the question of the extent of mast cell heterogeneity in man. As discussed above, there is some histological evidence for the existence of two types of mast cell in human gut[16], but enzymically dispersed and purified mast cells from the human gastrointestinal mucosa do not appear to differ from similarly prepared mast cells from lung parenchyma in their mediator content, ultrastructure or secretory characteristics[4, 24, 25]. Clearly, any differences are much more subtle than in the rat. However, accumulating evidence indicates that there may be significant differences in the mast cells from human skin. These cells show some affinity for safranin on sequential staining[18], while the lung and intestinal cells do not, and, unlike the latter, the cutaneous cells release histamine on stimulation with morphine, substance P, polylysine and compound 48/80[10, 24]. The full extent of mast cell heterogeneity in man thus remains to be determined, and the situation in human lung is discussed further below.

Responsiveness towards anti-allergic drugs

The widespread involvement of mast cells and basophils in a diversity of allergic disorders has naturally led to attempts to develop drugs that suppress the function of these cells. Such drugs would represent an obvious therapeutic development, since agents which prevent the release of inflammatory mediators should attenuate the very earliest stages of the allergic response. However, there are a number of problems inherent in this approach, not least being the recognition that many allergic diseases are complex inflammatory processes involving a large number of different cell types. More relevantly for the present article, however, is the fact that many potential anti-allergic drugs show a high degree of mast cell selectivity in their action. Again, this topic has been recently reviewed by the present author[19, 28-30] and some representative examples will be discussed in outline here.

The introduction of the prototype anti-allergic drug, disodium cromoglycate, provided a major advance in the treatment and prophylaxis of asthma and other allergic conditions. The clinical utility of the drug is undoubtedly complex but has been generally attributed, at least in part, to its ability to inhibit mediator release from tissue mast cells. In fact, the chromone provides a particularly striking example of the selectivity of given mast cell stabilizing compounds. As is well known, the drug is a very potent

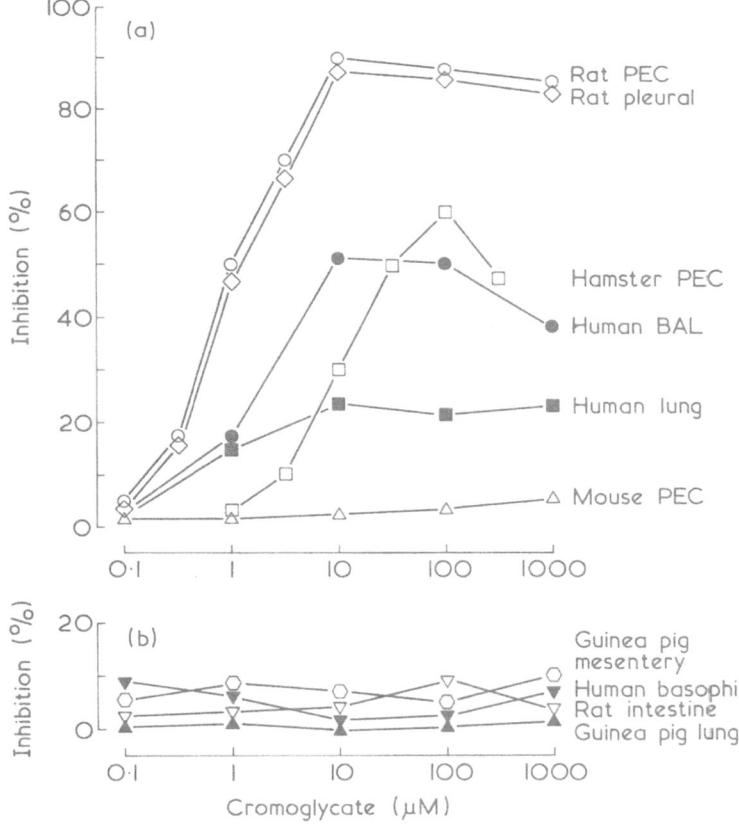

Figure 6.2 Inhibition by disodium cromoglycate of anaphylactic histamine release from isolated mast cells from various sources. Results are based on at least four experiments and error bars are omitted for clarity. For further details, see legend to Figure 6.1. Taken from Pearce[29] and reproduced with the permission of Raven Press, New York

inhibitor of immunologically induced histamine release from rat peritoneal and pleural mast cells (Figure 6.2a). In contrast, the compound is significantly less active against peritoneal cells from the hamster and totally ineffective against those cells from the mouse. The chromone is similarly inactive against tissue mast cells of the guinea pig, mucosal mast cells from the rat intestine and human basophils (Figure 6.2b). The situation in human lung is discussed further below, but the drug shows limited activity against pulmonary mast cells isolated from lung parenchyma while being significantly more reactive against airway cells recovered by bronchoalveolar lavage (Figure 6.2a).

The effect of a variety of inhibitors on histamine release from rat connective tissue and gut mucosal mast cells, human mast cells from lung and intestine and human basophils is summarized in Table 6.5. As discussed above, cromoglycate is most active against rat serosal mast cells. The compound shows modest activity in human lung, and unlike the rat, in human intestine[31], but is ineffective against the basophil. In total contrast, the naturally occurring flavonoid quercetin (3,5,7,3',4'-pentahydroxyflavone), which is structurally related to cromoglycate, is equipotent against all five cell types. This may indicate that the two drugs have distinct modes of action.

Elevated intracellular concentrations of cyclic AMP (cAMP) are generally considered to inhibit histamine release from mast cells, and analogues of the nucleotide such as 8-bromo-cyclic AMP suppress secretion from all the cell types so far examined (Table 6.5). However, pharmaco-logical agents which potentially raise cAMP levels by activation of adenylate cyclase or by inhibition of cyclic nucleotide phosphodiesterase show differential effects. Thus, the sympathomimetic agent isoprenaline is an effective inhibitor of mediator release from the human cells, provided that the reaction is 'staged' in the basophil[24], but inactive against the rat cells, possibly indicating the absence of functionally coupled β-adrenoceptors in the latter.

Table 6.5 Effect of various inhibitors on human basophils and mast cells (MC) from different sources

			Cell type		
Inhibitor	Rat peritoneal MC	Rat intestinal MC	Human lung MC	Human intestinal MC	Human basophil
Cromoglycate	+ + +	—	+	+	—
Quercetin	+ + +	+ + +	+ + +	+ + +	+ + +
Br-cAMP	+ + +	+ + +	+ + +	?	+ + +
Isoprenaline	—	—	+ + +	?	+ + +
Theophylline	+ + +	—	+ + +	+ + +	+ + +
H₂-agonists	—	?	—	?	+ + +
BPB	+ + +	?	+ + +	?	+ + +
ETYA	+ + +	?	+ + +	?	+ + +
Corticosteroids	+ + +	?	—	?	+ + +

The ability of various inhibitors to block histamine secretion from various mast cells and basophils is subjectively graded. For discussion and explanation of abbreviations, see text and for sources of original data, see Table 6.4

The phosphodiesterase inhibitor, theophylline, is active against all of the histaminocytes, with the singular exception of the rat intestinal mast cell. The latter may thus possibly possess a unique phosphodiesterase isozyme which is insensitive to the action of the methylxanthine. Of the histaminocytes studied, the human basophil appears to be unique in possessing a functional histamine H_2-receptor. The latter seems to be coupled to adenylate cyclase, and thereby provides a negative feedback mechanism for the automodulation of histamine release.

The phospholipase A_2 inhibitor *p*-bromophenacylbromide (BPB) and the combined cyclooxygenase-lipoxygenase inhibitor 5,8,11,14-eicosatetraenoic acid (ETYA) inhibit activation of all the mast cells so far studied, possibly indicating the importance of the release and oxidative metabolism of arachidonic acid in the stimulus–secretion coupling process itself.

The effect of corticosteroids on mediator release from mast cells has been the subject of conflicting reports in the literature, but recent investigations have shown that overnight incubation with pharmacological concentrations of glucocorticoids attenuates secretion from rat serosal mast cells and human basophils. The relative activities of a series of steroids correlates well with their anti-inflammatory activity *in vivo*. In sharp contrast, the same studies failed to show any effect of these drugs on isolated human lung mast cells. It should be noted, however, that we have recently found (unpublished work) that high-dose steroid therapy markedly reduces the reactivity of mast cells recovered by bronchoalveolar lavage of asthmatic subjects, perhaps indicating the potential problems of extrapolating from *in vivo* data to the clinical situation.

The above results then show that the differential reactivity of mast cells towards secretory stimuli clearly extends also to anti-allergic drugs. As before, there are major functional differences between serosal and intestinal mast cells in the rat, but not in man. Again, the major differences in the latter case appear to exist between tissue mast cells and peripheral blood basophils.

HUMAN LUNG MAST CELLS

Human bronchial asthma is characterized by a widespread and variable intrathoracic airflow obstruction caused, at least in part, by the release of chemical mediators from mast cells and other inflammatory cells. Mast cells are widely distributed throughout the human respiratory tract and are found in large numbers in the walls of the alveoli and airways. Most mast cells in the conducting airways are located between the bronchial epithelium and the basement membrane, but appreciable numbers of cells are found intercalated between the epithelial cells and adjacent to the surface of the lumen. Since bronchoconstriction occurs within minutes of antigen-challenge in allergic subjects, it seems unlikely that macromolecular or large particulate antigens would normally penetrate small airways and cross the mucosa to release mediators from parenchymal mast cells within this space of time. However, cells lying superficially within the mucosa of the airways would be in an ideal position to mediate rapid bronchial reactions, and might be expected to be of major importance in modulating the initial phases of the allergic response. These cells would come into immediate contact with both inhaled antigens and potentially useful drugs, and would release their mediators directly onto the airway surface. More deeply situated mast cells and other cell types may then become progressively involved in the development of the chronic disease as damage to the mucosal surface and respiratory epithelium allows an increased penetration of inhaled antigen. Superficially located mast cells may be recovered directly from human lung by bronchoalveolar lavage (BAL)[18, 34–37] whereas, as discussed, parenchymal mast cells may be obtained by enzymic dissociation of the intact tissue. We then felt it was of obvious interest to examine in detail the properties of these two cell types, particularly in view of the potentially novel properties of mast cells recovered from mucosal surfaces.

Nature of the cells recovered from dispersed lung and by BAL

The majority (80–90%) of the cells obtained by BAL of normal subjects are alveolar macrophages, but appreciable numbers of lymphocytes, neutrophils and eosinophils are also recovered. In our hands[34, 38], mast cells comprise 0.25–0.5% of the total nucleated population, although lower values have been obtained by other authors[18]. Macrophages again predominate (~ 80%) in suspensions of cells obtained by enzymic dissociation of whole lung, but these preparations again contain significant numbers of lymphocytes and neutrophils and an increased proportion of mast cells (~ 3–5%) relative to the BAL fluid. In our studies[38], the BAL mast cell was found to have a significantly lower histamine content than the dispersed lung cell (~ 1 and 3 pg/cell, respectively) although this observation has not been confirmed by others[18]. Both BAL and parenchymal lung mast cells are sensitive to formalin fixation and stain orthochromatically with alcian blue, and do not counterstain with safranin[18, 34, 38]. As discussed above, these histochemical characteristics seem to be general for human mast cells.

Dispersed lung and BAL mast cells appear to differ somewhat in their ultrastructure[39, 40]. The cytoplasm of the parenchymal lung cell is dominated by secretory granules. A few of these are amorphous, but the majority contain crystalline structures. The latter are typified by whorls or scrolls, although gratings and lattices are also seen. All three patterns may be observed in the same granule. The BAL cell broadly resembles that from the parenchyma, but there are fewer granules, some of which appear to be incompletely formed or disrupted, and numerous lipid bodies and cytoplasmic folds and projections. In total, the cell appears to be partially activated.

The lavage fluid of extrinsic asthmatic subjects contains a significantly higher proportion of both eosinophils and mast cells than normal controls (Figure 6.3). The histamine content of the lavage increases in parallel with the number of mast cells. The forced expiratory volume in one second (FEV_1), forced vital capacity (FVC), and the histamine concentration required to produce a 20% reduction in FEV_1 (PC_{20} histamine) has also been determined in these patients[35]. Strikingly, there is a highly significant, inverse correlation between the percentage of mast cells in the lavage fluid and both

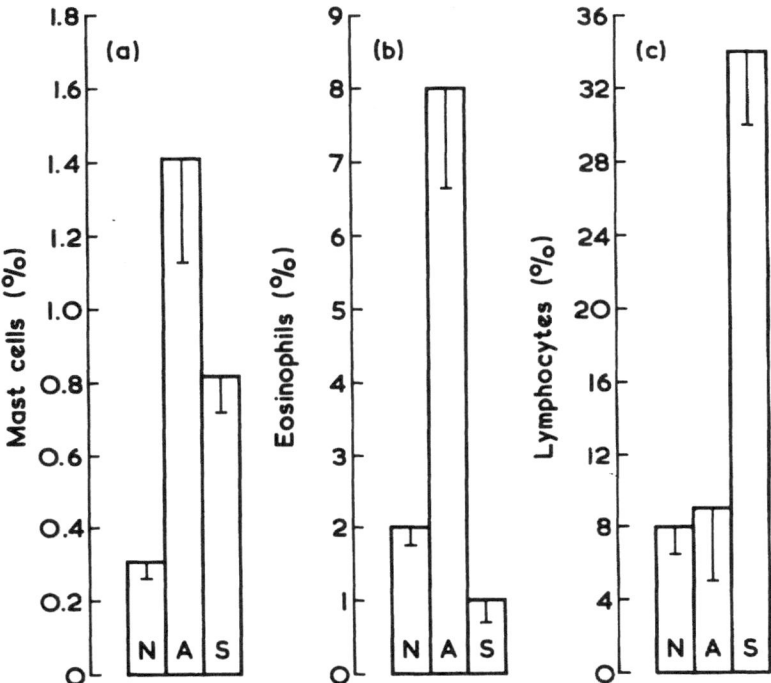

Figure 6.3 Percentage of mast cells, eosinophils and lymphocytes in the fluid recovered by BAL of subjects with extrinsic asthma (A, $n = 10$), sarcoidosis (S, $n = 36$) and normal controls (N, $n = 20$). Values are means ± SEM and taken from the data of Pearce *et al.*[38]

the FEV_1 (expressed as a percentage of the predicted) and the FEV_1/FVC ratio. A similar inverse correlation is seen between histamine content and these parameters of pulmonary function. There is also significant inverse correlation between the percentage of mast cells and the PC_{20} histamine.

There is a similarly increased proportion of mast cells, and of lymphocytes, in the BAL fluid of patients with biopsy proven sarcoidosis (Figure 6.3)[36]. The increase in mast cells is greatest in subjects with positive gallium scans and in those with radiological evidence of pulmonary lesions, but is not correlated with the percentage recovery of lymphocytes, the duration or the radiographic stage of the disease.

Immunologically induced histamine release

The mast cells obtained by BAL of subjects with extrinsic asthma and sarcoidosis have identical fixation and staining properties and the same histamine content as normal controls. However, the spontaneous release of histamine from the cells of asthmatic subjects is significantly greater than the other two populations[38], indicating that these cells may be inherently unstable.

187

Mast cells obtained by BAL of normal subjects release histamine in a dose-dependent fashion on challenge with anti-human IgE[34]. Most interestingly, mast cells obtained by BAL of asthmatic subjects[35] and sarcoids[36] show an enhanced reactivity towards anti-IgE, and exhibit a greater release of histamine at all effective dilutions of the antiserum. This effect is confined to the BAL cells, and is not apparent in the basophil leukocytes of these individuals which behave identically to the controls. Specific antigen also leads to histamine release from BAL cells and basophils of asthmatic subjects, but not controls. The accentuation of histamine release from the BAL cells of sarcoids is significantly greater in patients with positive gallium scans, and correlates directly with the percentage of lymphocytes in the lavage fluid[36]. The increase is particularly noted in patients with greater than 20% of lymphocytes in the fluid.

Peripheral blood basophils generally respond to lower dilutions of antiserum than BAL cells, and exhibit an enhanced maximum release, but display a characteristic, bell-shaped dose-response curve[38]. The rates of histamine release from the BAL and dispersed lung cells are comparable, and secretion is essentially complete within 2–5 min. However, release from the basophil is much slower, and requires at least 20 min for completion.

Release of arachidonic acid metabolites

In addition to histamine, anti-IgE induces a dose-dependent release of immunoreactive PGD_2 and LTC_4 from both BAL and parenchymal lung cells (Table 6.6). Anti-IgE is more effective in inducing PGD_2 production than histamine release from the BAL cells, and measurable amounts of the prostanoid are generated at lower dilutions of the antiserum. Liberation of PGD_2 is significantly correlated with the percentage of histamine release, implying that both mediators are derived from the mast cell, although it is of course impossible to determine unambiguously the origin of released mediators in mixed cell populations. The spontaneous generation of LTC_4 is variable and higher concentrations of anti-IgE are required to evoke the *de novo* production of the eicosanoid. No correlation is observed between

Table 6.6 Immunologically induced release of mediators from BAL and dispersed lung (DL) cells

Anti-IgE (dilution)	Histamine (% release)		LTC_4 (ng/10^6 mast cells)		PGD_2 (ng/10^6 mast cells)	
	BAL	DL	BAL	DL	BAL	DL
100	39.0 ± 6.2	49.5 ± 6.5	18.2 ± 3.5	16.1 ± 5.0	242 ± 50	145 ± 49
300	34.8 ± 5.7	41.0 ± 9.0	10.5 ± 3.5	11.8 ± 3.2	251 ± 60	139 ± 39
1000	31.9 ± 4.9	31.7 ± 7.3	7.0 ± 2.5	8.8 ± 2.9	219 ± 47	142 ± 30
10 000	17.1 ± 10.2	10.0 ± 5.0	2.2 ± 1.2	2.9 ± 1.8	127 ± 34	63 ± 20
100 000	0 ± 2.0	0.5 ± 0.5	—	0.6 ± 0.3	61 ± 33	36 ± 20

All values are means ± SEM for 10 (BAL) or 8 (DL) experiments, and are corrected for the spontaneous releases in the absence of inducer. Spontaneous releases for the BAL and DL cells, respectively, were: histamine 11.5 ± 2.0 and 4.4 ± 1.4, LTC_4 11.0 ± 7.3 and 1.8 ± 0.6, and PGD_2 55 ± 10 and 20 ± 14. Taken from Leung *et al.*[41] and reproduced with the permission of Birkhauser Verlag AG, Basel

the percentage of histamine release and the generation of LTC_4 by BAL cells, suggesting either that this relationship may be obscured by the high spontaneous release of the leukotriene or that cells other than mast cells are also involved in its production. BAL cells spontaneously release more PGD_2 than dispersed lung cells and possibly rather more of the prostanoid following immunological challenge when the data are corrected for the relative numbers of mast cells in the preparations (Table 6.6). However, the production of histamine, PGD_2 and LTC_4 are all significantly intercorrelated for the parenchymal cells. As might be expected, the rates of release of the newly generated mediators are slower than for histamine for both BAL and dispersed lung cells, and require 10–15 min for completion.

Despite the uncertainties involved in the interpretation of these experiments, it is however clear that human BAL cells do not represent a distinct subpopulation analogous to the tissue culture derived mouse 'mucosal' mast cell which preferentially produces LTC_4 upon immune activation. It may then be the case that all human mast cells, as has been established for purified preparations of intestinal and lung parenchymal cells, are capable of generating significant amounts of both lipoxygenase and cyclooxygenase products of arachidonic acid metabolism (Table 6.3). This of course contrasts with the rat peritoneal mast cell which, as discussed, produces almost entirely PGD_2.

Hyperosmolar release of histamine

In some 70–80% of asthmatic subjects vigorous exercise leads, within 10 min, to a pronounced airflow obstruction. This phenomenon is known as exercise-induced asthma (EIA). The precise mechanisms involved in the induction of EIA remain to be resolved, but considerable evidence suggests that the initiating event may be respiratory water loss resulting in an increase in the osmolarity of the fluid lining the epithelium of the airways[42]. This hyperosmolar stimulus may in turn lead to the activation of pulmonary mast cells. Consistently, increases in circulating levels of mast cell markers have been demonstrated during EIA[42], and incubation in a hyperosmolar buffer *in vitro* triggers histamine release from human basophils and potentiates immunological mediator release from isolated human lung cells[43]. In our hands, varying the osmolarity of the incubation medium from 280 to 1270 mosm/kg by adding increasing concentrations of mannitol (0.1–1 mol/l) leads to a dose-dependent release of histamine from both BAL and dispersed lung cells[38]. The kinetics of the process are complex. There is an initial, fairly rapid release of the amine which reaches a plateau after about 10 min. Thereafter, the release increases slowly and progressively over a 60 min period. After 10 min of incubation, the BAL cells are significantly more reactive than the dispersed lung cells, the two populations releasing ~ 12% and 3% of their total histamine, respectively. Under the same conditions, isolated basophils are even more responsive, and release in excess of 50% of their histamine content. Interestingly, sodium cromoglycate attenuates the hyperosmolar release from the BAL cells with a maximum inhibition of ~ 40% at a concentration of 10 μmol/l.

Table 6.7 Effect of various anti-allergic drugs on histamine release from human pulmonary mast cells

	IC_{30}^{*} (μmol/l)	
Drug	BAL cells	Dispersed lung
Cromoglycate	3	200
Nedocromil	0.3	5
Salbutamol	0.02	0.1
Theophylline	500	300

IC_{30}^{*} denotes the concentration of drug required to produce 30% inhibition of immunologically induced histamine release. Taken from Pearce et al.[38] and reproduced with the permission of S. Karger AG, Basel

Inhibition of histamine release

Immunologically induced histamine release from both BAL and dispersed lung cells is significantly inhibited by sodium cromoglycate, its more potent congener nedocromil, the β-adrenoceptor agonist, salbutamol, and the phosphodiesterase inhibitor, theophylline (Table 6.7). The latter compounds show comparable activity against both cell types, but cromoglycate and nedocromil are strikingly more effective against the BAL cells. In addition, nedocromil is at least one order of magnitude more effective than cromoglycate in suppressing histamine release from both BAL and parenchymal lung cells. The kinetics of the inhibition are also different: the activity of nedocromil and cromoglycate on the BAL cells increases following preincubation of the cells with the drugs, whereas tachyphylaxis is observed with the dispersed lung cells[37]. The former observation is, of course, more in keeping with the clinical utility of the drugs which are ideally administered prophylactically prior to antigen exposure.

CONCLUDING REMARKS

In total, the above studies show that there are subtle but distinct differences between human pulmonary mast cells obtained by BAL and from lung parenchyma. Increased numbers of mast cells are recovered by BAL of asthmatic subjects and these cells are hyperresponsive to immunological challenge and exhibit a higher spontaneous release of histamine. Most importantly, there is a significant correlation between the percentage of mast cells in the BAL fluid of asthmatics and the severity of the disease as assessed by measured indices of both airway obstruction and bronchial hyperreactivity. This association considerably strengthens the hypothesis that these cells may play a central role in the pathogenesis of the disorder. BAL mast cells show a similarly increased reactivity to hyperosmolar challenge, suggesting that they may be directly involved in the precipitation of EIA.

Increased numbers of mast cells are also found in the BAL fluid of patients with pulmonary sarcoidosis, suggesting that they may also play a role in the pathology of this condition. The reactivity of these cells correlates directly with the proportion of lymphocytes in the lavage and the possible role of lymphokines in the activation of human mast cells clearly requires further study.

In addition to histamine, immunological activation of BAL and dispersed lung cells leads to the release of the newly generated mediators PGD_2 and LTC_4. Clearly, the generation of these potent inflammatory and broncho-constrictor agents in response to IgE-dependent challenge by cells lying superficially within the lung is likely to have profound effects *in vivo*.

The most striking difference between the BAL and parenchymal cells is in their response to the anti-allergic drugs cromoglycate and nedocromil sodium. Given the location of the BAL cells immediately adjacent to the luminal surface, and their consequently greater exposure to inhaled drugs, this finding may have considerable clinical significance. In total, in view of their particular properties and strategic position within the airways, BAL mast cells may provide an especially good model for the study of immediate hypersensitivity reactions in the lung and for screening novel drugs for their treatment.

Acknowledgements

Work from the author's laboratories was supported by grants from The Asthma Research Council, Fisons Pharmaceuticals Ltd., MRC, NATO, SERC and The Wellcome Trust.

References

1. Halim, H. J., Fischer, B. and Schmutzler, W. (1982). Centrifugal elutriation studies in mast cells from rats, guinea pigs and man. *Agents and Actions*, **12**, 189–91
2. Ali, H. and Pearce, F. L. (1985). Isolation and properties of cardiac and other mast cells from the rat and guinea pig. *Agents and Actions*, **16**, 138–40
3. Befus, A. D., Pearce, F. L., Gauldie, J., Horsewood, P. and Bienenstock, J. (1982). Mucosal mast cells. I. Isolation and functional characteristics of rat intestinal mast cells. *J. Immunol.*, **128**, 2475–80
4. Fox, C. C., Dvorak, A. M., Peters, S. P., Kagey-Sobotka, A. and Lichtenstein, L. M. (1985). Isolation and characterization of human intestinal mucosal mast cells. *J. Immunol.*, **135**, 483–91
5. Ennis, M. (1982). Histamine release from human pulmonary mast cells. *Agents and Actions*, **12**, 60–3
6. Schulman, E. S., MacGlashan, D. W., Peters, S. P., Schleimer, R. P., Newball, H. H. and Lichtenstein, L. M. (1982). Human lung mast cells: purification and characterization. *J. Immunol.*, **129**, 2662–7
7. Barrett, K. E., Ennis, M. and Pearce, F. L. (1983). Mast cells isolated from guinea pig lung: characterization and studies on histamine secretion. *Agents and Actions*, **13**, 122–5
8. Pearce, F. L. and Ennis, M. (1980). Isolation and some properties of mast cells from the mesentery of the rat and guinea pig. *Agents and Actions*, **10**, 124–31
9. Barrett, K. E., Ali, H. and Pearce, F. L. (1985). Studies on histamine secretion from enzymically dispersed cutaneous mast cells of the rat. *J. Invest. Dermatol.*, **84**, 22–6
10. Benyon, R. C., Church, M. K., Clegg, L. S. and Holgate, S. T. (1986). Dispersion and characterisation of mast cells from human skin. *Int. Arch. Allergy Appl. Immunol.*, **79**, 332–4

191

11. Church, M. K., Mageed, R. A. K. and Holgate, S. T. (1983). Human tonsillar mast cells. Characteristics of histamine secretion and methods of dispersion. *Int. Arch. Allergy Appl. Immunol.*, **72**, 188–90
12. Enerbäck, L. (1981). The gut mucosal mast cell. *Monog. Allergy*, **17**, 222–32
13. Pearce, F. L., Befus, A. D., Gauldie, J. and Bienenstock, J. (1982). Mucosal mast cells. II. Effects of anti-allergic compounds on histamine secretion by isolated intestinal mast cells. *J. Immunol.*, **128**, 2481–6
14. Okuda, M., Ohnishi, M. and Ohtsuka, H. (1985). The effects of cromolyn sodium on the nasal mast cells. *Ann. Allergy*, **55**, 721–3
15. Strobel, S., Miller, H. R. P. and Ferguson, A. (1981). Human intestinal mucosal mast cells: evaluation of fixation and staining techniques. *J. Clin. Pathol.*, **34**, 851–8
16. Befus, D., Goodacre, R., Dyke, N. and Bienenstock, J. (1985). Mast cell heterogeneity in man. I. Histologic studies in the intestine. *Int. Arch. Allergy Appl. Immunol.*, **76**, 232–6
17. Greenwood, B. (1985). The histology of mast cells. In Engström, I. and Lindholm, N. (eds.) *Current Views on Bronchial Asthma*, pp. 143–9. (Stockholm: Fisons Sweden AB)
18. Agius, R. M., Howarth, P. H., Robinson, C. and Holgate, S. T. (1986). Human broncho-alveolar mast cells and their mediators. In Kay, A. B. (ed.) *Asthma: Clinical Pharmacology and Therapeutic Progress*, pp. 274–85. (Oxford: Blackwell Scientific Publications)
19. Pearce, F. L. (1986). On the heterogeneity of mast cells. *Pharmacology*, **32**, 61–71
20. Lewis, R. A. and Austen, K. F. (1981). Mediation of local homeostasis and inflammation by leukotrienes and other mast-cell dependent compounds. *Nature (London)*, **293**, 103–8
21. Razin, E., Mencia-Huerta, J.-M., Stevens, R. L., Lewis, R. A., Liu, F.-T., Corey, E. J. and Austen, K. F. (1983). IgE-mediated release of leukotriene C₄, chondroitin sulphate E proteoglycan, β-hexosaminidase, and histamine from cultured bone marrow derived mouse mast cells. *J. Exp. Med.*, **157**, 189–201
22. Schulman, E. S., MacGlashan, D. W., Schleimer, R. P., Peters, S. P., Kagey-Sobotka, A., Newball, H. H. and Lichtenstein, L. M. (1983). Purified human basophils and mast cells: current concepts of mediator release. *Eur. J. Resp. Dis.*, **64** (Suppl. 128), 53–61
23. MacGlashan, D. W., Schleimer, R. P., Peters, S. P., Schulman, E. S., Adams, G. K., Sobotka, A. K., Newball, H. H. and Lichtenstein, L. M. (1983). Comparative studies of human basophils and mast cells. *Fed. Proc.*, **42**, 2504–9
24. Lichtenstein, L. M., Fox, C. C., Schleimer, R. P., Proud, D., Naclerio, R. M. and Kagey-Sobotka, A. (1986). Heterogeneity in human histamine-containing cells. In Befus, A. D., Bienenstock, J. and Denburg, J. A. (eds.) *Mast Cell Differentiation and Heterogeneity*, pp. 331–45. (NY: Raven Press)
25. Fox, C. C., Kagey-Sobotka, A., Schleimer, R. P., Peters, S. P., MacGlashan, D. W. and Lichtenstein, L. M. (1985). Mediator release from human basophils and mast cells from lung and intestinal mucosa. *Int. Arch. Allergy Appl. Immunol.*, **77**, 130–6
26. Mencia-Huerta, J. M. and Benhamou, M. (1986). PAF-acether (platelet activating factor): an update. (1986). In Kay, A. B. (ed.) *Asthma: Clinical PHarmacology and Therapeutic Progress*, pp. 237–50. (Oxford: Blackwell Scientific Publications)
27. Page, C. P., Archer, C. B., Paul, W. and Morley, J. (1984). PAF-acether: a mediator of inflammation and asthma. *Trends Pharmacol. Sci.*, **5**, 1–3
28. Pearce, F. L. (1986). Mast cell heterogeneity: an overview. In Kay, A. B. (ed.) *Asthma: Clinical Pharmacology and Therapeutic Progress*, pp. 251–64. (Oxford: Blackwell Scientific Publications)
29. Pearce, F. L. (1986). Functional differences between mast cells from various locations. In Befus, A. D., Bienenstock, J. and Denburg, J. (eds.) *Mast Cell Differentiation and Heterogeneity*, pp. 215–22. (NY: Raven Press)
30. Pearce, F. L., Ali, H., Barrett, K. E., Befus, A. D., Bienenstock, J., Brostoff, J., Ennis, M., Flint, K. C., Hudspith, B., Johnson, N. McI., Leung, K. B. P. and Peachell, P. T. (1985). Functional characteristics of mucosal and connective tissue mast cells of man, the rat and other animals. *Int. Arch. Allergy Appl. Immunol.*, **77**, 724–6
31. Befus, D., Lee, T., Goto, T., Goodacre, R., Shanahan, F. and Bienenstock, J. (1986). Histologic and functional properties of mast cells in rats and humans. In Befus, A. D., Bienenstock, J. and Denburg, J. (eds.) *Mast Cell Differentiation and Heterogeneity*, pp. 205–13. (NY: Raven Press)

192

32. Ali, H., Leung, K. B. P., Pearce, F. L., Hayes, N. A. and Foreman, J. C. (1986). Comparison of the histamine releasing action of substance P on mast cells and basophils from different species and tissues. *Int. Arch. Allergy Appl. Immunol.*, **79**, 413–18

33. Pearce, F. L. (1982). Functional heterogeneity of mast cells from different species and tissues. *Klin. Wochenschr.*, **60**, 954–7

34. Flint, K. C., Leung, K. B. P., Pearce, F. L., Hudspith, B. N., Brostoff, J. and Johnson, N. McI. (1985). Human mast cells recovered by bronchoalveolar lavage: their morphology, histamine release and the effects of sodium cromoglycate. *Clin. Sci.*, **68**, 427–32

35. Flint, K. C., Leung, K. B. P., Hudspith, B. N., Brostoff, J., Pearce, F. L. and Johnson, N. McI. (1985). Bronchoalveolar mast cells in extrinsic asthma: a mechanism for the initiation of antigen specific bronchoconstriction. *Br. Med. J.*, **291**, 923–6

36. Flint, K. C., Leung, K. B. P., Hudspith, B. N., Brostoff, J., Pearce, F. L., Geraint-James, D. and Johnson, N. McI. (1986). Bronchoalveolar mast cells in sarcoidosis: increased numbers and accentuation of mediator release. *Thorax*, **41**, 94–9

37. Leung, K. B. P., Flint, K. C., Brostoff, J., Hudspith, B. N., Johnson, N. McI. and Pearce, F. L. (1986). A comparison of nedocromil sodium and sodium cromoglycate on human lung mast cells obtained by bronchoalveolar lavage and by dispersion of lung fragments. *Eur. J. Resp. Dis.*, **69** (Suppl. 147), 223–6

38. Pearce, F. L., Flint, K. C., Leung, K. B. P., Hudspith, B. N., Seager, K., Hammond, M. D., Brostoff, J., Geraint-James, D. and Johnson, N. McI. (1987). Some studies on human pulmonary mast cells obtained by bronchoalveolar lavage and by enzymic dissociation of whole lung tissue. *Int. Arch. Allergy Appl. Immunol.*, **82**, 507–12

39. Caulfield, J. P., Lewis, R. A., Hein, A. and Austen, K. F. (1980). Secretion in dissociated human pulmonary mast cells. *J. Cell Biol.*, **85**, 299–301

40. Holgate, S. T., Hardy, C., Robinson, C., Agius, R. M. and Howarth, P. H. (1986). The mast cell as a primary effector cell in the pathogenesis of asthma. *J. Allergy Clin. Immunol.*, **77**, 275–82

41. Leung, K. B. P., Flint, K. C., Hudspith, B. N., Brostoff, J., Johnson, N. McI., Seager, K., Hammond, M. D. and Pearce, F. L. (1987). Some further properties of human pulmonary mast cells recovered by bronchoalveolar lavage and enzymic dispersion of lung tissue. *Agents and Actions*, **20**, 213–15

42. Lee, T. H. (1986). Heat loss, osmolarity and the respiratory epithelium. In Kay, A. B. (ed.) *Asthma: Clinical Pharmacology and Therapeutic Progress*, pp. 393–400. (Oxford: Blackwell Scientific Publications)

43. Eggleston, P. E., Kagey-Sobotka, A., Schleimer, R. P. and Lichtenstein, L. M. (1984). Interaction between hyperosmolar and IgE-mediated histamine release from basophils and mast cells. *Am. Rev. Resp. Dis.*, **130**, 86–91

7
Stimulus–Secretion Coupling in Mast Cells and Basophils

R. C. BENYON

INTRODUCTION

Secretory granules are an outstanding feature of mast cell and basophil morphology, and their mediator contents represent major products of the cellular biosynthetic machinery. For example, human lung mast cell tryptase and rat mast cell neutral proteases constitute >20% of total cell protein[1-3]. An optimal secretory stimulus is capable of releasing >60% of the total granule contents, and yet this secretory event may have been initiated by the bridging of only several hundred to a thousand IgE-receptors at the cell surface[4]. The mechanism whereby a very small stimulus acting at the cell periphery is translated into the fusion of granules with each other and the plasma membrane with the resulting secretion of mediators is termed stimulus–secretion coupling.

In this chapter, I will briefly discuss some of the early changes in mast cell and basophil biochemistry detectable following IgE-dependent and non-immunological stimulation, and the possible role of such biochemical perturbations in stimulus–secretion coupling. This area of research is rapidly expanding, but there are two recent reviews to which I draw the reader's attention[5,6]. The potential physiological and pathological roles of released mast cell and basophil mediators are not described here, these being discussed by Dr Schwartz in Chapter 4.

AGGREGATION OF IgE-Fc RECEPTORS

Over the past 20 years, much evidence has accumulated, particularly from the studies of T. Ishizaka and K. Ishizaka, suggesting that aggregation of IgE-receptors is the initiating stimulus of IgE-dependent histamine secretion. In 1968, these workers demonstrated that intracutaneous injection of preformed allergen–IgE complexes provoked a mast cell-dependent erythema-weal reaction in normal human individuals when two or more antibody molecules were present in the complexes, i.e. the allergen was at least divalent[7]. Identical biological activities to these complexes were present in polymerized IgE molecules, without the requirement for antigen. Subsequently, Segal *et al.*[8] demonstrated that, in the rat, dimers of IgE could induce similar skin reactions. Such studies suggest that mast cell activation is initiated by the formation of cross-linkages between pairs of IgE molecules (and hence IgE-receptors). This hypothesis was further tested by Ishizaka and Ishizaka[9] who prepared purified anti-IgE receptor (anti-RBL) antibodies and, by enzymatic procedures, generated Fab monomer fragments with only one receptor recognition site. In support of the hypothesis, these fragments did not release histamine even though they bound to the mast cell surface. Dimerization of IgE-receptors is a sufficient secretory stimulus in human basophils also[10], although in these and RBL-cells, receptor trimerization is a more effective stimulus[11, 12]. Although studies with rat mast cells[13], rat basophil leukaemia cells[14], human lung mast cells[15] and human basophils[16] have demonstrated that IgE can bind to a total of 10^4–10^6 high affinity ($K = 10^8$–10^{10} l/mol) receptors per cell, it is probable that only a few percent of total cell-surface IgE-receptors need be aggregated to initiate substantial histamine release. In human basophils[4], histamine secretion is detectable following aggregation of less than 1%, i.e. typically a few hundred IgE-receptors, whilst optimum secretion required occupancy of 10–15% of antigen binding sites. Biochemical changes consequent upon receptor aggregation are also detectable following a very small stimulus. Maeyama *et al.*[17] studied the breakdown of phosphoinositides in RBL cells following stimulation by IgE trimers and detected significant phospholipid breakdown following aggregation of about 100 receptors.

Although it has long been known that some portion of the Fc-fragment of IgE is involved in receptor binding[18, 19], the precise site involved is still uncertain. Recent studies suggest that a region near the C2–C3 junction on each epsilon heavy-chain constitutes the binding site[20, 21]. Although the mast cell/basophil receptor is highly specific in its binding of IgE rather than any other class of immunoglobulin, binding can occur between IgE and receptors of different species. For example, human basophils can bind rodent IgE[22].

The mechanism whereby IgE-receptor aggregation triggers the associated biochemical changes discussed later is unknown. Perhaps some clues as to receptor function will be derived from studies of receptor structure. Due to the ready availability of rat basophil leukaemia (RBL) cells in homogeneous culture, it is not surprising that we know most about the structure of the IgE-receptor of this cell. Progress in the study of this receptor has been the subject of several recent reviews[6, 23, 24]. Available evidence suggests that the receptor contains four polypeptide chains consisting of a single α-chain containing the IgE binding site, a single β-chain and two identical γ-chains linked covalently by disulphide bonds. The receptor may therefore be represented as $\alpha\beta\gamma_2$. The α-chain is rich in carbohydrate (30% by weight). Proteolytic cleavage studies suggest that the α- and β-chains each consist of two domains. With regard to the topology of the receptor within the membrane, labelling studies suggest that the α-chain is readily accessible at the cell-surface, whilst the β- and

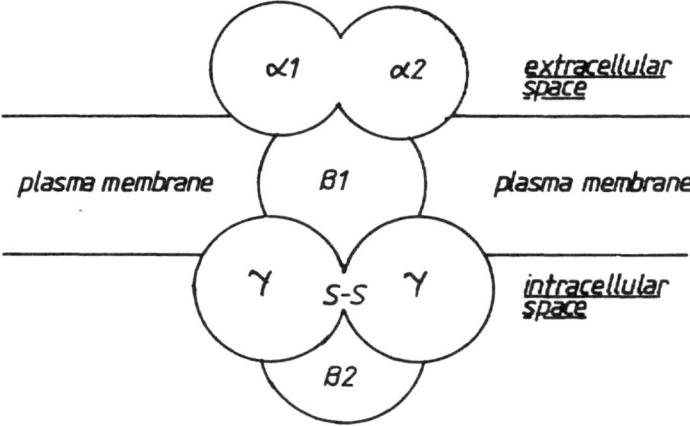

Figure 7.1 Proposed relationship between subunits of the RBL cell IgE-receptor

γ_2-chains are not, and may be buried within the plasma membrane. A schematic diagram showing the proposed relationship between receptor subunits and the plasma membrane is shown in Figure 7.1.

Although we know that the IgE-receptor has a complex structure, information on the role of the various subunits in signal transduction across the plasma membrane is lacking. It is conceivable that receptors in the aggregated state may themselves gain some catalytic activity or form an ion channel. Alternatively, aggregates may activate some enzyme or ion channels separate from the receptor. These two distinct mechanisms (i.e. intrinsic and extrinsic receptor activity) have previously been discussed by Metzger[23]. So far, the only catalytic activity that has been ascribed to IgE-receptors is autophosphorylation of tyrosine residues in both β- and γ-chains[6]. Interestingly, the appearance of tyrosine kinase activity occurs in the epidermal growth factor receptor following aggregation by anti-receptor antibodies, possibly due to a conformational change in the extracellular (ligand-binding) domain of the receptor[25]. Certain other receptors, such as the insulin receptor and the platelet-derived growth factor receptor also have intrinsic tyrosine kinase activity[26]. However, whether such enzymatic activity has any role in IgE-dependent stimulus–secretion coupling is yet to be determined. Hempstead et al.[27] reported that antigen stimulation of rat mast cells causes phosphorylation of the α-chain of the IgE receptor. However, this effect was mimicked by calcium ionophore[28], suggesting that phosphorylation was not a consequence of receptor activation itself but was a secondary effect perhaps mediated by increased intracellular calcium. In contrast, in aggregated RBL cell IgE-receptors, Perez-Montfort et al.[29] demonstrated increased phosphorylation of tyrosine in β- and γ-chains, but not α-chains. IgE-receptors from these cells have also been reported to incorporate phosphate into serine, a reaction possibly mediated by protein kinase C[30].

Stanworth and co-workers consider that receptor-bound IgE itself plays a more important role in the effector function of cross-linked receptors than previously considered. Their observation that a basic peptide consisting of a short sequence of 10 amino acids (Lys–Thr–Lys–Gly–Ser–Gly–Phe–Phe–Val–Phe) of the C4 region of IgE ('IgE-decapeptide') could initiate histamine secretion from rat mast cells[31, 32] has led to the proposition that crosslinkage of mast cell receptor-bound IgE by antigen brings about a conformational change in the antibody thus exposing the decapeptide sequence for interaction with a second type of receptor present on the plasma membrane[33]. Activation of this second receptor would be responsible for the initiation of histamine secretion, with the IgE-receptor functioning only as a 'carrier' for IgE. In support of this hypothesis, peptides such as substance P and adrenocorticotrophic hormone, which have certain structural similarities to the active C4 decapeptide, are histamine releasers in rat mast cells. However, not all the available evidence supports the proposed mechanism of Stanworth and co-workers. Firstly, rat mast cells can be activated by antibodies to IgE-receptors[9] without the involvement of cell-bound IgE. Secondly, human lung mast cells are unresponsive to the IgE-decapeptide, although anti-IgE (which, presumably, functions like antigen in cross-linking IgE) is an effective stimulus[34]. Thirdly, IgE-decapeptide-induced 5-hydroxytryptamine release from rat mast cells is much more rapid than that by antigen, and the peptide stimulus only is blocked by benzalkonium chloride[35], suggesting that these two stimuli have distinct mechanisms of cell activation. Major differences between peptide and immunological stimuli have also been observed in human skin mast cells[36].

To summarize, histamine release from mast cells and basophils is initiated by the formation of small aggregates (dimers, trimers) of IgE-receptors at the plasma membrane. Whether receptor aggregation allows the expression of intrinsic enzymatic activity of receptors or promotes the interaction of receptors with separate effector proteins is uncertain.

ACTIVATION OF SERINE ESTERASES

Activation of one or more proteolytic enzymes might constitute an early step in stimulus–secretion coupling in mast cell and basophils. Austen and co-workers have demonstrated that diisopropylfluorophosphonate (DFP), an irreversible inhibitor of serine esterases, prevented IgE-dependent histamine release from guinea pig chopped lung[37], rat mast cells[38, 39] and human lung[40]. Histamine release was inhibited only when inhibitors were present at the time of challenge. When cells or tissues were preincubated with DFP, which was then washed out immediately before challenge, the inhibitory effect was greatly diminished, suggesting that the serine esterase in resting cells is not present in the active form. The observation that DFP is ineffective when added after challenge suggests it is involved in the initiation of the secretory response. The findings of Pruzansky and Patterson[41] suggest that a DFP-inhibitable protease is also involved in the initiation of histamine release in human basophils, probably in the calcium-independent activation stage[5].

These various findings are consistent with the hypothesis that IgE-dependent activation of mast cells and basophils leads to activation of a serine esterase necessary for histamine secretion, the pro-esterase being non-inhibitable by DFP. In further support of this hypothesis, α-chymotrypsin[42, 43] and rat mast cell chymase[44] activate mediator secretion from rat mast cells. Chymase-induced secretion of preformed and newly-generated mediators has a similar time-course to that initiated by anti-IgE and, as with IgE-dependent stimulation, is associated with a monophasic increase in cyclic AMP (cAMP) concentrations at 15–45 s after cell stimulation. However, mediator secretion by these two stimuli is differently modulated by pharmacological agents[45], suggesting that chymase and anti-IgE do not share an identical secretory mechanism. Stimulus–secretion coupling in mouse mast cells induced by the proteolytic enzyme, glycosylation-enhancing factor (GEF, a kallikrein-like enzyme) and bradykinin shares several features with that initiated by anti-IgE, in that both activate phospholipid methylation and adenylate cyclase and increase ^{45}Ca accumulation[46]. In support of the hypothesis that proteolytic cleavage of some as yet unknown substrate is involved in IgE-dependent histamine secretion, Ishizaka and Ishizaka[5] have demonstrated that trypsin and chymotrypsin inhibitors block IgE-dependent increases in phospholipid methylation and cAMP accumulation in rat mast cells. The observation that these two biochemical events were also blocked by serine esterase inhibitors in anti-IgE challenged mast cell plasma membranes suggests that the protease is associated with this cell fraction.

In summary, the observations of several independent workers indicate that activation of one or more serine esterases is involved in IgE-dependent histamine release. However, the protease involved has not yet been identified, nor has the mechanism of its activation or its substrate. These are important points to consider, as the protease appears to be involved in a very early stage of stimulus–secretion coupling.

BREAKDOWN OF PHOSPHOINOSITIDES

In a large number of systems it has been demonstrated that activation of cell-surface receptors ultimately linked to calcium mobilization enhances the breakdown of phosphoinositides[47–49]. In earlier studies, phosphatidyl-inositol (PI) breakdown to diacylglycerol was measured experimentally by analysing the incorporation of radiolabelled precursors such as [^{32}P]phosphate and [^{3}H]inositol into phosphatidic acid and PI derived from the newly-generated diacylglycerol (the 'PI cycle') (Figure 7.2). In rat mast cells, several workers[50–52] have demonstrated that various secretagogues including anti-IgE, compound 48/80, concanavalin A, calcium ionophore A23187 and chymotrypsin cause an accumulation of [^{32}P]phosphate into mast cell PI, suggestive of increased activity of the PI cycle. More recently, Ishizaka et al.[53] demonstrated enhanced [^{32}P]phosphate incorporation into various phospholipids consequent upon IgE-dependent-activation of human cultured basophils. With regard to the temporal relationship between enhanced phospholipid metabolism and histamine secretion, Kennerly et al.[50] demonstrated

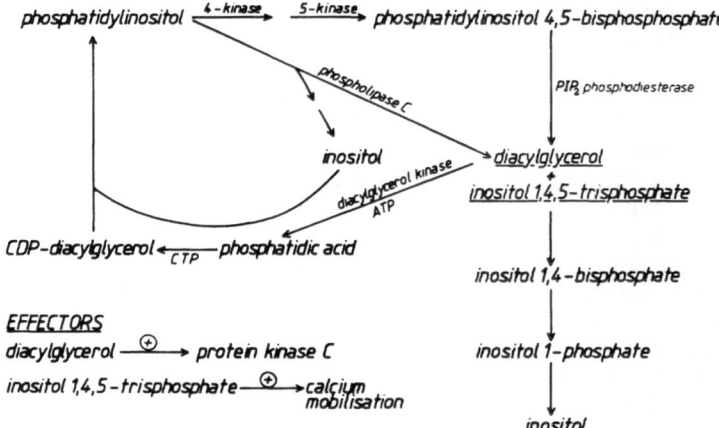

Figure 7.2 Stimulus-dependent breakdown of phosphatidylinositol and phosphoinositides and generation of secondary messengers. Abbreviations: CTP, cytidine triphosphate; CDP, cytidine diphosphate; ATP, adenosine triphosphate; PIP₂, phosphatidylinositol 4,5-bisphosphate

that [^{32}P]phosphate incorporation into phosphatidic acid occurred within 3 s of challenge with anti-IgE, whilst Ishizuka and Nozawa[54] demonstrated that antigen-induced breakdown of [^{3}H]glycerol-labelled PI occurred in parallel with histamine secretion. Thus, stimulus-dependent PI turnover can occur rapidly enough to play a role in signal transduction prior to calcium mobilization and, furthermore, the observation that PI breakdown can occur at the low levels of intracellular calcium normally found in unactivated rat mast cells suggests that it is not itself a secondary effect of increased cytosolic calcium[51].

More recently, interest has shifted to the potential role of polyphosphoinositide (PPI) breakdown in calcium mobilization. Phosphorylation of inositol hydroxyl groups by specific kinase enzymes results in the sequential formation of phosphatidylinositol-4-phosphate (PIP) and phosphatidyl-inositol-4,5-bisphosphate (PIP₂) (Figure 7.2)[55, 56]. The PPI are normally present as a minor proportion of eukaryotic cell PI[57]. A number of independent workers have demonstrated that, in various cells, PIP₂ breakdown follows activation of receptors linked to calcium mobilization[49]. This breakdown is mediated by phospholipase C-type enzymes (PIP₂ phosphodiesterases) with the resulting formation of diacylglycerol (DAG) and inositol-1,4,5-trisphosphate (IP₃). The mechanism whereby receptor activation leads to PIP₂ phosphodiesterase stimulation is uncertain. Recent evidence indicates that in some cells, including mast cells, the phosphodiesterase might be regulated by guanine nucleotide regulatory proteins (G-proteins) related to the inhibitory (Ni) G-protein involved in hormonal regulation of adenylate cyclase and cGMP phosphodiesterase[58–62]. However, whether such regulatory proteins are involved in the coupling of IgE-receptor activation to PIP₂ breakdown is unknown. Breakdown of IP₃ and termination of its ability to mobilize calcium from intracellular stores can occur either by direct removal of the 5-phosphate[63] or by conversion to inositol-(1,3,4,5)-tetrakisphosphate and 5-dephosphorylation[64].

In support of a role of PPI breakdown in histamine release, antigen activation of RBL-2H3 cells increases levels of inositol phosphates within 2–4 min of challenge[65, 66]. The degree of inositol phosphate accumulation correlated with the number of receptors aggregated[17], and occurred concurrently with increases in intracellular calcium and histamine secretion. However, unlike stimulus-dependent phosphoinositide breakdown in mast cells[51], this pathway in RBL cells shows a requirement for extracellular calcium[65] and is stimulated by calcium ionophore[67], presumably due to increased intracellular calcium. The relationships between PIP_2 breakdown and calcium ion fluxes in mast cells and basophils may be further complicated by observations that PIP_2 phosphodiesterase activity, at least in neutrophils, might be modulated by changes in calcium ion concentration[68]. However, other studies have demonstrated that PIP_2 hydrolysis can occur at submicromolar calcium ion concentrations[69].

Little is known about PPI hydrolysis in IgE-dependent mediator secretion from mast cells, as certain methodological difficulties have been encountered[66]. However, Ishizuka *et al.*[70] have demonstrated a rapid breakdown of PI 4-phosphate in rat mast cells within 5 s of antigen stimulation.

The relationship between stimulus-dependent PIP_2 breakdown observed in RBL cells and PI turnover in rat mast cells[50–52, 54] is uncertain. Increased [^{32}P]phosphate or [^{3}H]inositol incorporation into PI need not reflect enhanced PI breakdown, but rather a generally increased level of DAG, which could arise from a variety of sources. From studies with thrombin-stimulated platelets, Wilson *et al.*[71] have suggested that although PIP_2 breakdown does occur in these cells, with the resultant generation of IP_3, a large amount of PI is also hydrolysed. This latter phospholipid might serve to generate DAG, a putative second messenger in secretion.

The products of PIP_2 breakdown have important properties which suggest they may have potential roles in signal transduction in mast cells and basophils. Hydrolysis of PIP_2 by phospholipase C-type enzymes results in the formation of IP_3 and DAG. The former product has been demonstrated to mobilize calcium from intracellular stores, probably mainly endoplasmic reticulum[63, 72]. Various studies using permeabilized cells have demonstrated that submicromolar concentrations of IP_3 are required for half-maximal calcium release from intracellular stores[73]. Whether IP_3 can also provide calcium flux across the plasma membrane is uncertain. Interestingly, inositol-1-phosphate, which would result from PI hydrolysis, appears to be unable to mobilize calcium[73].

The other product of PI or PIP_2 breakdown, diacylglycerol, is known to be an activator of protein kinase C (C-kinase)[74]. This enzyme appears to be ubiquitously distributed in mammalian organs and various phyla[75]. Diacylglycerol activates C-kinase, in the presence of phospholipid, by reversibly increasing its affinity for calcium ions such that it can be activated at submicromolar concentrations of this cation[76, 77]. Diacylglycerol, derived from the hydrolysis of membrane phospholipids, could thus serve as a second messenger to activate protein phosphorylation. Experimentally, the effects of DAG on C-kinase can be mimicked by phorbol esters such as phorbol myristate acetate (PMA)[78, 79]. Several observations suggest that C-kinase activation may have a role in mast cell and basophil stimulus–secretion coupling. Firstly, in rat mast cells[54], mouse cultured mast cells[80] and human cultured basophils[53], IgE-dependent stimulation causes a rapid accumulation of DAG which precedes or is concurrent with histamine secretion. Secondly, White et al.[80] have demonstrated that antigen-activation of mouse cultured mast cells stimulates C-kinase activity associated with the cell particulate fraction. Kinase activation was maximal 30 s after challenge and preceded histamine secretion, and both enzyme activation and histamine release were similarly dependent on antigen concentration. Thirdly, phorbol esters at low concentrations (< 10 ng/ml) are poor histamine releasers alone, but potentiate histamine secretion activated by sub-optimal concentrations of IgE- and calcium ionophore stimuli in human basophils[81, 82], rat peritoneal mast cells[83, 84] and RBL cells[85]. With regard to the effector function of C-kinase, in rat mast cells, Katakami et al.[83] demonstrated that TPA induces phosphorylation of four endogenous cytosolic proteins of molecular weight 22 000, 31 000, 34 000 and 60 000 Daltons, this pattern of phosphorylation being mimicked by concanavalin A. Heiman and Crews[84] demonstrated stimulus-dependent phosphorylation of proteins of molecular weight 48 000, 55 000, 59 000 and 78 000 Daltons within one minute of stimulation with various stimuli. Compound 48/80, A23187, anti-IgE and concanavalin A showed a different pattern of protein phosphorylation, but the most consistent and largest changes occurred in the 48 000 Dalton fraction which was also the one most affected by TPA. However, although TPA potentiated A23187-induced histamine secretion, the effect on A23187-induced 48 000 Dalton fraction phosphorylation was no more than additive, demonstrating a poor correlation between phosphorylation of the 48 000 Dalton protein and mediator secretion.

The interactions between phorbol esters and other secretagogues suggest that C-kinase has a positive modulatory role in histamine secretion. Such a conclusion is supported by the findings that, in a variety of other cell types, C-kinase activation potentiates responses to calcium-mobilizing stimuli[73, 86]. The two products of PIP_2 breakdown, i.e. IP_3 and DAG, may therefore represent two limbs of a secondary messenger pathway which positively interact with each other. However, that C-kinase can also negatively modulate secretion is suggested by observations with RBL cells. Sagi-Eisenberg et al.[87] demonstrated that TPA at < 10 ng/ml potentiated antigen-induced serotonin release but, in contrast, completely blocked the intracellular calcium increase normally associated with this secretagogue. Analysis of the time-course of antigen-induced secretion in the presence of TPA demonstrated that TPA inhibited serotonin secretion during the early phase of secretion, but enhanced secretion thereafter, there being a net enhancement over the whole time-course. These workers suggested that TPA stimulated both an 'off' signal early in stimulus–secretion coupling and an 'on' signal later in the sequence. With higher concentrations of TPA, the 'off' signal predominated, with a net reduction of antigen-dependent serotonin secretion. The concept of C-kinase as a negative modulator of signal transduction is further supported by observations that, in mast cells[88] and a variety of other cell types[89–91], phorbol esters can inhibit phosphoinositide breakdown and calcium mobilization. This suggests that DAG normally formed during PIP_2 hydrolysis can exert a negative feedback effect, limiting receptor-mediated signals.

In conclusion, receptor-mediated breakdown of PIP_2 in mast cells and basophils can generate products with potential secondary messenger roles. Inositol-1,4,5-trisphosphate might serve to mobilize calcium from intracellular stores, whilst DAG can activate C-kinase, with subsequent protein phosphorylation. Studies of the potential roles of PIP_2 hydrolysis in mast cells and basophils are in their infancy, and our present theories draw heavily for support on what is known of this pathway and its products in other cell systems.

METHYLATION OF PHOSPHOLIPIDS

Cross-linkage of IgE-receptors occurs within the environment of the plasma membrane and, therefore, it might be expected that the earliest observable biochemical events in mast cells and basophils activated through these receptors would involve membrane components. In this regard, a variety of stimuli which activate mast cells and basophils via IgE-receptors have been reported to increase the methylation of the major membrane phospholipid phosphatidylethanolamine (PE). The pathway of PE methylation was first described in liver microsomes[92, 93]. By this pathway, a maximum of three methyl groups are incorporated into the ethanolamine moiety of PE, with the sequential formation of phosphatidyl-N-monomethyl-PE, phosphatidyl-N,N-dimethyl-PE and phosphatidylcholine. The enzyme catalysing these lipid conversions, PE N-methyltransferase, utilizes S-adenosylmethionine (AdoMet) as methyl donor and, in common with other AdoMet-dependent methyltransferases, is competitively inhibited by S-adenosylhomocysteine formed from AdoMet during transmethylation (Figure 7.3)[94, 95]. Adenosine and some of its analogues such as 3-deazaadenosine (DZA) inhibit methylation by promoting the accumulation of S-adenosylhomocysteine and other nucleosidyl-homocysteines. Liver microsomes are a particularly rich source of PE methyltransferase, and up to 40% of the total phosphatidylcholine of rat hepatocytes derives from this pathway[96]. However, the activity of this enzyme in other cell types, including mast cells, has been calculated to be 100- to 1000-fold lower[97].

Evidence for a central role of PE methylation in mast cell and basophil activation has derived from two lines of study. Firstly, radiolabelling studies have shown increased transfer of [³H-methyl] groups from [³H-methyl] AdoMet into cell lipids to occur rapidly following IgE-receptor cross-linkage. Secondly, pharmacological agents which inhibit AdoMet-dependent methylation also inhibit various biochemical changes associated with cell activation. Stimulus-dependent increases in lipid radiolabelling have been reported in rat peritoneal mast cells activated with concanavalin A[98], anti-IgE and anti-RBL[99], C3a and C5a[100]; in mouse mast cells activated with anti-IgE[101], antigen[102] and bradykinin[46]; in human lung mast cells activated with antigen

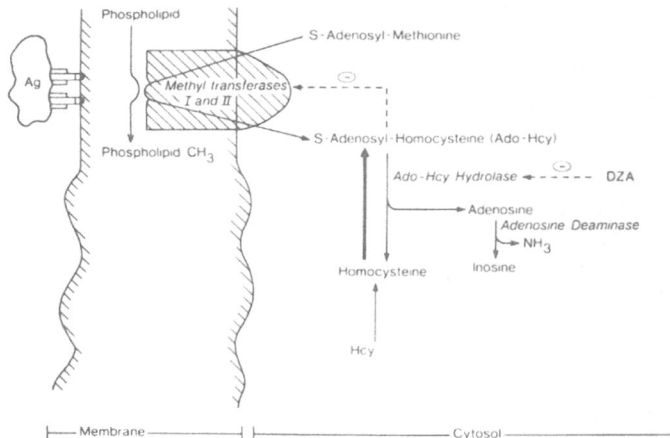

Figure 7.3 Proposed involvement of IgE-dependent phospholipid methylation in mast cells and inhibitory actions of 3-deazaadenosine and homocysteine thiolactone. Abbreviations: Ag, antigen binding at IgE-receptor; phospholipid CH_3, methylated phospholipid; DZA, 3-deaza-adenosine; Hcy, homocysteine thiolactone

and anti-IgE[103]; in human cultured basophils activated with anti-IgE[53] and in RBL-2H3 cells activated with antigen[104]. In each preparation, increased [^{3}H-methyl] incorporation into chloroform/methanol extracted lipids (used as an indicator of PE methylation) was transient, reaching a maximum at 15–30 s after stimulation in rat, mouse and human cells and 5 min in RBL cells. Levels of methylated lipids declined thereafter to baseline levels within 1–2 min (20 min in RBL cells) after challenge. The peak of stimulated lipid labelling varied from 2-fold[98] to > 120-fold[99] of that in unstimulated cells and preceded, or was concurrent with, stimulus-dependent increases in ^{45}Ca accumulation, cAMP synthesis, phosphoinositide metabolism and histamine secretion[5, 53]. The observation that increased lipid methylation is one of the earliest changes detectable in activated mast cells, coupled with the observations that methylation inhibitors such as DZA and homocysteine inhibit the later biochemical changes at similar concentrations to those which inhibit PE methylation, has led to the suggestion that phospholipid methylation is an essential process in signal transduction initiated through the IgE-receptor[5, 105].

However, recent studies have cast serious doubt on both the experimental and theoretical basis of the hypothesis that PE methylation is involved in signal transduction in mast cells and basophils. Several workers have been unable to confirm that IgE-dependent stimulation of these cells increases [^{3}H-methyl] incorporation into PE, no changes in lipid radiolabelling having been detected in rat mast cells stimulated with concanavalin A, antigen or anti-IgE[66, 106, 107], RBL-2H3 cells stimulated with antigen[66] or human lung mast cells stimulated with anti-IgE (Figure 7.4). These studies have also highlighted the potential inadequacy of using [^{3}H-methyl] incorporation into chloroform/methanol-extracted lipids as a measurement of PE

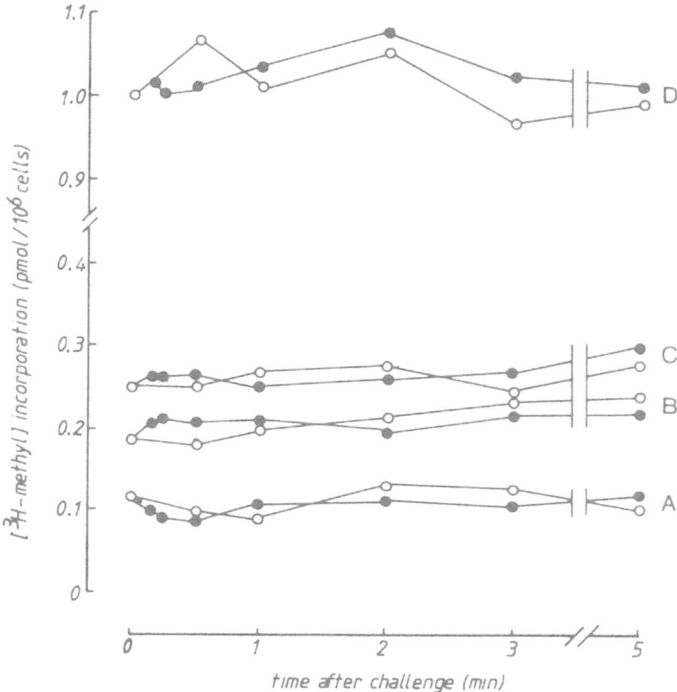

Figure 7.4 Lack of effect of anti-IgE stimulation on [³H-methyl] incorporation into chloroform/methanol-extracted lipids of mast cell-enriched human dispersed lung cells. Four preparations of lung cells containing A. 58%, B. 42%, C. 50%, and D. 55% mast cells were incubated for 30 minutes with L-[³H-methyl]methionine prior to activation with epsilon-chain-specific anti-IgE 25 μg/ml (O) or non-immune goat IgG (). Lipid methylation was measured as described in reference 103. Results are the means of duplicate determinations at each time point. Spontaneous and net anti-IgE-induced histamine releases were A. 5.8 and 42.2%, B. 13.2 and 29.1%, C. 6.7 and 22.3%, D. 10.1 and 25.6%, respectively. Thin layer chromatography of lipid extracts of two further preparations confirmed the absence of anti-IgE-dependent changes in radiolabelling of phosphatidylethanolamine

methylation[53, 98, 99, 103, 104], as typically only 30% of the total label in crude lipid extracts is associated with methyl derivatives of PE, the largest radio-labelled fraction being neutral lipids[66, 106, 107]. Analysis of rat mast cell[107] and human lung mast cell (unpublished observations) lipid extracts by thin-layer chromatography and high-pressure liquid chromatography[66] confirmed the absence of any stimulus-dependent changes in the formation of methylated PE derivatives.

Recent studies with methyltransferase inhibitors also cast doubt on the proposed role of stimulus-dependent PE methylation in activating adenylate cyclase[55, 103, 108] as the methyltransferase inhibitors DZA and homocysteine thiolactone (Hcy) do not diminish anti-IgE-dependent increases in cAMP in rat mast cells[107], human lung mast cells[109] or human basophils[110] at concentrations which inhibit histamine secretion by >50%. Indeed, in each cell type, these drugs increased both basal and stimulus-increased levels of cAMP, these effects being particularly marked in basophils. This may possibly reflect inhibition of cAMP phosphodiesterase by these compounds[111, 112]. As increased levels of cAMP are generally inhibitory to mediator secretion[113], these findings suggest an alternative mechanism whereby these commonly-used methyltransferase inhibitors might decrease mast cell and basophil secretion. The observation that DZA and Hcy inhibit histamine release from human lung mast cells activated with calcium ionophore[114], a secretagogue with which PE methylation has not previously been associated, is also inconsistent with the view that these drugs inhibit mast cell histamine secretion solely through effects on PE methylation. It remains possible that in human lung mast cells, methylation of as yet uncharacterized substrates might be involved in stimulus–secretion coupling distal to calcium influx, although this appears not to be the case in rat mast cells and human basophils in which DZA/Hcy inhibit only IgE-dependent secretion[115, 116]. Due to the wide spectrum of activity of DZA and Hcy as methyltransferase inhibitors, studies with these compounds are likely to yield little information about the nature of methylation reactions putatively involved in histamine secretion and merely demonstrate that the overall integrity of cellular transmethylation is necessary for secretion.

The precise mechanism whereby an increased formation of methylated phospholipids in mast cells/basophils might modulate the activity of calcium channels, adenylate cyclase and the enzymes of phosphoinositide breakdown has not been investigated. With regard to the control of adenylate cyclase activity, it has been postulated that increased methylation of PE increases membrane fluidity within the environment of this enzyme, perhaps facilitating its interaction with GTP regulatory proteins[108]. Although changes in membrane fluidity have never been measured in activated mast cells, such a hypothesis is supported by the observations of Hirata and co-workers that increases in the levels of methylated PE (particularly monomethyl derivative) in rat erythrocyte ghosts were associated with dramatic changes in membrane fluidity[117]. These workers have postulated that altered membrane fluidity was a consequence of transbilayer movement ('flip–flop') of PE during methylation[105, 118]. The basis for this postulate derives from the findings of these workers in several cell types[118–120] which suggest that PE methylation is catalysed by two distinct enzymes. The enzyme catalysing the first methylation is situated within the cytoplasmic leaflet of the plasma membrane and acts on PE within that leaflet catalysing its conversion to monomethyl-PE. By an unknown mechanism linked to this conversion, monomethyl-PE is then translocated across the bilayer to become a substrate for the second enzyme, situated within the extracellular-facing leaflet of the bilayer. This enzyme then catalyses the conversion of monomethyl-PE to dimethyl-PE and phosphatidylcholine. The 'flip–flop' of PE is, therefore, driven by the asymmetric distribution of the methyltransferases in the bilayer[105]. However, although the genetic studies of McGivney et al.[121] support the hypothesis that conversion of PE to phosphatidylcholine requires two enzymes in RBL cells, Audubert and Vance[122] have argued that in a variety of other cells only one enzyme is required, and several groups have demonstrated that the rat liver

PE methyltransferase is a single enzyme[123, 124]. In the light of these findings, as the number of enzymes involved in PE methylation in mast cells is unknown, it is probably too early to ascribe any functions to PE methylation such as modulation of membrane fluidity which are considered to be a consequence of an asymmetric distribution of two enzymes.

Regardless of the number of enzymes involved in their synthesis, the role of methylated PE derivatives in controlling membrane fluidity has been questioned. Firstly, Vance and de Kruijff[97] have calculated that the extremely small amounts of monomethyl PE formed in the rat erythrocyte preparations of Hirata and Axelrod[117] constituted $< 0.0012\%$ conversion of total plasma membrane PE, and concluded that this would be insufficient to cause the relatively large observed changes in membrane fluidity. Secondly, several workers[125-127] have failed to detect increased fluidity in membranes greatly enriched in monomethyl PE. Whether experimental manipulations which increase levels of methylated PE derivatives in mast cell membranes have any effects on membrane fluidity remains to be determined.

In summary, studies using methyltransferase inhibitors having a wide spectrum of activity suggest that the overall integrity of mast cell and basophil methylation is required for IgE-dependent secretion of histamine. Although evidence presented by Ishizaka and co-workers, suggests that, under certain circumstances, cross-linkage of IgE-receptors activates PE methylation, the observations of various other workers cast doubt on the importance of such lipid conversions to stimulus–secretion coupling.

CALCIUM ACCUMULATION

For some time it has been appreciated that calcium ions play an important role in secretion[128-130]. Evidence from some of the older studies supporting this hypothesis in mast cell secretion has been reviewed by Pearce[129] and will be briefly discussed.

Firstly, IgE-dependent histamine secretion from mast cells is dependent on, or greatly enhanced by, the inclusion of calcium ions (0.05–2 mmol/l) in the extracellular medium. Secondly, calcium ionophores such as A23187 and ionomycin activate mast cells and basophils for histamine release in calcium-containing media[131]. Mediator release by low concentrations ($< 10 \mu mol/l$) of A23187 is non-cytotoxic and induces morphological changes similar to IgE-directed stimuli. This might demonstrate that the mast cell secretory mechanism is always intact and only awaits an increase in intracellular calcium to initiate mediator release. Thirdly, calcium ions injected directly into rat mesentery mast cells by micropipette induces histamine secretion[132]. Fourthly, lanthanide ions, which have an ionic radius similar to that of calcium and which displace calcium ions from membrane binding sites, competitively inhibit IgE-dependent histamine release from rat mast cells[133].

Whilst these various studies demonstrate a general requirement of secretion for calcium ions, they give no information on changes in calcium disposition during or preceding secretion. Attempts have been made to measure changes in mast cell cytosolic calcium concentration following IgE-dependent stimulation by monitoring the accumulation of ^{45}Ca from the extracellular medium[99, 134, 135]. Foreman et al.[134] observed that accumulation of ^{45}Ca by rat mast cells was complete within 1 min of activation with antigen, concanavalin A or dextran, and roughly paralleled the time-course of histamine secretion. The observations that ^{45}Ca accumulation and histamine secretion were both similarly dependent on secretagogue concentration, similarly affected by pharmacological agents and that ^{45}Ca accumulation could be diminished by only 33% by metabolic inhibitors (which completely blocked secretion) suggested to these workers that radiolabel accumulation reflected calcium uptake in response to stimuli. ^{45}Ca uptake has been extensively used by Ishizaka and co-workers to measure calcium signals in activated mast cells and basophils of other species apart from rat, including human lung mast cells and basophils[53, 103] and mouse mast cells[46, 101]. In each case, increased accumulation of ^{45}Ca preceded or was concurrent with histamine secretion. However, the studies of various workers[136–138] suggest that mast cell accumulation of ^{45}Ca is poorly related to secretion, and a significant component of this accumulation reflects non-specific binding to granule membranes exposed during exocytosis. It has been calculated by Ishizaka and Ishizaka[5] that only 40% of observed ^{45}Ca accumulation reflects true calcium influx across the plasma membrane.

More recently, White et al.[102] used the fluorescent tetracarboxylate calcium chelator quin-2[139] to demonstrate that cytosolic calcium ion concentrations are increased in rat mast cells activated with antigen or A23187. Increases in fluorescence, which reached a maximum at 20–30 seconds following activation (in comparison with 1–2 min using ^{45}Ca), were related to the antigen concentration. A reduced, but detectable, increase in quin-2 calcium binding (and histamine secretion) was obtained following antigen activation in the absence of extracellular calcium ions, possibly demonstrating that this stimulus can release calcium ions from intracellular stores.

However, exposure of cells to high concentrations of quin-2, such as those used in this study (100 μmol/l), has been associated with cytotoxicity[66], which was not assessed in the studies of White et al.[102]. This fluorescent probe, at lower concentrations, has been used successfully to monitor calcium changes in stimulated RBL cells[65, 66, 140]. In these studies, antigen activation resulted in increases of up to 12-fold in internal calcium ion concentration from basal levels of approximately 100 nmol/l, within 3 min of activation. Increases in intracellular calcium were coincident with the initiation of histamine and arachidonate release and the hydrolysis of phosphoinositides. After an initial rapid increase, levels of intracellular calcium ions decreased only slowly as long as IgE-receptors remained cross-linked, but decreased rapidly when the linkages were disrupted. Further studies by Maeyama et al.[17] demonstrated that levels of intracellular calcium were directly related to the degree of IgE-receptor cross-linkage until all receptors were aggregated, whereas histamine release reached a maximum at sub-maximal levels of receptor aggregation. These findings suggest that histamine secretion is not limited by the availability of intracellular calcium.

What is the mechanism by which the calcium signal is generated? The numerous studies of Hirata and Ishizaka and their co-workers[5, 105] suggest that stimulus-dependent increases in phospholipid methylation have an important role in the opening of calcium channels in mast cells and basophils. The evidence for this postulate derives from several observations. Firstly, they have observed that a brief, monophasic increase in phospholipid methylation precedes ^{45}Ca accumulation following IgE-receptor cross-linkage in mast cells and basophils of a variety of species; secondly, inhibitors of cellular methylation block stimulus-dependent increases in ^{45}Ca accumulation; thirdly, phosphatidylserine, which reportedly activates phospholipid methyltransferase[98], enhances IgE-dependent ^{45}Ca accumulation[134] and quin-2 fluorescence[102] in rat mast cells. It has, therefore, been suggested[104] that increased phospholipid methylation increases plasma membrane fluidity in the environment of calcium channels facilitating their opening. However, as discussed later, several practical and theoretical considerations argue against this proposed role of phospholipid methylation.

A radically different mechanism of calcium gating has been proposed by Mazurek and co-workers who have suggested that the calcium gate is the cromolyn-binding protein (CBP) isolated by them from RBL cells[141, 142]. This 60 000 Dalton protein was undetectable in certain RBL variants which, although able to bind IgE, are unable to secrete histamine following IgE-dependent stimulation[143]. These variants regained their responsiveness when isolated CBP was subsequently implanted into their plasma membranes[144]. In planar bilayers reconstituted with both purified IgE-receptors and CBP, the addition of specific antigen or anti-IgE caused a marked change in ion conductance, as did the addition of anti-CBP antibodies to bilayers containing CBP (but not receptors) alone[145, 146]. These studies suggest that close juxtaposition of CBP within the plasma membrane allows the expression of calcium channel activity. Little is known about the interaction of CBP and the IgE-receptor, so the mechanism whereby receptor cross-linkage causes CBP aggregation is uncertain. So far CBP is the only effector system identified as directly interacting with the IgE-receptor. However, there are several serious faults with this attractively simple model which have been discussed by Metzger et al.[6].

Yet another calcium mobilization mechanism has been described in mast cells, the effectors being inositol phosphates, particularly inositol-1,4,5-trisphosphate. This has been discussed in detail in the section on phosphoinositide hydrolysis.

To summarize, a number of independent studies have demonstrated that IgE-dependent activation of mast cells and basophils increases intracellular concentrations of calcium ions. However, despite intensive research over the past decade the precise mechanism whereby IgE-receptor aggregation is linked to this calcium signal remains uncertain.

ADENYLATE CYCLASE AND PROTEIN KINASE ACTIVATION

Cross-linkage of IgE-receptors of rat mast cells[107, 108, 147–150], human basophils[53, 110, 151, 152] and human lung mast cells[103] is associated with increases in cellular cAMP concentrations. In each cell preparation, the early increase in cAMP is transient, reaching a maximum at 15–45 s following challenge, and declining to baseline in 2–3 min. Maximum accumulation of cAMP precedes or is concurrent with the onset of ^{45}Ca accumulation and histamine release, but follows stimulus-associated changes in phospholipid methylation. The possible relationship between phospholipid methylation and adenylate cyclase activation has been discussed in a previous section. A later rise in cAMP in rat mast cells at 2–3 min after stimulation can be suppressed by indomethacin, unlike the early rise, and is probably due to adenylate cyclase stimulation by mast cell-derived prostaglandin D_2[148]. It is, therefore, considered that only the early changes in cAMP may be involved in stimulus–secretion coupling.

The mast cell adenylate cyclase complex has been manipulated pharmacologically to determine whether the function of the transient rise in cAMP is to facilitate or inhibit mediator release. It has long been appreciated that agents which alter mast cell and basophil cAMP levels modulate mediator release. In early studies in guinea pig lung, high doses of adrenaline were shown to inhibit antigen-induced histamine secretion[153]. Similarly, in human lung fragments, mediator release is inhibited by agents which elevate cAMP[154], or enhanced by agents which decrease cellular cAMP[155]. Similar results have been obtained with human dispersed lung mast cells[156–158] and human basophils[159–163]. Such findings would suggest that the IgE-dependent increase in cAMP is inhibitory to secretion, possibly constituting a negative feedback mechanism. However, in rat serosal mast cells, in which the relationship between cyclic nucleotide changes and mediator secretion has been most thoroughly investigated, there appears to be no consistent relationship between changes in cAMP levels caused by various agents and inhibition of mediator secretion. For example, β-adrenoceptor agonists cause little or no inhibition of IgE-dependent mediator secretion despite raising cAMP levels[164–166]. However, some, but not all[167], inhibitors of cAMP phosphodiesterase, such as theophylline or 3-isobutyl-1-methyl-xanthine, which prevent the breakdown of endogenous cAMP, decrease mediator secretion by both IgE-dependent and non-immunological stimuli[168–171]. The studies of Holgate et al.[170] further demonstrate the complex relationship between cAMP levels and mediator secretion. These workers found that neither prostaglandin (PG) D_2 nor PGI_2 alone inhibited IgE-dependent mediator secretion despite raising cAMP 2–3-fold, whereas theophylline alone produced a dose-related inhibition of mediator release that was inversely correlated to mast cell levels of cAMP. Although theophylline enhanced PGD_2-dependent increases in cAMP, IgE-dependent histamine release was inhibited no more than with theophylline alone. On the basis of these results, it was suggested that several physical pools of adenylate cyclase may exist in rat mast cells which are differentially affected by stimuli and drugs, and only some of which are linked to the modulation of mediator secretion. Changes in cAMP of these different pools might be differently coupled to effector proteins, i.e. protein kinases. In rat mast cells, the early rise in cAMP is associated with the activation of cAMP-dependent protein kinases. These proteins constitute >94% of total cytosolic rat mast cell kinase activity, with type I kinase and type II kinase being present in the ratio

1.5:1. IgE-dependent activation induced a maximal increase in protein kinase activity at 60 s after challenge[172], with both isozymes being approximately equally activated. Theophylline, which both increased cAMP and inhibited IgE-dependent secretion, activated protein kinase, whereas prostaglandin D_2 raised cAMP but had little effect on secretion or kinase activation[173]. When added together, these agents increased kinase activity and decreased mediator release no more than theophylline alone, demonstrating a correlation between kinase activation and inhibition of mediator release.

In contrast, other observations suggest that increases in cAMP might facilitate secretion. Firstly, Holgate et al.[174] demonstrated that the ability of purine and ribose modified analogues of adenosine to inhibit or enhance IgE-dependent increases in cAMP paralleled their ability to inhibit or enhance mediator secretion. However, these studies are complicated by the ability of adenosine to enhance mediator secretion by a cAMP-independent mechanism[150]. Secondly, in human basophils[175] and rat mast cells[176], 2',5'-dideoxy-adenosine (DDA) inhibits IgE-dependent increases in cAMP and mediator secretion.

Studies using pharmacological agents to manipulate adenylate cyclase, therefore, give apparently discordant findings, in that agents which either enhance (e.g. phosphodiesterase inhibitors) or diminish (e.g. DDA) IgE-dependent changes in rat mast cell cAMP and protein kinase activity inhibit mediator secretion. It has, therefore, been postulated that the time-course of changes in drug-induced cAMP content relative to challenge might decide the final effect on mediator secretion. In support of this, in rat mast cells, the β-adrenoceptor agonist salbutamol or the adenylate cyclase activator forskolin inhibit antigen-dependent secretion when added 2–5 min prior to challenge, enhance secretion when added simultaneously with challenge, or have no effect when added after challege[177]. Similarly in human lung mast cells and basophils, adenosine has different effects depending on whether it is added before (inhibits secretion) or after (enhances secretion) IgE-dependent challenge[157, 163].

Sustained elevations of cAMP prior to challenge might inhibit secretion by prematurely activating protein kinases, leaving these enzymes in a non-activatable state at the time of subsequent challenge. This would be the case with phosphodiesterase inhibitors which are commonly added several minutes before challenge. However, stimulation of adenylate cyclase by salbutamol/forskolin added at challenge would coincide with and enhance the immunological stimulation of this enzyme. Added after challenge these drugs would stimulate adenylate cyclase too late in stimulus–secretion coupling to have any effect. A similar mechanism might explain the biphasic effects of adenosine in human lung mast cells[157] and basophils[163] in which addition of drug before or after IgE-dependent challenge inhibits or potentiates histamine secretion, respectively.

There are several potential mechanisms by which cAMP might inhibit mediator secretion. Firstly, in cells such as smooth muscle and platelets, increased levels of cAMP are associated with enhanced sequestration of calcium into intracellular stores secondary to phosphorylation of membrane proteins, e.g. sarcolemmal phospholamban[178–180]. Decreased cytoplasmic

211

availability of calcium ions would be expected to inhibit secretion. Secondly, protein kinase-dependent phosphorylation of myosin light-chain kinase[181] could potentially inhibit cytoskeletal changes associated with secretion[182]. Thirdly, increased levels of cAMP inhibit IgE-dependent increases in phospholipid turnover in rat mast cells[183], and thereby could decrease availability of diacylglycerol which, as described in a previous section, has a potential role as a second messenger for activation of protein kinase C. Fourthly, it has been demonstrated that theophylline[108] or isoprenaline[5] treatment of rat mast cells depresses IgE-dependent phospholipid methylation. According to the theories of Ishizaka and co-workers[5] decreased activity of this pathway would result in inhibition of mediator secretion.

Mechanisms by which cAMP might enhance secretion are less clear. In rat heart some agents which elevate cAMP activate a slow calcium channel following phosphorylation of a 23 000 Dalton sarcolemmal protein (calciductin)[184] which is thought to enhance the cytoplasmic accumulation of calcium. If a similar mechanism operated in mast cells, then agents which raise cAMP could enhance IgE-dependent calcium influx.

Despite these various pharmacological and biochemical observations, it is possible that IgE-dependent increases of cAMP have no important role in histamine secretion. Firstly, in RBL-2H3 cells, although there is a functional adenylate cyclase, IgE-dependent stimulation does not increase cAMP[5] although increases in phosphoinositide breakdown and calcium influx are evident[65]. Secondly, in human lung mast cells some workers[185, 186] have been unable to demonstrate IgE-dependent accumulation of cAMP, in contrast to the previous findings of Ishizaka et al.[103]. Thirdly, non-immunological agents which are effective secretagogues in rat mast cells do not increase cellular cAMP[149, 168, 187]. This latter observation would suggest that, if cAMP has any role in IgE-dependent secretion, then this occurs at an early stage in stimulus–secretion coupling which is not shared by these other stimuli.

With the recent appreciation that GTP-regulatory proteins might mediate the breakdown of phosphoinositides, it has been suggested that activation of adenylate cyclase by IgE-dependent stimuli might be a side effect of the liberation of stimulatory α-subunits of such proteins[177]. However, the observations that immunological stimuli also promote phosphoinositide breakdown but do not activate adenylate cyclase is not in accord with this. Alternatively, adenylate cyclase activation might be secondary to stimulus-dependent calcium accumulation in the cytoplasm[188].

In summary, despite intensive study for over a decade, the function of cAMP in mast cell and basophil secretion is poorly understood, there being evidence that supports a positive modulatory role, a negative modulatory role or no role for this cyclic nucleotide. A unifying hypothesis remains elusive.

PROTEIN PHOSPHORYLATION FOLLOWING STIMULATION

Several mast cell proteins are radiolabelled following activation of [^{32}P] phosphate loaded cells by both IgE-dependent and non-immunological stimuli. Challenge with anti-IgE, compound 48/80, ionophore A23187 and the peptide hormone somatostatin is associated with a calcium-dependent phosphorylation of up to four proteins of molecular weight 42 000, 59 000, 68 000 and 78 000 Dalton[189-193]. Compound 48/80-induced phosphorylation of the 42 000, 59 000 and 68 000 Dalton proteins was rapid in onset, peaking at 30 seconds, whilst phosphorylation of the 78 000 Dalton protein occurred more slowly reaching a maximum at 120 s and persisting until 300 s[189]. These time-course characteristics coupled with the observations that pharmacologically-induced phosphorylation of 78 000 Dalton protein inhibits secretion[190, 193], has led to the proposal that phosphorylation of the 42 000, 59 000 and 68 000 Dalton proteins is involved in the onset and/or continuation of secretion, whilst that of the 78 000 Dalton protein is involved in cessation of secretion. Whilst the nature of the protein kinases which modify these proteins are unknown, the evidence of Wells and Mann[193] suggests that the 78 000 Dalton protein is phosphorylated by a cGMP-dependent kinase. It should be noted that the four proteins reported by Sieghart and co-workers to be phosphorylated are of a different molecular weight from those modified following activation of rat mast cell protein kinase C[83] (see above). However, two proteins phosphorylated in the activated cell preparations of Heiman and Crews[84] are identical in molecular weight (59 000, 78 000 Dalton) to two of the proteins identified by Sieghart and co-workers.

ACTIVATION BY NON-IgE-DEPENDENT STIMULI

A large variety of compounds induce non-cytotoxic histamine secretion from rat serosal mast cells (reviewed in Reference 194). These include polybasic agents (compound 48/80, poly-L-lysine, poly-L-arginine), neuropeptides (substance P, somatostatin, vasoactive intestinal polypeptide), anaphlatoxins C3a and C5a, drugs (morphine, D-tubocurarine) and calcium ionophores (A23187, ionomycin). Whilst human basophils are stimulated by formyl methionyl-leucyl-phenylalanine[195], polylysine and polyarginine[196] and C5a[197], mast cells dispersed from human tissues secrete histamine only in response to calcium ionophore A23187 of various non-immunological stimuli so far tested[34, 198], with the notable exception of human skin mast cells which are responsive to substance P, poly-L-lysine, compound 48/80 and morphine[36, 199] (Table 7.1). Mast cell and basophil receptors for non-immunological stimuli have not been isolated as yet. Several stimuli, such as substance P, compound 48/80, poly-L-lysine and morphine may interact with a common, low-specificity receptor on human skin mast cells as the substance P antagonist (D-Pro^4, D-Trp$^{7, 9, 10}$)-substance P fragment 4-11 peptide[200] antagonizes histamine release by all these agents but not that by anti-IgE (unpublished observations). Whether this peptide actually inhibits binding at a receptor or is a functional antagonist is uncertain. A low-specificity receptor capable of binding a number of basic/neuropeptide secretagogues may also exist on rat serosal mast cells[201, 202].

The mechanism of stimulus-secretion coupling used by these non-immunological stimuli has not been as extensively investigated as that of IgE-dependent stimuli, but several observations suggest that the two types of

Table 7.1 Histamine release from human lung mast cells, skin mast cells and basophils in response to a variety of stimuli. $(+)$ = release, $(-)$ = no release

	Lung mast cell	Skin mast cell	Basophil
Stimulation			
Antigen	+	+	+
A23187	+	+	+
Co 48/80	−	+	−
Subs P	−	+	?
Morphine	−	+	−
Poly-L-lysine	−	+	+
FMLP	−	−	+

stimuli utilize different secretory pathways. Firstly, in both rat serosal[203] and human skin[36] mast cells, histamine release activated by substance P or compound 48/80 is very rapid, being complete in < 20 s, whilst that by anti-IgE requires > 3 min for completion. Secondly, histamine secretion by polybasic agents is either partially dependent (in human)[36] or independent (in rat)[129] on the presence of extracellular calcium ions, whereas IgE-dependent stimuli are much less effective in the absence of this cation. This suggests that the two stimuli utilize different calcium pools for secretion. Thirdly, the acidic lipid phosphatidylserine (PS) enhances the response of certain rodent mast cells to IgE-dependent but not non-immunological stimuli[204]. However, it should be noted that human mast cells show no enhanced response to IgE-dependent stimuli in the presence of phosphatidylserine[205]. The PS effect in rat mast cells may be intimately related to calcium requirement, as PS is known to facilitate both IgE-dependent accumulation of ^{45}Ca[134] and enhancement of quin-2 fluorescence[102] in rat mast cells. Fourthly, immunological stimulation of histamine secretion in the absence of calcium does not inhibit subsequent secretion by non-immunological stimulus, i.e. these stimuli do not exhibit cross-desensitization[196, 206, 207]. Fifthly, in human skin mast cells, although anti-IgE induces release of prostaglandin D_2 (40 ng/10^6 mast cells), concentrations of substance P which stimulate similar histamine secretion generate much less of this eicosanoid (3.5 ng/10^6 mast cells) (unpublished observations). Taken together, these five lines of evidence support the hypothesis that non-immunological stimuli have a secretory mechanism distinct from IgE-dependent stimuli.

However, with regard to the biochemistry of mediator secretion, research has so far been concentrated on the immunological stimulus, and little is known about stimulus–secretion coupling activated by any of the non-immunological stimuli. In rat mast cells, calcium ionophore and compound 48/80, like anti-IgE, stimulate phosphoinositide metabolism[50, 52] but do not stimulate phospholipid methylation[207]. This latter pathway is, however, activated by C3a and C5a[100] and the proteolytic enzyme glycosylation-enhancing factor[46]. Non-immunological stimuli also differ from IgE-dependent in failing to promote accumulation of cAMP in rat mast cells[149, 168, 187]. However, compound 48/80 does enhance ^{45}Ca accumulation by these cells[208, 209]. This latter observation does not seem to be in accord with the idea that compound 48/80 has no requirement for extracellular calcium ions for secretion. However, the relationship between stimulus-dependent ^{45}Ca accumulation and the calcium signal for secretion might be tenuous, as previously discussed above, and a better insight into the calcium pools utilized by non-immunological stimuli awaits the use of the new generation calcium indicators such as fura-2[210].

To summarize, compared to IgE-dependent stimuli, little is known about the receptors, secretory mechanism or released spectrum of mediators, associated with non-immunological stimuli. The discovery that human skin mast cells[36, 211, 212] and synovial mast cells[213] respond to non-immunological stimuli points to a potentially important physiological and pathological mechanism for mast cell activation distinct from the immediate allergic mechanism, and which will probably have different requirements for its pharmacological modulation.

CONCLUSIONS

Cross-linkage of mast cell or basophil high-affinity IgE-receptors causes several changes in cellular biochemistry considered to play a role in the release of preformed and newly-generated mediators of inflammation. Several of the earliest changes observed involve membrane phospholipids. Data accumulated over several years by Dr T. Ishizaka and co-workers suggest that PE methylation is a crucial event being intimately linked with calcium influx across the plasma membrane, adenylate cyclase activation and increased PI metabolism. However, there is presently a great deal of uncertainty about the role of this pathway in stimulus–secretion coupling. The other pathway involving phospholipids, the breakdown of phosphoinositides, generates products which can both increase membrane permeability to calcium ions (inositol-1,4,5-trisphosphate) and promote covalent modification of proteins (diacylglycerol activation of protein kinase C). Increased accumulation of cAMP, with resultant activation of protein kinases, represents another means of modifying the activity of a different spectrum of proteins through phosphorylation. Although a number of proteins have been identified as substrates for both cAMP-dependent and Ca^{2+}-phospholipid-dependent protein kinases in mast cells and basophils, as yet no role has been ascribed to them. With regard to the involvement of serine esterases in secretion, activation of enzymes by proteolytic cleavage has been known for many years to be involved in amplification cascades such as complement fixation and blood coagulation. It is interesting to speculate that serine esterases thought to be activated following mast cell activation might be involved in a similar amplification cascade. Whatever the role of such proteases, along with protein kinase they represent another means of modifying protein function.

There are still many gaps in our understanding of stimulus–secretion coupling, particularly the mechanism whereby IgE-receptor aggregation is linked to activation of the various phospholipid-modifying enzymes, serine esterases and adenylate cyclase. Recent studies demonstrating that GTP-regulatory proteins are able to modify the activity of adenylate cyclase[214] and polyphosphoinositide phosphodiesterase[61] make these proteins good candidates for second messenger molecules, translating the receptor aggregation signal to activation of enzyme systems.

In conclusion, the field of signal transduction in mast cells and basophils is expanding rapidly and, invariably, reviews of the subject become quickly outdated. However, the various pathways of lipid and protein biochemistry believed to be involved in stimulus–secretion coupling should be considered not in isolation but rather as an integrated system, the understanding and control of which, both physiologically and pharmacologically, is our ultimate goal.

References

1. Schwartz, L. B., Riedel, C., Caulfield, J. P., Wasserman, S. I. and Austen, K. F. (1981). Cell association of complexes of chymase, heparin proteoglycan and protein after degranulation by rat mast cells. *J. Immunol.*, **126**, 2071–8
2. Schwartz, L. B., Lewis, R. A., Seldin, D. and Austen, K. F. (1981). Acid hydrolases and tryptase from secretory granules of dispersed lung mast cells. *J. Immunol.*, **126**, 1290–4
3. Schwartz, L. B., Riedel, C., Schratz, J. J. and Austen, K. F. (1982). Localization of carboxypeptidase A to the macromolecular heparin proteoglycan–protein complex in secretory granules of rat serosal mast cells. *J. Immunol.*, **128**, 1128–33
4. MacGlashan, D. W. and Lichtenstein, L. M. (1983). Studies of antigen binding on human basophils. I. Antigen binding and functional consequences. *J. Immunol.*, **130**, 2330–6
5. Ishizaka T. and Ishizaka, K. (1984). Activation of mast cells for mediator release through IgE receptors. *Prog. Allergy*, **34**, 188–235
6. Metzger, H., Alcarez, G., Hohman, R., Kinet, J.-P., Pribluda, V. and Quarto, R. (1986). The receptor with high affinity for immunoglobulin E. *Ann. Rev. Immunol.*, **4**, 419–70
7. Ishizaka, K. and Ishizaka, T. (1968). Induction of erythema wheal reactions by soluble antigen – IgE antibody complexes in man. *J. Immunol.*, **101**, 68–78
8. Segal, D. M., Taurog, J. D. and Metzger, H. (1977). Dimeric immunoglobulin E serves as a unit for mast cell degranulation. *Proc. Natl. Acad. Sci. USA*, **74**, 2993–7
9. Ishizaka, T. and Ishizaka, K. (1978). Triggering of histamine release from rat mast cells by divalent antibodies against IgE receptors. *J. Immunol.*, **120**, 800–5
10. Siraganian, R. P., Hook, W. A. and Levine, B. B. (1975). Specific *in vitro* histamine release from basophils by divalent haptens: Evidence for activation by simple bridging of membrane-bound antibody. *Immunochemistry*, **12**, 149–57
11. Fewtrell, C. and Metzger, H. (1980). Larger oligomers of IgE are more effective than dimers in stimulating rat basophilic leukemia cells. *J. Immunol.*, **125**, 701–10
12. Kagey-Sobotka, A., Dembo, M., Goldstein, B., Metzger, M. and Lichtenstein, L. M. (1981). Qualitative characteristics of histamine release from human basophils by covalently cross-linked IgE. *J. Immunol.*, **127**, 2285–91
13. Conrad, D. H., Bazin, H., Sehon, A. H. and Froese, A. (1975). Binding parameters of the interaction between rat IgE and rat mast cell receptors. *J. Immunol.*, **114**, 1688–91
14. Kulczycki, A. Jr. and Metzger, H. (1974). The interaction of IgE with rat basophilic leukaemia cells. II Quantitative aspects of the binding reaction. *J. Exp. Med.*, **140**, 1676–95
15. Coleman, J. W. and Godfrey, R. C. (1981). The number and affinity of IgE receptors on dispersed human lung mast cells. *Immunology*, **44**, 859–63
16. Malveaux, F. J., Conroy, M. C., Adkinson, N. F. and Lichtenstein, L. M. (1978). IgE receptors on human basophils: relationship to serum IgE concentration. *J. Clin. Invest.*, **62**, 176–81

17. Maeyama, R., Hohman, R. J., Metzger, H. and Beaven, M. A. (1985). IgE receptor cross linking, phosphatidylinositol (PI) breakdown and histamine release in rat basophil leukemia cells: enhanced response with D20 (Abstr.). *Fed. Proc.*, **44**, 1917

18. Stanworth, D. R., Humphrey, J. H., Bennich, H. and Johansson, S. G. O. (1968). Inhibition of Prausnitz–Kustner reaction by proteolytic-cleavage fragments of a human myeloma protein of immunoglobulin class E. *Lancet*, **2**, 17–18

19. Ishizaka, K., Ishizaka, T. and Lee, E. H. (1970). Biologic functions of the Fc fragments of E myeloma protein. *Immunochemistry*, **7**, 687–702

20. Perez-Montfort, R. and Metzger, H. (1982). Proteolysis of soluble IgE-receptor complexes: Localization of sites on IgE which interact with the Fc receptor. *Mol. Immunol.*, **19**, 1113–25

21. Baird, B. and Holowka, D. (1985). Structural mapping of Fc receptor-bound immunoglobulin E: Proximity to the membrane surface of the antibody combining site and another site in the Fab segments. *Biochemistry*, **24**, 6252–9

22. Ishizaka, T. and Conrad, D. H. (1983). Binding characteristics of human IgE receptors and initial triggering events in human mast cells for histamine release. *Monogr. Allergy*, **18**, 14–24

23. Metzger, H. (1983). The receptor on mast cells and related cells with high affinity for IgE. In Inman, F. P. and Kindt, T. J. (eds.) *Contemporary Topics in Molecular Immunology*, pp. 115–45. (NY: Plenum)

24. Froese, A. (1984). Receptors for IgE on mast cells and basophils. *Prog. Allergy*, **34**, 142–87

25. Heffetz, D. and Zick, Y. (1986). Receptor aggregation is necessary for activation of the soluble insulin receptor kinase. *J. Biol. Chem.*, **261**, 889–94

26. Ramachandran, J. and Ullrich, A. (1987). Hormonal regulation of protein tyrosine kinase activity. *Trends Pharmacol. Sci.*, **8**, 28–31

27. Hempstead, B. L., Parker, C. W. and Kulczycki, A. (1983). Selective phosphorylation of the IgE receptor in antigen-stimulated rat mast cells. *Proc. Natl. Acad. Sci. USA*, **80**, 3050–3

28. Hempstead, B. L., Kulczycki, A. and Parker, C. W. (1981). Phosphorylation of the IgE-receptor from ionophore A23187 stimulated intact rat mast cells. *Biochem. Biophys. Res. Commun.*, **98**, 815–22

29. Perez-Montfort, R., Fewtrell, C. and Metzger, H. (1983). Changes in the receptor for immunoglobulin E coincident with receptor-mediated stimulation of basophilic leukemia cells. *Biochemistry*, **22**, 5733–7

30. Teshima, R., Ikebuchi, H. and Terao, T. (1984). Ca++ dependent and phorbol ester activating phosphorylation of a 36 K-dalton protein of rat basophilic leukaemia cell membranes and immunoprecipitation of the phosphorylated protein with IgE-anti-IgE system. *Biochem. Biophys. Res. Commun.*, **125**, 867–74

31. Stanworth, D. R., Kings, M., Roy, P. D., Moran, J. M. and Moran, D. M. (1979). Synthetic peptides comprising sequences of human immunoglobulin E heavy chain capable of releasing histamine. *Biochem. J.*, **180**, 665–8

32. Stanworth, D. R., Coleman, J. W. and Khan, Z. (1984). Essential structural requirements for triggering of mast cells by a synthetic peptide comprising a sequence in the C$_\epsilon$4 domain of human IgE. *Mol. Immunol.*, **21**, 243–7

33. Stanworth, D. R. (1984). The role of non-antigen receptors in mast cell signalling processes. *Mol. Immunol.*, **21**, 1183–90

34. Church, M. K., Pao, G. J.-K. and Holgate, S. T. (1982). Characterization of histamine secretion from dispersed human lung mast cells: effects of anti-IgE, calcium ionophore A23187, compound 48/80 and basic polypeptides. *J. Immunol.*, **129**, 2116–21

35. Coleman, J. W., Holgate, S. T., Church, M. K. and Godfrey, R. C. (1981). Immunoglobulin E decapeptide induced 5-hydroxytryptamine release from rat peritoneal mast cells: comparison with corticotropin-(1-24)-peptide, polyarginine, polylysine and antigen. *Biochem. J.*, **198**, 615–19

36. Benyon, R. C., Lowman, M. A. and Church, M. K. (1987). Human skin mast cells: their dispersion, purification and secretory characterization. *J. Immunol.*, **138**, 861–7

37. Austen, K. F. and Brocklehurst, W. E. (1960). Anaphylaxis in chopped guinea pig lung. 1. Effect of peptidase substrates and inhibitors. *J. Exp. Med.*, **113**, 521–39

38. Becker, E. L. and Austen, K. F. (1966). Mechanisms of immunologic injury of rat peritoneal mast cells. I The effect of phosphonate inhibitors on the homocytotropic antibody-mediated histamine release and the first component of rat complement. *J. Exp. Med.*, **124**, 379–95
39. Austen, K. F. and Becker, E. L. (1966). Mechanisms of immunologic injury of rat mast cells. II Complement requirement and phosphonate ester inhibition of release of histamine by rabbit anti-rat gamma globulin. *J. Exp. Med.*, **124**, 397–405
40. Kaliner, M. and Austen, K. F. (1973). A sequence of biochemical events in the antigen-induced release of chemical mediators from sensitized human lung tissues. *J. Exp. Med.*, **138**, 1077–94
41. Pruzansky, J. J. and Patterson, R. (1975). The diisopropylfluorophosphate inhibitable step in antigen-induced histamine release from human leukocytes. *J. Immunol.*, **114**, 939–43
42. Uvnas, B. and Antonsson, J. (1963). Triggering action of phosphatidase A and chymo-trypsins on degranulation of rat mesentery mast cells. *Biochem. Pharmacol.*, **12**, 867–73
43. Lagunoff, D., Chi, E. Y. and Wan, H. (1975). Effects of chymotrypsin and trypsin on rat peritoneal mast cells. *Biochem. Pharmacol.*, **24**, 1573–8
44. Schick, B., Austen, K. F. and Schwartz, L. B. (1984). Activation of rat serosal mast cells by chymase, an endogenous secretory granule protease. *J. Immunol.*, **132**, 2571–7
45. Schick, B. and Austen, K. F. (1985). Pharmacological modulation of activation-secretion of rat serosal mast cells by chymase, an endogenous secretory granule protease. *Immunology*, **56**, 513–22
46. Ishizaka, T., Iwata, M. and Ishizaka, K. (1985). Release of histamine and arachidonate from mouse mast cells induced by glycosylation-enhancing factor and bradykinin. *J. Immunol.*, **134**, 1880–7
47. Michell, R. H. (1975). Inositol phospholipids and cell surface receptor function. *Biochim. Biophys. Acta*, **415**, 81–147
48. Farese, R. V. (1983). The phosphatidate–phosphoinositide cycle: an intracellular messenger system in the action of hormones and neurotransmitters. *Metabolism*, **32**, 628–41
49. Berridge, M. J. (1984). Inositol trisphosphate and diacylglycerol as second messengers. *Biochem. J.*, **220**, 345–60
50. Kennerly, D. A., Suilivan, T. J. and Parker, C. W. (1979). Activation of phospholipid metabolism during mediator release from stimulated rat mast cells. *J. Immunol.*, **122**, 152–9
51. Cockcroft, S. and Gomperts, B. D. (1979). Evidence for a role of phosphatidylinositol turn-over in stimulus–secretion coupling. Studies with rat peritoneal mast cells. *Biochem. J.*, **178**, 681–7
52. Schellenberg, R. R. (1980). Enhanced phospholipid metabolism in rat mast cells stimulated to release histamine. *Immunology*, **41**, 123–9
53. Ishizaka, T., Conrad, D. H., Huff, T. F., Metcalfe, D. D., Stevens, R. L. and Lewis, R. A. (1985). Unique features of human basophilic granulocytes developed in *in vitro* culture. *Int. Arch. Allergy Appl. Immunol.*, **77**, 137–43
54. Ishizuka, Y. and Nozawa, Y. (1983). Concerted stimulation of PI turnover, Ca^{2+} influx and histamine release in antigen activated rat mast cells. *Biochem. Biophys. Res. Commun.*, **117**, 716–27
55. Hawthorne, J. N. and Pickard, M. R. (1979). Phospholipids in synaptic function. *J. Neurochem.*, **32**, 5–14
56. Downes, C. and Michell, R. H. (1982). Phosphatidylinositol-4-phosphate and phos-phatidylinositol 4,5-bisphosphate; Lipids in search of a function. *Cell Calcium*, **3**, 467–502
57. Majerus, P. W., Neufeld, E. J. and Wilson, D. B. (1984). Production of phosphoinositide-derived messengers. *Cell*, **37**, 701–3
58. Rodbell, M. (1980). The role of hormone receptors and GTP-regulatory proteins in mem-brane transduction. *Nature*, **284**, 17–22
59. Manning, D. R. and Gilman, A. G. (1983). The regulatory components of adenylate cyclase and transducin. *J. Biol. Chem.*, **258**, 7059–63
60. Gomperts, B. D. (1983). Involvement of guanine nucleotide binding protein in the gating of calcium by receptors. *Nature*, **306**, 64–6

61. Cockcroft, S. and Gomperts, B. D. (1985). Role of guanine nucleotide binding protein in the activation of polyphosphoinositide phosphodiesterase. *Nature*, **314**, 534–6
62. Nakamura, T. and Ui, M. (1985). Simultaneous inhibitions of inositol phospholipid breakdown, arachidonic acid release, and histamine secretion in rat mast cells by islet-activating protein, pertussis toxin. *J. Biol. Chem.*, **260**, 3584–93
63. Berridge, M. J. and Irvine, R. F. (1984). Inositol trisphosphate, a novel second messenger in cellular signal transduction. *Nature*, **312**, 315–21
64. Irvine R. F., Letcher, A. J., Heslop, J. P. and Berridge, M. J. (1986). The inositol tris/ tetrakisphosphate pathway – demonstration of Ins(1,4,5)P3 3-kinase activity in animal tissues. *Nature*, **320**, 631–4
65. Beaven, M. A., Moore, J. P., Smith, G., Hesketh, T. R. and Metcalfe, J. C. (1984). The calcium signal and phosphatidyl-inositol turnover in 2H3 cells. *J. Biol. Chem.*, **259**, 7137–42
66. Moore, J. P., Johannsson, A., Hesketh, T. R., Smith, G. A. and Metcalfe, J. C. (1984). Calcium signals and phospholipid methylation in eukaryotic cells. *Biochem. J.*, **221**, 675–84
67. Lo, T. N., Saul, W. and Beaven, M. A. (1987). Ionophore-induced secretion from rat leukemic basophil (2H3) cell requires cellular ATP and hydrolysis of inositol phospholipids. *Fed. Proc.*, **46**, 930 (Abstr.)
68. Cockcroft, S., Baldwin, J. M. and Allan, D. (1984). The Ca²⁺-activated polyphosphoinositide phosphodiesterase of human and rabbit neutrophil membranes. *Biochem. J.*, **221**, 477–82
69. Irvine, R. F., Letcher, A. J. and Dawson, R. M. C. (1984). Phosphatidylinositol-4,5-bisphosphate phosphodiesterase and phosphomonoesterase activities of rat brain. *Biochem. J.*, **218**, 177–85
70. Ishizuka, Y., Imai, A. and Nozawa, Y. (1984). Polyphosphoinositide turnover in rat mast cells stimulated by antigen: rapid and preferential breakdown of phosphatidylinositol-4-phosphate (DPI). *Biochem. Biophys. Res. Commun.*, **123**, 875–81
71. Wilson, D. B., Neufeld, E. J. and Majerus, P. W. (1985). Phosphoinositide interconversion in thrombin-stimulated human platelets. *J. Biol. Chem.*, **260**, 1046–51
72. Streb, H., Irvine, R. F., Berridge, M. J. and Schutz, I. (1983). Release of calcium from a nonmitochondrial intracellular store in pancreatic acinar cells by inositol-1,4,5 trisphosphate. *Nature*, **306**, 67–9
73. Berridge, M. J. (1986). Inositol trisphosphate: a new second messenger. In Schou. J. S., Geisler, A., Norn, S. (eds.) *Drug Receptors and Dynamic Processes in Cells (Alfred Benzon Symposium)*, pp. 99–104. (Copenhagen: Munksgaard)
74. Kishimoto, A., Takai, Y., Mori, T., Kikkawa U. and Nishizuka, Y. (1980). Activation of calcium and phospholipid-dependent protein kinase by diacylglycerol and its possible relation to phosphatidylinositol turnover. *J. Biol. Chem.*, **255**, 2272–6
75. Kuo, J. F., Andersson, R. C. G., Wise, B. C., Mackerlova, L., Salomonsson, I., Brackett, N. L., Katoh, N., Shoji, M. and Wrenn, R. W. (1980). Calcium-dependent protein kinase: widespread occurrence in various tissues and phyla of the animal kingdom and comparison of effects of phospholipid, calmodulin and trifluoperazine. *Proc. Natl. Acad. Sci. USA*, **77**, 7039–43
76. Takai, Y., Kishimoto, A., Kikkawa, U., Mori, T. and Nishizuka, Y. (1979). Unsaturated diacylglycerol as a possible messenger for the activation of calcium activated phospholipid dependent protein kinase system. *Biochem. Biophys. Res. Commun.*, **91**, 1218–24
77. Kaibuchi, K., Takai, Y. and Nishizuka, Y. (1981). Cooperative roles of various membrane phospholipids in the activation of calcium activated, phospholipid-dependent protein kinase. *J. Biol. Chem.*, **256**, 7146–9
78. Castagna, M., Takai, Y., Kaibuchi, K., Sano, K., Kikkawa, U. and Nishizuka, Y. (1982). Direct activation of calcium-activated, phospholipid-dependent protein kinase C by tumor-promoting phorbol esters. *J. Biol. Chem.*, **257**, 7847–51
79. Niedel, J. E., Kuhn, L. J. and Vandenbark, G. R. (1983). Phorbol diester receptor co-purifies with protein kinase C. *Proc. Natl. Acad. Sci. USA*, **80**, 36–40
80. White, J. R., Plaznik, D. H., Ishizaka, K. and Ishizaka, T. (1985). Antigen-induced increase in protein kinase C activity in plasma membranes of mast cells. *Proc. Natl. Acad. Sci. USA*, **82**, 8193–7
81. Schleimer, R. P., Gillespie, E. and Lichtenstein, L. M. (1981). Release of histamine from

human leukocytes stimulated with the tumour-promoting phorbol diesters. 1 Characterization of the response. *J. Immunol.*, **126**, 570–4

82. Schleimer, R. P., Gillespie, E., Daiuta, R. and Lichtenstein, L. M. (1982). Release of histamine from human leukocytes stimulated with the tumour-promoting phorbol esters: 2. Interactions with other stimuli. *J. Immunol.*, **128**, 136–40

83. Katakami, Y., Kaibuchi, K., Sawamura, M., Takai, Y. and Nishizuka, Y. (1984). Synergistic action of protein kinase C and calcium for histamine release from rat peritoneal mast cells. *Biochem. Biophys. Res. Commun.*, **121**, 573–8

84. Heiman, A. S. and Crews, F. T. (1985). Characterization of the effects of phorbol esters on rat mast cell secretion. *J. Immunol.*, **134**, 548–55

85. Sagi-Eisenberg, R. and Pecht, I. (1984). Protein kinase C, a coupling element between stimulus and secretion of basophils. *Immunol. Lett.*, **8**, 237–41

86. Knight, D. E. and Baker, P. F. (1983). The phorbol ester TPA increases the affinity of exocytosis for calcium in 'leaky' adrenal medullary cells. *FEBS Lett.*, **160**, 98–100

87. Sagi-Eisenberg, R., Lieman, H. and Pecht, I. (1985). Protein kinase C regulation of the receptor-coupled calcium signal in histamine-secreting rat basophilic leukaemia cells. *Nature*, **313**, 59–60

88. Okano, Y., Takagi, H., Nakashima, S., Tohmatsu, T. and Nozawa, Y. (1985). Inhibitory action of phorbol myristate acetate on histamine secretion and polyphosphoinositide turnover induced by compound 48/80 in mast cells. *Biochem. Biophys. Res. Commun.*, **132**, 110–17

89. Watson, S. P. and Lapetina, E. G. (1985). 1,2 Diacylglycerol and phorbol esters inhibit agonist-induced formation of inositol phosphates in human platelets: possible implications for negative feedback regulation of inositol phospholipid hydrolysis. *Proc. Natl. Acad. Sci. USA*, **82**, 2623–6

90. Orellana, S. A., Solski, P. A. and Brown, J. H. (1985). Phorbol ester inhibits phosphoinositide hydrolysis and calcium mobilization in cultured astrocytoma cells. *J. Biol. Chem.*, **260**, 5236–9

91. Gold, M. R. and DeFranco, A. L. (1987). Phorbol esters and dioctanoylglycerol block anti-IgM-stimulated phosphoinositide hydrolysis in the murine B cell lymphoma WEH1-231. *J. Immunol.*, **138**, 868–76

92. Bremer, J., Figard, P. H. and Greenberg, D. M. (1960). The biosynthesis of choline and its relation to phospholipid metabolism. *Biochim. Biophys. Acta*, **43**, 477–88

93. Bremer, J. and Greenberg, D. M. (1961). Methyl transferring enzyme system of microsomes in the biosynthesis of lecithin (phosphatidylcholine). *Biochim. Biophys. Acta*, **46**, 205–16

94. Cantoni, G. L. and Scarano, E. (1954). The formation of S-adenosylhomocysteine in enzymatic transmethylation reactions. *J. Am. Chem. Soc.*, **76**, 4744

95. Borchardt, R. T. (1977). Synthesis and biological activity of analogs of adenosylhomocysteine as inhibitors of methyltransferases. In Salvatore, F., Borek, E., Zappia, V., Williams-Ashman, H. G. and Schlenk, F. (eds.) *The Biochemistry of S-Adenosylmethionine*, pp. 151–71. (NY: Columbia Univ. Press)

96. Sundler, R. and Akesson, B. (1975). Regulation of phospholipid biosynthesis in isolated rat hepatocytes. Effect of different substrates. *J. Biol. Chem.*, **250**, 3359–67

97. Vance, D. E. and de Kruijff, B. (1980). The possible functional significance of phosphatidylethanolamine methylation. *Nature*, **288**, 277–8

98. Hirata, F., Axelrod, J. and Crews, F. T. (1979). Concanavalin A stimulates phospholipid methylation and phosphatidylserine decarboxylation in rat mast cells. *Proc. Natl. Acad. Sci. USA*, **76**, 4813–16

99. Ishizaka, T., Hirata, F., Ishizaka, K. and Axelrod, J. (1980). Stimulation of phospholipid methylation, Ca^{2+} influx, and histamine release by bridging of IgE receptors on rat mast cells. *Proc. Natl. Acad. Sci. USA*, **77**, 1903–6

100. Ishizaka, T. (1983). Methylation of membrane phospholipid in mast cell activation. In Hadden, J. W. (ed.) *Advances in Immunopharmacology*, pp. 623–8. (Oxford: Pergamon)

101. Daeron, M., Sterk, A. R., Hirata, F. and Ishizaka, T. (1982). Biochemical analysis of glucocorticoid-induced inhibition of IgE-mediated histamine release from mouse mast cells. *J. Immunol.*, **129**, 1212–18

102. White, J. R., Ishizaka, T., Ishizaka, K. and Sha'afi, R. I. (1984). Direct demonstration of increased intracellular concentration of free calcium as measured by quin-2 in stimulated rat peritoneal mast cell. *Proc. Natl. Acad. Sci. USA*, **81**, 3978–82

103. Ishizaka, T., Conrad, D. H., Schulman, E. S., Sterk, A. R. and Ishizaka, K. (1983). Biochemical analysis of initial triggering events of IgE-mediated histamine release from human lung mast cells. *J. Immunol.*, **130**, 2357–62

104. Crews, F. T., Morita, Y., McGivney, A., Hirata, F., Siraganian, R. P. and Axelrod, J. (1981). IgE-mediated histamine release in rat basophilic leukaemia cells: receptor activation, phospholipid methylation, Ca flux, and release of arachidonic acid. *Arch. Biochem. Biophys.*, **212**, 561–71

105. Hirata, F. and Axelrod, J. (1980). Phospholipid methylation and biological signal transduction. *Science*, **209**, 1082–90

106. Boam, D. S. W., Stanworth, D. R., Spanner, S. G. and Ansell, G. B. (1984). Is the stepwise methylation of phosphatidyl ethanolamine relevant to the release of histamine from the mast cell? *Biochem. Soc. Trans.*, **12**, 782–3

107. Benyon, R. C., Church, M. K. and Holgate, S. T. (1986). IgE-dependent activation of mast cells is not associated with enhanced phospholipid methylation. *Biochem. Pharmacol.*, **35**, 2535–44

108. Ishizaka, T., Hirata, F., Sterk, A. R., Ishizaka, K. and Axelrod, J. A. (1981). Bridging of IgE receptors activates phospholipid methylation and adenylate cyclase in mast cell plasma membranes. *Proc. Natl. Acad. Sci. USA*, **78**, 6812–16

109. Benyon, R. C., Church, M. K., Holgate, S. T. and Hughes, P. J. (1985). Methyltransferase inhibitors may inhibit histamine released by elevating cyclic AMP in mast cells and basophils (Abstr.). *Br. J. Pharmacol.*, **86** (Proceedings Suppl.), 407P

110. Hughes, P. J., Benyon, R. C. and Church, M. K. (1987). Adenosine inhibits IgE-dependent histamine secretion from human basophil leukocytes by two independent mechanisms. *J. Pharmacol. Exp. Ther.*, **242**, 1064–70

111. Zimmerman, T. P., Schmitges, C. J., Wolberg, G., Deeprose, R. D., Duncan, G. S., Cuatrecasas, P. and Elion, G. B. (1980). Modulation of cyclic AMP metabolism by S-adenosylhomocysteine and S-3-deazaadenosylhomocysteine in mouse lymphocytes. *Proc. Natl. Acad. Sci. USA*, 77, 5639–43

112. Schanche, J.-S., Ogreid, D., Doskeland, S. O., Refsnes, M., Sand, T. E., Ueland, P. M. and Christoffersen, T. (1982). Evidence against a requirement for phospholipid methylation in adenylate cyclase activation by hormones. Methyltransferase inhibitors do not impair cyclic AMP accumulation induced by glucagon or β-adrenergic agents in rat hepatocytes. *FEBS Lett.*, **138**, 167–72

113. Winslow, C. M. and Austen, K. F. (1984). Role of cyclic nucleotides in the activation-secretion response. *Prog. Allergy*, **34**, 236–70

114. Benyon, R. C., Church, M. K. and Holgate, S. T. (1984). The effect of methyltransferase inhibitors on histamine release from human dispersed lung mast cells activated with anti-human IgE and calcium ionophore. *Biochem. Pharmacol.*, **33**, 2881–6

115. Morita, Y. and Siraganian, R. P. (1981). Inhibition of IgE-mediated histamine release from rat basophil leukaemia cells and rat mast cells by inhibitors of transmethylation. *J. Immunol.*, **127**, 1339–44

116. Morita, Y., Chiang, P. K. and Siraganian, R. P. (1981). Effect of inhibitors of transmethylation on histamine release from human basophils. *Biochem. Pharmacol.*, **30**, 785–91

117. Hirata, F. and Axelrod, J. (1978). Enzymatic methylation of phosphatidylethanolamine increases erythrocyte membrane fluidity. *Nature*, **275**, 219–20

118. Hirata, F. and Axelrod, J. (1978). Enzymatic synthesis and rapid translocation of phosphatidylcholine by two methyltransferases in erythrocyte membranes. *Proc. Natl. Acad. Sci. USA*, **75**, 2348–52

119. Hirata, F., Viveros, O. H., Diliberto, E. J. Jr. and Axelrod, J. (1978). Identification and properties of two methyltransferases in the conversion of phosphatidylethanolamine to phosphatidylcholine. *Proc. Natl. Acad. Sci. USA*, **75**, 1718–21

120. Crews, F. T., Hirata, F. and Axelrod, J. (1980). Identification and properties of two methyltransferases that synthesise phosphatidylcholine in rat brain synaptosomes. *J. Neurochem.*, **34**, 1491–8

121. McGivney, A., Crews, F. T., Hirata, F., Axelrod, J. and Siraganian, R. P. (1981). Rat basophilic leukaemia cell lines defective in phospholipid methyltransferase enzymes: reconstitution by hybridisation of IgE-mediated phospholipid methylation and histamine release. *Proc. Natl. Acad. Sci. USA*, **78**, 6176–80

122. Audubert, F. and Vance, D. E. (1983). Pitfalls and problems in studies on the methylation of phosphatidylethanolamine. *J. Biol. Chem.*, **258**, 10695–701

123. Schneider, W. J. and Vance, D. E. (1979). Conversion of phosphatidylethanolamine to phosphatidylcholine in rat liver. Partial purification and characterization of the enzymatic activities. *J. Biol. Chem.*, **254**, 3886–91

124. Pajares, M. A., Villalba, M. and Mato, J. M. (1986). Purification of phospholipid methyltransferase from rat liver microsomal fraction. *Biochem. J.*, **237**, 699–705

125. McKenzie, R. C. and Brophy, P. J. (1983). Isoproterenol stimulates lipid methylation in C6 cells without affecting membrane fluidity. *FEBS Lett.*, **164**, 244–6

126. McKenzie, R. C. and Brophy, P. J. (1984). Lipid composition and physical properties of membranes from C-6 glial cells with altered phospholipid polar headgroups. *Biochim. Biophys. Acta*, **769**, 357–62

127. Mio, M., Okamoto, M., Akagi, M. and Tasaka, K. (1984). Effect of N-methylation of phosphatidylethanolamine on the fluidity of phospholipid bilayers. *Biochem. Biophys. Res. Commun.*, **120**, 989–95

128. Berridge, M. J. (1982). Calcium as a trigger for cellular events. Precautions regarding the interpretation of ^{45}Ca fluxes in connection with histamine release in rat mast cells. In Cheung, W. Y. (ed.) *Calcium and Cell Function*, Vol. III, pp. 1–36. (NY: Academic Press)

129. Pearce, F. L. (1982). Calcium and histamine secretion from mast cells. *Prog. Med. Chem.*, **19**, 59–109

130. Case, R. M. (1984). The role of calcium stores in secretion. *Cell Calcium*, **5**, 89–110

131. Bennett, J. P., Cockcroft, S. and Gomperts, B. P. (1979). Ionomycin stimulates mast cell histamine secretion by forming a lipid soluble calcium complex. *Nature*, **282**, 851–3

132. Kanno, T., Cochrane, D. E. and Douglas, W. W. (1973). Exocytosis (secretory granule extrusion) induced by injection of calcium into mast cells. *Can. J. Physiol. Pharmacol.*, **51**, 1001–4

133. Pearce, F. L., Ennis, M., Truneh, A. and White, J. R. (1981). The role of intra- and extracellular calcium in histamine release from rat peritoneal mast cells. *Agents Actions*, **11**, 51–4

134. Foreman, J. C., Hallett, M. B. and Mongar, J. L. (1977). The relationship between histamine secretion and ^{45}calcium uptake by mast cells. *J. Physiol. (Lond.)*, **271**, 193–214

135. Ishizaka, T., Foreman, J. C., Sterk, A. R. and Ishizaka, K. (1979). Induction of calcium flux across the rat mast cell membrane by bridging IgE receptors. *Proc. Natl. Acad. Sci. USA*, **76**, 5858–62

136. Grosman, N. and Diamant, B. (1978). Binding of ^{45}calcium to isolated rat mast cells in connection with histamine release. *Agents Actions*, **8**, 338–46

137. Barrett-Bee, K. (1981). Antigen-induced histamine release from sensitized tissue and the measurement of calcium ion fluxes. *Biochem. Biophys. Res. Commun.*, **98**, 397–403

138. Grosman, N. and Diamant, B. (1984). Histamine secretion from mast cells and basophils. *Trends Pharmacol. Sci.*, **5**, 183–4

139. Tsien, R. Y. (1981). A non-disruptive technique for loading calcium buffers and indicators into cells. *Nature*, **290**, 527–8

140. Beaven, M. A., Rogers, J., Moore, J. P., Hesketh, T. R., Smith, G. A. and Metcalfe, J. C. (1984). The mechanism of the calcium signal and correlation with histamine release in 2H3 cells. *J. Biochem. Chem.*, **259**, 7129–36

141. Mazurek, N., Berger, G. and Pecht, I. (1980). A binding site on mast cells and basophils for the antiallergic drug cromolyn. *Nature*, **286**, 722–3

142. Mazurek, N., Bashkin, P. and Pecht, I. (1982). Isolation of a basophilic membrane protein binding the anti-allergic drug cromolyn. *EMBO J.*, **1**, 585–90

143. Mazurek, N., Bashkin, P., Petrauk, A. and Pecht, I. (1983). Basophil variants with impaired cromoglycate binding do not respond to an immunological degranulation stimulus. *Nature*, **303**, 528–30

144. Mazurek, N., Baskin, P., Loyter, A. and Pecht, I. (1983). Restoration of the calcium influx and degranulation capacity of variant RBL-2H3 cells upon implantation of isolated cromolyn binding protein. *Proc. Natl. Acad. Sci. USA*, **80**, 6014–18
145. Mazurek, N., Schindler, H., Schurholz, T. L. and Pecht, I. (1984). The cromolyn binding protein constitutes the calcium channel of basophils opening upon immunological stimulus. *Proc. Natl. Acad. Sci. USA*, **81**, 6841–5
146. Pecht, I., Dulic, V., Rivnay, B. and Corcia, A. (1986). Transmembrane signalling in basophils: Ion conductance measurements on planar bilayers reconstituted with purified Fc receptors and the cromolyn binding protein. In Befus, A. D., Denburg, J. A. and Bienenstock, J. (eds.) *Mast Cell Differentiation and Heterogeneity*, pp. 301–11. (NY: Raven Press)
147. Sullivan, T. J., Parker, K. L., Kulczycki, A. and Parker, C. W. (1976). Modulation of cyclic AMP in purified rat mast cells: III Studies on the effects of concanavalin A and anti-IgE during histamine release. *J. Immunol.*, **117**, 713–16
148. Lewis, R. A., Holgate, S. T., Roberts, L. J., Maguire, J. F., Oates, J. A. and Austen, K. F. (1979). Effects of indomethacin on cyclic nucleotide levels and histamine release from rat serosal mast cells. *J. Immunol.*, **123**, 1663–8
149. Burt, D. S. and Stanworth, D. R. (1983). Changes in cellular levels of cyclic AMP in rat mast cells during secretion of histamine induced by immunoglobulin E decapeptide and ACTH (1–24) peptide. Comparison with immunological and ionophore triggers. *Biochim. Biophys. Acta*, **762**, 458–65
150. Church, M. K., Hughes, P. J. and Vardey, C. J. (1986). Studies on the receptor mediating cyclic AMP-independent enhancement by adenosine of IgE-dependent mediator release from rat mast cells. *Br. J. Pharmacol.*, **87**, 233–42
151. Lichtenstein, L. M., Kagey-Sobotka, A., Malveaux, F. L. and Gillespie, E. (1978). IgE-induced changes in human basophil cyclic AMP levels. *Int. Arch. Allergy Appl. Immunol.*, **56**, 473–8
152. Hughes, P. J., Holgate, S. T., Roath, S. T. and Church, M. K. (1983). The relationship between cyclic AMP changes and histamine release from basophil-enriched human leucocytes. *Biochem. Pharmacol.*, **32**, 2557–63
153. Schild, H. O. (1936). Histamine release and anaphylactic shock in isolated lungs of guinea pigs. *Q. J. Exp. Physiol.*, **26**, 165–79
154. Orange, R. P., Austen, W. G. and Austen, K. F. (1971). Immunologic release of histamine and slow reacting substance of anaphylaxis from human lung. 1. Modulation by agents influencing cellular levels of cyclic 3',5'-adenosine monophosphate. *J. Exp. Med.*, **134** (Suppl.), 136S–48S
155. Kaliner, M., Orange, R. P. and Austen, K. F. (1972). Immunological release of histamine and SRS-A from human lung. IV. Enhancement by cholinergic and alpha-adrenergic stimulation. *J. Exp. Med.*, **136**, 556–67
156. Schulman, E. S., MacGlashan, D. W., Peters, S. P., Schleimer, R. P., Newball, H. H. and Lichtenstein, L. M. (1982). Human lung mast cells: purification and characterization. *J. Immunol.*, **129**, 2662–7
157. Hughes, P. J., Holgate, S. T. and Church, M. K. (1984). Adenosine inhibits and potentiates IgE-dependent histamine release from human lung mast cells by an A2-purinoceptor mediated mechanism. *Biochem. Pharmacol.*, **33**, 3847–52
158. Church, M. K. and Hiroi, J. (1987). Inhibition of IgE-dependent histamine release from human dispersed lung mast cells by anti-allergic drugs and salbutamol. *Br. J. Pharmacol.*, **90**, 421–9
159. Bourne, H. R., Melmon, K. L. and Lichtenstein, L. M. (1971). Histamine augments leukocyte cyclic AMP and blocks antigenic histamine release. *Science*, **173**, 743–4
160. Lichtenstein, L. M. and Margolis, S. (1968). Histamine release *in vitro*: inhibition by catecholamines and methylxanthines. *Science*, **161**, 902–3
161. Plaut, M., Marone, G., Thomas, L. L. and Lichtenstein, L. M. (1980). Cyclic nucleotides in immune responses and allergy. *Adv. Cyclic Nucleotide Res.*, **12**, 161–72
162. Tung, R., Kagey-Sobotka, A., Plaut, M. and Lichtenstein, L. M. (1982). H2 antihistamines augment antigen-induced histamine release from human basophils *in vitro*. *J. Immunol.*, **129**, 2113–15
163. Church, M. K., Holgate, S. T. and Hughes, P. J. (1983). Adenosine inhibits and

potentiates IgE-dependent histamine release from human basophils by an A2-receptor mediated mechanism. *Br. J. Pharmacol.*, **80**, 719–26

164. Johnson, A. R. and Moran, N. C. (1970). Inhibition of the release of histamine from rat mast cells: the effect of cold and adrenergic drugs on release of histamine by compound 48/80 and antigen. *J. Pharmacol. Exp. Ther.*, **175**, 632–40

165. Johnson, A. R., Moran, N. C. and Mayer, S. E. (1974). Cyclic AMP content and histamine release in rat mast cells. *J. Immunol.*, **112**, 511–19

166. Marquardt, D. L. and Wasserman, S. I. (1982). Characterization of rat mast cells by radioligand binding. *J. Immunol.*, **129**, 2122–7

167. Sydbom, A., Fredholm, B. B. and Uvnas, B. (1979). Evidence against a role of cyclic nucleotides in the regulation of anaphylactic histamine release in isolated rat mast cells. *Acta Physiol. Scand.*, **112**, 47–56

168. Sullivan, T. J., Parker, K. L., Eisen, S. A. and Parker, C. W. (1975). Modulation of cyclic AMP in purified rat mast cells. II Studies on the relationship between intracellular cyclic AMP concentrations and histamine release. *J. Immunol.*, **114**, 1480–5

169. Hayashi, H., Ichikawa, K., Saito, T. and Tomita, K. (1976). Inhibitory role of cyclic adenosine 3',5'-monophosphate in histamine release from rat peritoneal mast cells *in vitro*. *Biochem. Pharmacol.*, **25**, 1907–13

170. Holgate, S. T., Lewis, R. A., Maguire, J. F., Roberts, L. J., Oates, J. A. and Austen, K. F. (1980). Effects of prostaglandin D2 on rat serosal mast cells: Discordance between immunologic mediator release and cyclic AMP levels. *J. Immunol.*, **125**, 1367–73

171. Sydbom, A. and Fredholm, B. B. (1982). On the mechanism by which theophylline inhibits histamine release from rat mast cells. *Acta Physiol. Scand.*, **114**, 243–51

172. Holgate, S. T., Lewis, R. A. and Austen, K. F. (1980). 3',5'-cyclic adenosine monophosphate dependent protein kinase of the rat serosal mast cell and its immunologic activation. *J. Immunol.*, **124**, 2093–9

173. Holgate, S. T., Winslow, C. M., Lewis, R. A. and Austen, K. F. (1981). Effects of prostaglandin D2 and theophylline on rat serosal mast cells: Discordance between increased cellular levels of cyclic AMP and activation of cyclic AMP-dependent protein kinase. *J. Immunol.*, **127**, 1530–3

174. Holgate, S. T., Lewis, R. A. and Austen, K. F. (1980). Role of adenylate cyclase in immunologic release of mediators from rat mast cells: agonist and antagonist effects of purine- and ribose-modified analogs. *Proc. Natl. Acad. Sci. USA*, **77**, 6800–4

175. Hughes, P. J. and Church, M. K. (1986). Inhibition of immunological and non-immunological histamine release from human basophils by adenosine analogues that act at P-sites. *Biochem. Pharmacol.*, **35**, 1809–16

176. Winslow, C. M., Lewis, R. A. and Austen, K. F. (1981). Mast cell mediator release as a function of cyclic AMP protein kinase activation. *J. Exp. Med.*, **154**, 1125–33

177. Church, M. K., Hughes, P. J. and Holgate, S. T. (1986). Can a compartment theory explain the inconsistent relationship between cyclic AMP and mast cell mediators secretion. In Schou, J. S., Geisler, A. and Norn, S. (eds.) *Drug Receptors and Dynamic Processes in Cells*, (Alfred Benzon Symposium No. 22), pp. 172–88. (Copenhagen: Munksgaard)

178. Tada, M., Kirchberger, M. A. and Katz, A. M. (1975). Phosphorylation of a 22 000 Dalton component of the cardiac sarcoplasmic reticulum by 3',5'-adenosine cyclic monophosphate dependent protein kinase. *J. Biol. Chem.*, **250**, 2640–7

179. Tada, M. and Katz, A. M. (1982). Phosphorylation of the sarcoplasmic reticulum and sarcolemma. *Ann. Rev. Physiol.*, **44**, 401–23

180. Kaser-Glanzmann, R., Jakabova, M., Gworge, J. N. and Luscher, E. F. (1977). Stimulation of calcium uptake in platelet membrane vesicles by adenosine 3'5'-cyclic monophosphate and protein kinase. *Biochim. Biophys. Acta*, **466**, 899–902

181. Hathaway, D. R., Eaton, C. R. and Adelstein, R. S. (1981). Regulation of human platelet myosin light chain kinase by the catalytic subunit of cyclic AMP-dependent protein kinase. *Nature*, **291**, 252–3

182. Caulfield, J. P., Lewis, R. A., Hein, A. and Austen, K. F. (1980). Secretion of dissociated human pulmonary mast cells: evidence for solubilization of granule contents before discharge. *J. Cell Biol.*, **85**, 299–311

183. Kennerly, D. A., Secosan, C. J., Parker, C. W. and Sullivan, T. J. (1979). Modulation

of stimulated phospholipid metabolism in mast cells by pharmacologic agents that increase cyclic 3'5'-adenosine monophosphate. *J. Immunol.*, **123**, 1519–24

184. Speralakis, N. (1984). Cyclic AMP and phosphorylation in regulation of Ca^{2+} influx into myocardial cells and blockade by calcium antagonistic drugs. *Am. Heart J.*, **107**, 347–67

185. Lichtenstein, L. M., Schleimer, R. P., MacGlashan, D. W., Peters, S. P., Schulman, E. S., Proud, D., Creticos, P. S., Naclerio, R. M. and Kagey-Sobotka, A. (1984). *In vitro* and *in vivo* studies of mediator release from human mast cells. In Kay, A. B., Austen, K. F. and Lichtenstein, L. M. (eds.) *Asthma: Physiology, Immunopharmacology and Treatment. Third International Symposium*, pp. 1–18. (London: Academic Press)

186. Peachell, P., MacGlashan, D., Lichtenstein, L. M. and Schleimer, R. P. (1987). Regulation of human lung mast cell and basophil function by cyclic AMP. *Fed. Proc.*, **46**, 4153 (Abstr.)

187. Leoutosakos, A., Truneh, A. and Pearce, F. L. (1985). Role of cyclic AMP in the induction of histamine secretion from mast cells. *Agents Actions*, **16**, 126–8

188. Alm, P. E. (1984). Modulation of mast cell cAMP levels. A regulatory function of calmodulin. *Int. Arch. Allergy Appl. Immunol.*, **75**, 375–8

189. Sieghart, W., Theoharides, T. C., Alper, S. E., Douglas, W. W. and Greengard, P. (1978). Calcium-dependent protein phosphorylation during secretion by exocytosis in the mast cell. *Nature*, **275**, 329–31

190. Theoharides, T. C., Seighart, W., Greengard, P. and Douglas, W. W. (1980). Antiallergic drug cromolyn may inhibit secretion by regulating phosphorylation of a mast cell protein. *Science*, **207**, 80–2

191. Sieghart, W., Theoharides, T. C., Douglas, W. W. and Greengard, P. (1981). Phosphorylation of a single mast cell protein in response to drugs that inhibit secretion. *Biochem. Pharmacol.*, **30**, 2737–8

192. Theoharides, T. C., Sieghart, W., Greengard, P. and Douglas, W. W. (1981). Somatostatin-induced phosphorylation of mast cell proteins. *Biochem. Pharmacol.*, **30**, 2735–6

193. Wells, E. and Mann, J. (1983). Phosphorylation of a mast cell protein in response to treatment with anti-allergic compounds. Implications for the mode of action of sodium cromoglycate. *Biochem. Pharmacol.*, **32**, 837–42

194. Lagunoff, D., Martin, T. W. and Read, G. (1983). Agents that release histamine from mast cells. *Ann. Rev. Pharmacol. Toxicol.*, **23**, 331–51

195. Siraganian, R. P. and Hook, W. A. (1978). Mechanisms of histamine release by formyl-methionine containing peptides. *J. Immunol.*, **119**, 2078–83

196. Foreman, J. C. and Lichtenstein, L. M. (1980). Induction of histamine secretion by polycations. *Biochim. Biophys. Acta*, **629**, 587–603

197. Siraganian, R. P. and Hook, W. A. (1976). Complement-induced histamine release from human basophils. II Mechanism of the histamine release reaction. *J. Immunol.*, **116**, 639–46

198. Church, M. K., Coleman, J. W., Holgate, S. T. Pao, G. J.-K. and Welch, M. T. (1981). The effects of polyamines, 48/80 and calcium ionophore on histamine release from human dispersed lung and adenoidal mast cells (Abstr.). *Br. J. Pharmacol.*, **74**, 979P–80P

199. Lowman, M. A., Rees, P. H., Benyon, R. C. and Church, M. K. (1987). Human mast cell heterogeneity: Histamine release from mast cells dispersed from skin, lung, adenoids, tonsils and intestinal mucosa in response to IgE-dependent and non-immunological stimuli. *J. Allergy Clin. Immunol.* (In press)

200. Piotrowski, W., Devoy, M. A. B., Jordan, C. C. and Foreman, J. C. (1984). The substance P receptor on rat mast cells and in human skin. *Agents Actions*, **14**, 420–3

201. Grosman, N. (1981). Histamine release from isolated rat mast cells: effect of morphine and related drugs and their interaction with compound 48/80. *Agents Actions*, **11**, 196–203

202. Foreman, J. C., Jordan, C. C. and Piotrowski, W. (1982). Interaction of neurotensin with the substance P receptor mediating histamine release from rat mast cells and the flare in human skin. *Br. J. Pharmacol.*, **77**, 531–9

203. Fewtrell, C. M., Foreman, J. C., Jordan, C. C., Oehme, P., Renner, H. and Stewart, J. M. (1982). The effects of substance P on histamine and 5-hydroxytryptamine release in the rat. *J. Physiol. (Lond.)*, **330**, 393–411

204. Baxter, J. H. and Adamik, R. (1978). Differences in requirements and actions of various histamine-releasing agents. *Biochem. Pharmacol.*, **27**, 497–503

205. Ennis, M. (1982). Histamine release from pulmonary mast cells. *Agents Actions*, **12**, 60–3
206. Theoharides, T. C., Betchaku, T. and Douglas, W. W. (1981). Somatostatin-induced histamine secretion in mast cells: characterization of the effect. *Eur. J. Pharm.*, **69**, 127–37
207. Rosengard, B. R., Mahalik, C. and Cochrane, D. E. (1986). Mast cell secretion: differences between immunologic and non-immunologic stimulation. *Agents Actions*, **19**, 133–40
208. Spataro, A. C. and Bosmann, H. B. (1976). Mechanism of action of disodium cromoglycate-mast cell calcium ion influx after a histamine-releasing stimulus. *Biochem. Pharmacol.*, **25**, 505–10
209. Narendranath, S. R. and Dhanani, N. (1980). Movement of calcium ions and release of histamine from rat mast cells. *Int. Arch. Allergy Appl. Immunol.*, **61**, 9–18
210. Grynkiewicz, G., Poenie, M. and Tsien, R. Y. (1985). A new generation of Ca indicators with greatly improved fluorescence properties. *J. Biol. Chem.*, **260**, 3440–50
211. Tharp, M. D., Suvunrungsi, R. T. and Sullivan, T. J. (1983). IgE-mediated release of histamine from human cutaneous mast cells. *J. Immunol.*, **130**, 1896–901
212. Clegg, L. S., Church, M. K. and Holgate, S. T. (1985). Histamine secretion from human skin slices induced by anti-IgE and artificial secretagogues and the effects of sodium cromoglycate and salbutamol. *Clin. Allergy*, **15**, 321–8
213. Gruber, B., Poznansky, M., Boss, E., Partin, J., Gorevic, P. and Kaplan, A. P. (1986). Characterisation and functional studies of rheumatoid synovial mast cells. *Arthritis Rheumatism*, **29**, 944–55
214. Gilman, A. G. (1984). G proteins and the dual control of adenylate cyclase. *Cell*, **36**, 577–9

8
Inflammatory Cells in Allergic Disease

A. B. KAY

INTRODUCTION

Allergic diseases (evoked totally, or in part, by IgE-mediated mechanisms) affect many organs and tissues, but in particular the upper and lower respiratory tract, the eyes, the gastro-intestinal tract and the skin. The rapid release of mast cell-associated mediators probably accounts almost entirely for the clinical manifestations of immediate hypersensitivity, i.e. rhinorrhoea, nasal blockage, sneezing, wheeze, pruritus, abdominal discomfort and diarrhoea. After a single exposure to allergen these symptoms are self-limiting and usually subside spontaneously (Figure 8.1). With repeated exposure, a prominent local inflammatory response develops. This is associated with more prolonged and protracted symptoms such as bronchial irritability or hyperresponsiveness, permanent nasal congestion, indurated skin lesions and chronic mucoid diarrhoea. It should be borne in mind that mucus hypersecretion is a characteristic feature of inflammation at all mucosal surfaces.

Inflammation is essentially the response of vascularized tissue to injury and serves to resolve and repair the effect of damage. The causes of inflammation, like those of cell injury, are diverse and include, in addition to immunological reactions such as allergy and auto-immunity, infectious (bacteria, viruses and parasites), physical (burns, radiation and trauma) and chemical agents (drugs, toxins and industrial agents). The histopathological features of inflammation consist of changes in vascular flow and the calibre of small blood vessels, followed by alterations in vascular permeability leading to white cell events. Acute inflammation is of short duration, characterized by exudation of fluid and plasma proteins (oedema) and leukocyte emigration, with neutrophils being prominent. In contrast, chronic inflammation is of longer duration with a dense infiltrate of lymphocytes and macrophages. These cell types are found together with proliferation of blood vessels and connective tissue. In allergy and helminthic parasitic disease, the eosinophil is a particularly prominent cell. Both acute and chronic

227

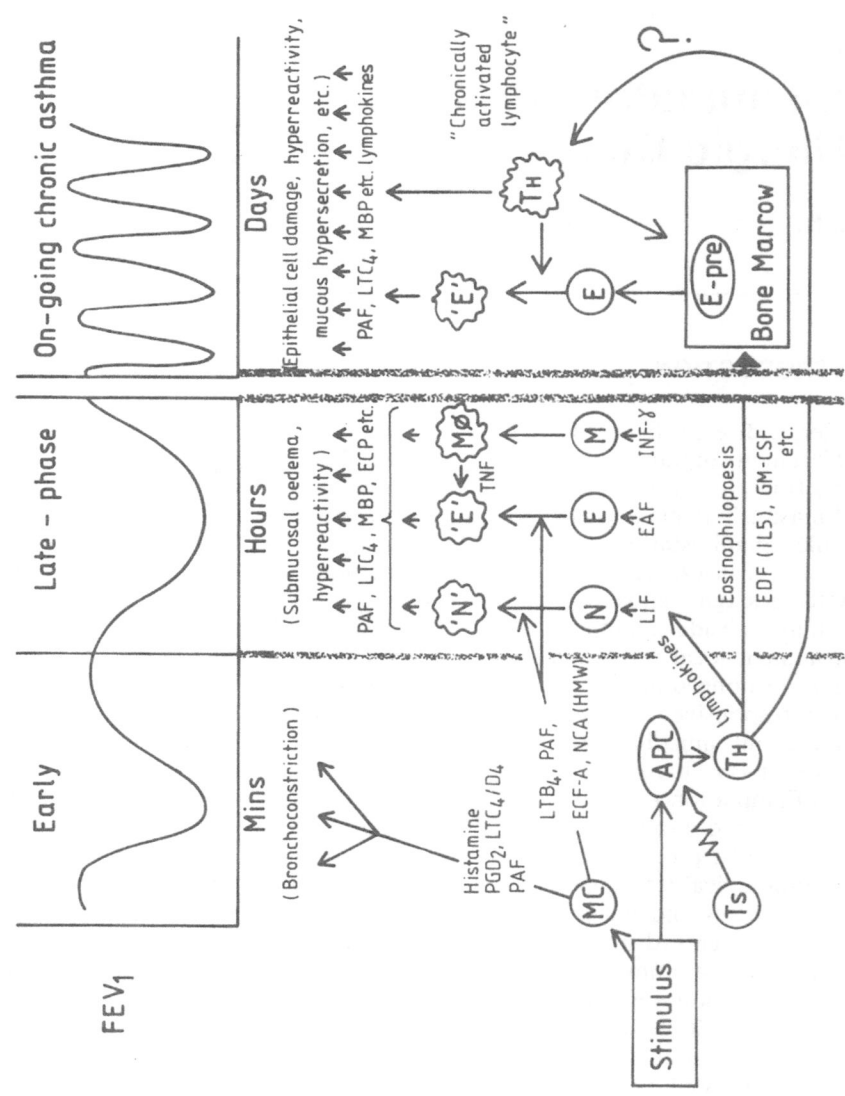

inflammation are associated with some degree of fibrin deposition with platelet adherence and the release of platelet products. The basophil is also an inflammatory cell, since it is prominent in certain forms of delayed-type hypersensitivity (particularly cutaneous basophil hypersensitivity) and is found in the upper airways in allergic rhinitis. At the present time there is no conclusive evidence that the basophil participates in pathological processes in the lung. Thus the cells emigrating from the blood vessels which contribute to inflammation in general, and allergic inflammation in particular, include the neutrophil, eosinophil, lymphocyte, macrophage and platelet, with the role of the basophil remaining uncertain. In addition, fixed tissue cells such as the mast cell, fibroblast and epithelial cell also participate in acute and chronic inflammation to a greater or lesser extent.

NEUTROPHILS

Neutrophils are non-dividing granule-containing cells which arise in the bone marrow and have a limited life span in the circulation. The neutrophil is traditionally considered to be a phagocytic cell with a particular role in the

---

Figure 8.1 A diagrammatic representation of the interactions between mediators of hypersensitivity and inflammatory cells in early-, late-phase, and ongoing asthma. For further explanation see text. Early-phase, or immediate reactions are largely the result of bronchoconstriction consequent to the release of mediators such as histamine, PGD_2, LTC_4/D_4 and PAF. The principal mediator cell (MC) is the mast cell (although other IgE receptor bearing cells such as the macrophage, eosinophil and platelet might also be involved in this immediate response). The stimulus for mediator cell activation may be either immunologic (IgE-dependent) or non-immunologic (i.e. changes in osmolarity as a result of the respiratory water loss associated with exercise-induced asthma). Late-phase reactions appear to be a consequence of infiltration with neutrophils (N), eosinophils (E) and macrophages (Mφ). These cells are recruited and activated either by mast cell-associated chemotactic factors [such as LTB_4, PAF, the eosinophil chemotactic factor of anaphylaxis (ECF-A) or high molecular weight neutrophil chemotactic activity (HMW-NCA)] and/or 'lymphokines' derived from T helper cells (T_H) which have been stimulated by antigen processed by the antigen processing cells (APC). These mononuclear cell interactions are under the control of regulatory T cells [T suppressor (T_S) cells for asthma] and it is speculated that the presence of these subsets may determine the magnitude of the late-phase response. Lymphokines and monokines which selectively activate neutrophils, eosinophils and monocytes include LIF, EAF and INF-gamma respectively. Macrophage-derived tumour necrosis factor (TNF) also amplifies the inflammatory response by its capacity to enhance eosinophil cytotoxicity. Eosinophil-derived agents such as PAF, LTC_4, MBP and ECP might be largely responsible for submucosal oedema and non-specific bronchial hyperreactivity which are characteristic features of late-phase reactions. T cell-derived lymphokines such as EDF (IL-5), together with GM-CSF, might lead to eosinophilopoiesis and account for the prolonged eosinophilia of ongoing chronic asthma. The T cell is prominent in the pathology of chronic asthma and possibly 'chronically activated'. Thus lymphocytes, driven by as yet undetermined 'antigens' (possibly viral) may perpetuate the inflammatory response in and around the bronchi. IL-5-like products from these putative activated lymphocytes might perpetuate (1) eosinophil production by the bone marrow, (2) its release into the circulation, (3) its migration into bronchial tissue and (4) activation to release PAF, LTC_4, MBP, etc. Lymphokines released directly from these T helper cells might also influence bronchial pathology. The end result is epithelial cell damage, amplification of hyperreactivity, together with mucus hypersecretion and total or partial plugging of small to medium size airways. The various aspects of this broad hypothesis are currently under investigation

ingestion and elimination of common pyogenic organisms. However, the neutrophil is also a secretory cell, especially when in contact with large non-phagocytosable surfaces, to which it adheres and secretes its granule enzymes by exocytosis[1]. The neutrophil has two forms of granules, primary (azurophilic) and secondary (specific). Primary granules contain myeloperoxidase, neutral proteases (cathepsin G, elastase and unspecific collagenase), acid hydrolases, lysozyme and cationic proteins. Secondary granules contain lactoferrin, vitamin B_{12} binding protein, C5 cleaving enzymes, specific collagenase and lysozyme. Following activation by agents such as the T cell-derived leukocyte inhibitory factor (LIF)[2] (Figure 8.1), secondary (and then primary granules) secrete their contents.

During inflammatory reactions, chemotactic stimuli from inflammatory loci lead to a series of changes in circulating white cells. For instance, mast cells elaborate a number of neutrophil chemotactic substances, which include leukotriene B_4 (LTB$_4$), platelet activating factor (PAF), and various peptides (largely uncharacterized) (Figure 8.1). The initial changes appear to be receptor mobilization with ruffling of the plasma membrane. For instance, increased expression of receptors for complement and IgG can be demonstrated when neutrophils, eosinophils and monocytes are incubated with chemotactic factors[3]. This appears to be an early event and is followed by partial degranulation with the release of enzymes from secondary specific granules. Leukocytes then deviate from their normal axial flow and aggregate and marginate on the endothelium. After disaggregation cells then migrate through the capillary endothelium. Outside the vessels the movement of cells in the tissue is thought to be under the influence of chemotactic and/or chemokinetic stimuli.

The neutrophil serves mainly to engulf opsonized invading micro-organisms, as well as releasing enzymes which limit the barrier presented by tissue planes, so allowing the emigration of other cell types such as eosinophils and mononuclear phagocytes.

It is well known that neutrophil infiltration is an early event in IgE-mediated reactions, particularly in the skin. Data obtained from models of asthma in experimental animals indicate that a similar situation exists in the lung[4]. The precise role of the neutrophil in asthma and allergic rhinitis is unclear, although there are a number of studies which suggest that alterations in this cell type occur during and after acute episodes of the disease, such as those evoked in the clinical laboratory under controlled conditions. For instance, after allergen-[5] or exercise-[6] induced asthma peripheral blood neutrophils are activated as determined by (1) increased membrane expression of complement receptors (CR) and (2) enhanced cytotoxicity of neutrophils for complement-coated targets (opsonized helminthic larvae)[7]. Similarly, after allergen-induced late-phase reactions there was a significant increase in the degree of neutrophil and monocyte activation as shown by the 'rosette' technique[8]. Preliminary experiments indicate that there are also functional alterations in peripheral blood neutrophils (i.e. increased cytotoxicity) after allergen-induced late-phase reactions (Figure 8.1). In the rabbit, neutrophils appear to have a direct role in the development of both late-phase reactions and heightened bronchial hyperresponsiveness[9].

More direct evidence for the involvement of the neutrophil has been obtained from asthmatic volunteers undergoing fibre-optic bronchoscopy and bronchoalveolar lavage (BAL) 6 h after inhalational challenge with either allergen or diluent control[10]. Those subjects who experienced dual (early- and late-phase) reactions (but not the single early responders) had a significant elevation in BAL neutrophils (as well as eosinophils and lymphocytes) on the allergen day, when compared to the control day.

The elaboration of a high molecular weight neutrophil chemotactic activity (HMW-NCA) into the circulation of patients after allergen- or exercise-induced early- and late-phase reactions is also well documented[11-14]. HMW-NCA was associated with molecules having a molecular size of approximately 600 K and a near neutral isoelectric point. This activity was recently identified in 'real asthma', i.e. from the serum of asthmatics admitted to hospital with acute severe disease (status asthmaticus)[15].

In a further study the number of neutrophils in bronchoalveolar lavage fluids from eight subjects with mild perennial asthma were compared to seasonal asthma, hayfever, and six non-atopic subjects who had no evidence of allergic disease[16]. Although there were no differences in the percentage of neutrophils between the groups, there were significantly more neutrophils in the small (20 ml) 'bronchial' wash compared to the larger (100 ml) 'broncho-alveolar' wash when the asthmatic and non-asthmatic groups were analysed together. In fact three of the normal subjects had neutrophil counts in the bronchial wash greater than 20%. Thus, although the neutrophil might be involved, to a greater or lesser extent, in the inflammatory process of asthma there is no evidence for believing that this cell plays a unique role in this disease.

EOSINOPHILS

Eosinophils are also bone marrow-derived 'end cells'. They are present in large numbers in the circulation and tissues in those conditions associated with raised IgE levels, such as hayfever, allergic asthma, allergic bronchopulmonary aspergillosis and helminth parasitic disease[17]. The cell is characterized by the presence of large intracytoplasmic granules which stain yellow–pink with eosin and other acid analine dyes. The granules are rich in peroxidase and three other basic proteins, major basic protein (MBP), eosinophil cationic protein (ECP) and eosinophil-derived neurotoxin. These proteins, especially MBP and ECP, are thought to be particularly important in allergic tissue damage where eosinophils are prominent. For instance, in severe chronic asthma large numbers of eosinophils infiltrate in and around the bronchi and release MBP. MBP is known to damage respiratory epithelial cells, as well as directly releasing histamine, and possibly other pharmacological agents from mast cells, thereby amplifying the allergic response.

Eosinophils bear receptors for IgG (Fc), IgE (Fc) and for activated complement fragments (CR1 and CR3). The eosinophil membrane has the potential for generating large quantities of leukotriene C_4[18] (one of the components of slow reacting substance of anaphylaxis), as well as PAF-acether[19] and

15-lipoxygenase products[20]. LTC_4 and PAF-acether are powerful constrictors of bronchial smooth muscle, and also induce mucus secretion from bronchial submucous glands. These agents, particularly PAF-acether, are potent chemotactic factors for the eosinophil itself.

Eosinophil maturation and differentiation from its precursor cell appear to be under the control of a 30 kD T cell-derived eosinophil differentiating factor[21] (EDF, interleukin-5) as well as granulocyte/monocyte-colony stimulating factor (Figure 8.1).

It is well known that a blood and sputum eosinophilia is often, but not invariably, found in association with mild or severe, acute or chronic asthma. Eosinophils are also very prominent cells in many of the histopathological sections obtained from asthma deaths. By the use of an immunofluorescent technique, MBP was prominent in the bronchial wall and in the mucus plugs of virtually all of these patients, even though only a few intact eosinophils were observed by routine light microscopy[22]. MBP concentrations are also raised in the sputum from asthmatics[23]. It is hypothesized that MBP, and possibly other granule-derived basic proteins, are directly responsible for the epithelial damage that is characteristic of the disease. In fact the characteristic pathology has been termed 'chronic eosinophilic desquamative bronchitis'.

There have been a number of studies relating eosinophils to allergen-invoked asthma. For instance, a blood eosinophilia accompanied late-phase, but not single early, asthmatic responses[24], and there was an inverse correlation between the blood eosinophil count and the degree of non-specific bronchial hyperreactivity as measured by the methacholine PC_{20}. The accumulation of eosinophils in the lungs of asthmatics undergoing late-phase responses was demonstrated by De Monchy et al.[25]. More recently Diaz et al.[10] confirmed these findings and, in addition, observed that numbers of BAL mast cells also decreased in late responders.

In a recent study bronchoalveolar lavage on 12 asthmatics (eight perennial, four seasonal) and nine non-asthmatic controls[26], there were significantly more eosinophils and epithelial cells in the asthmatic group compared with the non-asthmatic group. There was a significant correlation between the percentage of eosinophils in the lavage fluid and the levels of MBP. In addition, the levels of MBP were significantly greater in the subjects with hyper-reactive airways compared with those subjects who had normo-reactive airways. Thus this study supported the previous observations on the relationship between blood eosinophil counts and bronchial hyperreactivity[24], and suggests that this increased responsiveness may be mediated by eosinophil granule-derived products. Thus it is tempting to speculate that eosinophils and their products may play a role in the hyperresponsiveness of smooth muscle to non-specific agents possibly as a result of damage to the bronchial epithelium.

In a placebo-controlled double-blind trial it was shown that the mast cell stabilizing agent, disodium cromoglycate, suppressed the local accumulation of eosinophils in bronchial mucus and BAL fluid, and that these reductions in lung eosinophils were related to clinical improvement[10]. Thus, all these studies taken together provide evidence that eosinophils play a direct role in the pathogenesis of asthma. The evidence, although persuasive, is not proven.

BASOPHILS

Basophils and mast cells share a number of properties. These include the presence of large intracytoplasmic metachromatic granules, receptors for immunoglobulin E, and the capacity to release pre-formed (granule-associated) and newly formed (membrane-derived) pharmacological mediators. In other respects they are distinct, i.e. in the ultrastructure of the granules, developmental origins and their responsiveness to drugs which influence the release of pharmacological mediators[27].

In man and most animals basophils are polymorphonuclear leukocytes which differentiate in the bone marrow and circulate in the peripheral blood. They are also 'end-cells' incapable of division, and which have a life span of 8–12 days. Basophils account for about 0.5–1% of the circulating leukocytes and 0.3% of nucleated cells in the bone marrow. In many animal species there is a striking inverse relationship between the total number of basophils and mast cells suggesting that these cells augment each other, since they have similar functions.

Basophils are the smallest of the human granulocytes and have a diameter of 10–14 μm. They have bright metachromatic cytoplasmic granules that are larger, fewer and more widely separated than those for the mast cell. Ultrastructurally, the basophil granules are round to angular, membrane-bound structures up to 1.2 μm in diameter. The granule-derived mediators include histamine, acid hydrolases and a basophil-derived kallikrein. The glucosaminoglycan backbone consists largely of chondroitin sulphate (type A), which is less sulphated than mast cell heparin. Basophils have some features in common with eosinophils such as the presence of MBP and eosinophil lysophospholipase (Charcot–Leyden crystal protein). The cytoplasm of mature basophils contains abundant glycogen deposits, a small Golgi apparatus, a few mitochondria, ribosomes, strands of rough endoplasmic reticulum and a complex vesicular system. The unique property of the basophil and mast cell membrane is its ability to firmly bind the Fc portion of immunoglobulin E.

Large numbers of basophils infiltrate the skin in the reaction known as cutaneous basophil hypersensitivity (CBH). CBH and Jones–Mote reactions (JMR) are delayed reactions that are induced without mycobacterial adjuvants. Both can be T cell-dependent or antibody-dependent. There is evidence to suggest that such reactions participate in resistance to ectoparasitic ticks[28].

Apart from myeloproliferative disorders, a blood basophilia is rare, although the counts may reach 1 or 2% in atopics during the pollen season. Basophils have been recognized in nasal secretions in patients with hay fever, but generally speaking there is a paucity of data on the precise role of basophils in other immediate-type reactions in man.

PLATELETS

Platelets are the smallest cellular elements in the blood. They are derived from megakaryocytes, are non-nucleated and contain a large number of granules. Although they play an essential role in blood clotting and the arrest of bleeding, the granules also contain a variety of substances which may act as mediators of inflammation[29]. In addition, platelets have the ability to generate membrane-derived arachidonic acid metabolites, such as prostaglandins and 5-lipoxygenase products. The α-granules of the platelets are lysozymal and contain proteolytic enzymes and cationic substances which increase vascular permeability. For instance the specific platelet markers, platelet factor 4 and β-thromboglobulin, are contained largely within α-granules. Other granules, called dense bodies, contain ADP and the vasoactive amine, 5-hydroxytryptamine (serotonin), which has similar properties to histamine and causes smooth muscle contraction and increased vascular permeability. The release of active substances from platelets is a complex process dependent on adherence and aggregation. Platelets can be activated by collagen, thrombin and ADP, as well as platelet activating factor (or PAF-acether) which is derived from basophils, mast cells, macrophages, eosinophils and probably other cell types. Antigen/antibody complexes also initiate the platelet release reaction. It was recently shown that platelets possess low affinity IgE receptors, suggesting that these cells might be specifically sensitized in allergic disease in a comparable fashion to mast cells, basophils and macrophages. The importance of this observation is unclear. Nevertheless, platelets may well amplify allergic inflammation since they can be activated by mast cell- and macrophage-derived PAF.

MACROPHAGES

Lung macrophages are derived from blood monocytes and are one of the family of mononuclear phagocytic cells which are found in virtually every organ and tissue. Macrophages secrete numerous enzymes and mediators which are thought to have importance in the initiation and regulation of inflammatory reactions[30]. The granules, for instance, contain proteinases (e.g. cathepsin) and hydrolases (e.g. glucosidases). There is an array of non-lysozymal agents which include plasminogen activators, elastases, collagenases, complement components, coagulation components, interleukin 1, interferon (α/β) and apolipoprotein. The macrophages are rich in the cell organelles required for manufacture of proteins, i.e. ribosomes and rough and smooth endoplasmic reticulum.

Macrophages have surface receptors for IgG (Fc), IgE (Fc) and possess CR1 and CR3 for the complement components C3b and C3bi, respectively. They also contain Ia antigens, and play an essential role in antigen presentation to lymphocytes. The T cell-derived lymphokine (interferon-gamma) is particularly effective at activating the macrophage (Figure 8.1). Macrophages also adhere to a number of sugar residues, as, for instance, found on a number of bacteria. This property might be associated with their ability to act as non-specific scavengers for a wide variety of organisms and particulate matter.

The role of the macrophage in the pathogenesis of allergy and asthma is the subject of considerable interest. The identification of low affinity receptors for IgE on cells of the monocyte/macrophage series indicated that these cells might participate in IgE-mediated events[31,32]. A macrophage-associated acid hydrolase (β-glucuronidase) was identified in lung lavage samples from asthmatic patients after local provocation testing[33]. Alveolar macrophages from asthmatic patients could also be stimulated *in vitro* for IgE-dependent, allergen-induced secretion of β-glucuronidase[34]. There are a number of ways in which macrophage-derived factors may contribute to various inflammatory events in asthma. For instance, a macrophage-derived eosinophil activating factor (EAF) was recently described by Veith and Butterworth (Figure 8.1)[35]. EAF is a 40 K ($\pm$7 K) protein released from cultured, unstimulated human monocytes which enhances the IgG-dependent eosinophil-mediated cytotoxicity of helminthic larvae. EAF was also shown to enhance IgG-dependent LTC_4 production by human eosinophils[36]. Thus there appears to be a clear association between monocytes, eosinophils and LTC_4. This may have relevance to mechanisms in chronic asthma, and it is intriguing to speculate that EAF (or EAF-like substances) might be released in greater amounts from the macrophages of patients with the severe form of asthma. In this context, it was of interest that macrophage activation (as assessed by complement rosettes) increased after allergen challenge in patients who developed late-phase asthmatic reactions[10].

LYMPHOCYTES

There are two broad categories of lymphocytes. Thymus-derived lymphocytes, or T cells, are concerned with cell-mediated immunity (also called delayed hypersensitivity), and bone marrow-derived lymphocytes, or B cells. B cells mature into antibody-forming plasma cells. Plasma cells secrete all immunoglobulin classes, including IgE, which participate in immediate hypersensitivity. B cells complete their differentiation within the bone marrow with final maturation taking place in the peripheral lymphoid organs such as the spleen, lymph node and gut-associated lymphoid tissues[37]. T cell maturation involves T cell progenitors which rise in the bone marrow. These undergo further differentiation in the thymus, under local influences, to give cells which proliferate and differentiate to produce mature T cells.

T cells are initially primed by recognizing the combination of antigen and 'self' on macrophages. Macrophages first process antigen and then present it, on their cell surface, in combination with HL-A antigens to T lymphocytes. This interaction leads to T cell differentiation and proliferation with the formation of T lymphoblasts and the secretion of soluble mediators termed lymphokines. Other antigen-presenting cells (APC – Figure 8.1) include B cells, endothelial cells and dendritic cells. It seems likely that T cells are adapted to recognize cell surface-associated antigens, and for this reason are important in resistance to fungi and parasites, rejection of transplanted tissues and tumour surveillance. Besides delayed hypersensitivity T cells there are other T cell subpopulations; these include killer or cytotoxic T cells, T helper cells and T suppressor cells. These separate T cell populations can be recognized by specific cell surface markers using monoclonal antibody and immunofluorescence techniques.

Antigen recognition by B cells is also dependent on surface receptor contact followed by proliferation and differentiation. The differentiated B lymphocyte secretes antibody and assumes the characteristic morphology of plasma cells. Plasma cells have the armamentarium for active protein secretion and will produce antibody of one immunoglobulin class. IgE-secreting plasma cells are located in the lung and gut-associated lymphoid organs and other lymphoid tissues which are situated around portals of entry.

The role of T lymphocytes in asthma is uncertain, although a number of investigators have observed a deficiency of concanavalin A-induced suppressor cell function in asthmatic subjects[38-42]. Although delayed-type skin reactions to pollen antigens are not a feature of allergic asthma, specifically sensitized cells can be readily demonstrated *in vitro* either by lymphocyte mitogenesis to pollen allergens or the production of lymphokines such as macrophage migration inhibition factor[43,44]. In a recent study it was shown that there was a selective loss of circulating helper (OKT4) T cells and an apparent increase in activated (Ia positive) T cells after allergen-induced asthma[45]. These changes were also associated with a raised blood eosinophil count, suggesting that T cells may be activated in these situations to produce eosinophil stimulating substances.

In a more detailed study involving lung lavage six patients with single early responses (SER) were compared to six patients with dual, early- and late-phase (LPR) reactions to inhaled allergens[46]. In these subjects the percentages of T_H (OKT4), and T suppressor (T_S) (OKT8), and the T4/T8 ratio in blood and bronchoalveolar lavage (BAL) fluid were measured 6 h after challenge with either antigen or diluent control. Each procedure was separated by an interval of 7–14 days. When antigen was compared to diluent there were significant increases in the percentages of T_H, decreases in T_S and increases in the T4/T8 ratio in the blood of subjects with SER, whereas there were no significant differences during LPR. In contrast, T_H were significantly decreased and T_S increased and the T4/T8 ratio depressed in BAL in SER. In LPR there were increases in both T_H and T_S in BAL. Thus the data indicate that T_S predominates in BAL in SER, whereas in LPR both T_S and T_H are recruited to the lungs. The findings support the view that the T_H/T_S ratio may influence inflammatory changes associated with LPR. Thus, these investigations, and those of others, raise the possibility that either a form of delayed cell-mediated hypersensitivity mechanisms plays a role in the pathogenesis of late-phase reactions and/or that regulatory T-cells influence the activity of mast cells, or other mediator cells for the clinical expression of these delayed-in-time reactions.

CONCLUSIONS

There is evidence for believing that neutrophils, eosinophils, macrophages, platelets and lymphocytes all participate in allergic inflammation. It is likely that the final clinical expression in allergy and asthma results from a number of interreactions between these various cell types. Distinction must also be made between the clinical models of allergic disease (such as allergen-induced asthma evoked in the laboratory under controlled conditions) and day-to-day rhinitis and asthma which have many different facets, i.e. mild or severe, episodic or chronic. The patterns of reactivity in the clinical models consist predominantly of single early responses or dual reactions. The single early response is probably the result of the release of an array of pharmacological mediators acting directly on target tissue. The complexities of the late-phase reaction are beginning to be unravelled. An infiltration of neutrophils and eosinophils with release of products from both the granule and the cell membrane may contribute to smooth muscle contraction, mucosal oedema and mucus hypersecretion. The mechanism by which these cells arrive at the reaction site is unclear, but chemotactic lymphokines and/or mast cell-derived agents might be involved. The macrophage is also activated during late-phase reactions, and this cell type might also play a role in the mobilization of granulocytes. Preliminary studies suggest that regulatory T cells might be involved in the regulation of late-phase reactions. Perhaps loss of control by T suppressor cells may be critical for the clinical expression of these delayed-in-time responses. The relationship between the changes observed in late-phase reactions to those which occur in day-to-day disease is the subject of much discussion and speculation. Late-phase reactions in the lung, nose and skin appear to be a useful model of the disease in so far as they are associated with bronchial hyperreactivity and local eosinophilia, both of which are cardinal features of ongoing disease. It seems possible that the severe asthmatic might have uncontrolled release of eosinophil activating factors, possibly derived from macrophages, via T lymphocyte-dependent mechanisms, which in turn leads to intense inflammatory cell infiltration, with eosinophils being prominent. The establishment of 'superactivated' macrophages, refractory to the effects of corticosteroids and located in and around the bronchi, is a scenario possibly worthy of consideration. Unfortunately, knowledge of the natural history of rhinitis, asthma and other allergy-associated diseases is still hampered by lack of basic detail of the pathology as it exists on a day-to-day basis.

References

1. Wright, D. G. (1982). The neutrophil as a secretory organ of host defence. In Gallin, J. I. and Fauci, A. S. (eds.) *Phagocytic Cells: Advances in Host Defense Mechanisms, Vol. 1*, pp. 75–110. (NY: Raven Press)
2. Borish, L., O'Reilly, D., Klempner, M. S. and Rocklin, R. E. (1986). Leukocyte inhibitory factor (LIF) potentiates neutrophil responses to formyl-methionyl-leucyl-phenylalanine. *J. Immunol.*, **137**, 1897–903
3. Kay, A. B., Glass, E. J. and Salter, D. McG. (1979). Leuco-attractants enhance complement receptors on human phagocytic cells. *Clin. Exp. Immunol.*, **38**, 294–99
4. Murphy, K. R., Irvin, C. G., Glezen, L. S., Marsh, W. R. and Larsen, G. L. (1985). The effect of polymorphonuclear leukocyte depletion on the late asthmatic response and changes in airways reactivity. *Am. Rev. Resp. Dis.*, **131**, A6
5. Carroll, M., Durham, S. R., Walsh, G. M. and Kay, A. B. (1985). Leukocyte activation in allergen- and histamine-induced bronchoconstriction. *J. Allergy Clin. Immunol.*, **75**, 290–6
6. Papageorgiou, N., Carroll, M., Durham, S. R., Lee, T. H., Walsh, G. M. and Kay, A. B. (1983). Complement receptor enhancement as evidence of neutrophil activation after exercise-induced asthma. *Lancet*, **2**, 1220–3

7. Moqbel, R., Durham, S. R., Shaw, R. J., Walsh, G. M., MacDonald, A. J., Mackay, J. A., Carroll, M. P. and Kay, A. B. (1986). Enhancement of leukocyte cytotoxicity after exercise-induced asthma. *Am. Rev. Resp. Dis.*, **133**, 609–13

8. Durham, S. R., Carroll, M., Walsh, G. M. and Kay, A. B. (1984). Leukocyte activation in allergen-induced late-phase reactions. *N. Engl. J. Med.*, **311**, 1398–402

9. Larsen, G. L., Wilson, M. C., Marsh, W. R., Haslett, C. and Murphy, K. R. (1987). Neutrophils and late-phase reactions. In Kay, A. B. (ed.) *Allergy and Inflammation*. (London: Academic Press) (In press)

10. Diaz, P., Gonzalez, C., Galleguillos, F., Ancic, P. and Kay, A. B. (1986). Eosinophils and macrophages in bronchial mucus and bronchoalveolar lavage during allergen-induced late-phase asthmatic reactions. *J. Allergy Clin. Immunol.*, **77**, 244

11. Atkins, P. C., Norman, M., Weiner, H. and Zweiman, B. (1977). Release of neutrophil chemotactic activity during immediate hypersensitivity reactions in humans. *Ann. Intern. Med.*, **86**, 415–18

12. Nagy, L., Lee, T. H. and Kay, A. B. (1982). Neutrophil chemotactic activity in antigen-induced late asthmatic reactions. *N. Engl. J. Med.*, **306**, 497–501

13. Lee, T. H., Nagy, L., Nagakura, T., Walport, M. J. and Kay, A. B. (1982). Identification and partial characterisation of an exercise-induced neutrophil chemotactic factor in bronchial asthma. *J. Clin. Invest.*, **69**, 889–99

14. Lee, T. H., Nagakura, T., Papageorgiou, N., Iikura, Y. and Kay, A. B. (1983). Exercise-induced late asthmatic reactions with neutrophil chemotactic activity. *N. Engl. J. Med.*, **308**, 1502–5

15. Buchanan, D. R., Cromwell, O. and Kay, A. B. (1986). Neutrophil chemotactic activity (NCA) in acute severe asthma. *J. Allergy Clin. Immunol.*, **77**, 183

16. Collins, J. V., Wardlaw, A. J., Cromwell, O. and Kay, A. B. (1986). Mast cells and neutrophils in bronchoalveolar lavage from asthmatics. *J. Allergy Clin. Immunol.*, **77**, 209

17. Kay, A. B. (1985). Eosinophils as effector cells in immunity and hypersensitivity disorders. *Clin. Exp. Immunol.*, **62**, 1–12

18. Shaw, R. J., Walsh, G. M., Cromwell, O., Moqbel, R., Spry, C. J. F. and Kay, A. B. (1985). Activated human eosinophils generate SRS-A leukotrienes following physiological (IgG-dependent) stimulation. *Nature*, **316**, 150–2

19. Lee, T. C., Lenihan, D. J., Malone, B., Ruddy, L. L. and Wasserman, S. I. (1984). Increased biosynthesis of platelet-activating factor in activated human eosinophils. *J. Biol. Chem.*, **259**, 5526–30

20. Turk, J., Maas, R. L., Brash, A. R., Roberts, L. J. and Oates, J. A. (1982). Arachidonic acid 15-lipoxygenase products from human eosinophils. *J. Biol. Chem.*, **257**, 7056–67

21. Sanderson, C. J., O'Garra, A., Warren, D. J. and Klaus, G. G. B. (1986). Eosinophil differentiation factor also has B-cell growth factor activity: proposed name interleukin 4. *Proc. Natl. Acad. Sci. USA*, **83**, 437–40

22. Filley, W. V., Holley, K. E., Kephart, G. M. and Gleich, G. J. (1982). Identification by immunofluorescence of eosinophil granule major basic protein in lung tissues of patients with bronchial asthma. *Lancet*, **2**, 11–16

23. Frigas, E., Loegering, D. A., Solley, G. O., Farrow, G. M. and Gleich, G. J. (1981). Elevated levels of the eosinophil granule major basic protein in the sputum of patients with bronchial asthma. *Mayo Clin. Proc.*, **56**, 345–53

24. Durham, S. R. and Kay, A. B. (1985). Eosinophils, bronchial hyperreactivity and late-phase asthmatic reactions. *Clin. Allergy*, **15**, 411–18

25. De Monchy, J. G. R., Kauffman, H. F., Venge, P., Köeter, G. H., Jansen, H. M., Sluiter, H. J. and De Vries, K. (1985). Bronchoalveolar eosinophilia during allergen-induced late asthmatic reactions. *Am. Rev. Resp. Dis.*, **131**, 373–6

26. Kay, A. B., Wardlaw, A. J., Collins, J. V., Dunnette, S. and Gleich, G. J. (1986). Eosinophil and major basic protein in bronchoalveolar lavage in asthma: relationship to non-specific hyperreactivity. *J. Allergy Clin. Immunol.*, **77**, 236

27. Galli, S. J., Dvorak, A. M. and Dvorak, H. F. (1984). Basophils and mast cells: morphologic insights into their biology, secretory patterns and function. In Ishizaka, K. (ed.) *Mast Cell Activation and Mediator Release*, pp. 1–187. (Basle: Karger)

28. Askenase, P. W., Bagnall, B. G. and Worms, M. J. (1982). Cutaneous basophil associated

resistance to ectoparasites (ticks). I. Transfer with immune serum or immune cells. *Immunology*, **45**, 501-11

29. Taussig, M. J. (1984). Inflammation. In *Processes in Pathology and Microbiology*, 2nd Edn. pp. 3-68. (Oxford: Blackwell Scientific Publications)

30. Jessup, W., Leoni, P. and Dean, R. T. (1985). The macrophage in inflammation. In Venge, P. and Lindbom, A. (eds.) *Inflammation: Basic Mechanisms, Tissue Injuring Principles and Clinical Models*, pp. 161-186. (Stockholm: Almquist and Wiksell International)

31. Joseph, M., Tonnel, A. B., Capron, A. and Voisin, C. (1980). Enzyme release and superoxide anion production by human alveolar macrophages stimulated with immunoglobulin E. *Clin. Exp. Immunol.*, **40**, 416-22

32. Joseph, M., Tonnel, A. B., Capron, A. and Dessaint, J.-P. (1981). The interaction of IgE-antibody with human alveolar macrophages and its participation in the inflammatory processes of lung allergy. *Agents Actions*, **11**, 619-22

33. Tonnel, A. B., Joseph, M., Gosset, P., Fournier, E. and Capron, A. (1983). Stimulation of alveolar macrophages in asthmatic patients after local provocation test. *Lancet*, **1**, 1406-8

34. Joseph, M., Tonnel, A., Torpier, G., Capron, A., Arnoux, B. and Benveniste, J. (1983). Involvement of immunoglobulin E in the secretory processes of alveolar macrophages from asthmatic patients. *J. Clin. Invest.*, **71**, 221-30

35. Veith, M. C. and Butterworth, A. E. (1983). Enhancement of human eosinophil-mediated killing of *Schistosoma mansoni* larvae by mononuclear cell products *in vitro*. *J. Exp. Med.*, **157**, 1828-43

36. Fitzharris, P., Moqbel, R., Thorne, K. J. I., Richardson, B. A., Butterworth, A. E., Hartnell, A., Cromwell, O. and Kay, A. B. (1986). Monocyte-derived eosinophil activating factor (EAF) enhances LTC4 production by human eosinophils. *J. Allergy Clin. Immunol*, **77**, 235

37. Holborow, E. J. and Papamichail, M. (1983). The lymphoid system and lymphocyte subpopulations. In Holborow, E. J. and Reeves, W. G. (eds.) *Immunology in Medicine*, 2nd Edn. pp. 17-34. (London/NY: Academic Press)

38. Harper, T. B., Gaumer, H. R., Waring, W., Brannon, R. B., Salvaggio, J. E. (1980). A comparison of cell-mediated immunity and suppressor T-cell function in asthmatic and normal children. *Clin. Allergy*, **10**, 555-63

39. Rola-Pleszczynski, M. and Blanchard, R. (1981). Suppressor cell function in respiratory allergy. *Int. Arch. Allergy Appl. Immun.*, **64**, 361-70

40. Rivlin, J., Kuperman, O., Freier, S. and Godfrey, S. (1981). Suppressor T-lymphocyte activity in wheezy children with and without treatment by hyposensitization. *Clin. Allergy*, **11**, 353-6

41. Hwang, K. C., Fikrig, S. M., Friedman, H. M. and Gupta, S. (1985). Deficient concanavalin A-induced suppressor-cell activity in patients with bronchial asthma, allergic rhinitis, and atopic dermatitis. *Clin. Allergy*, **15**, 67-72

42. Ilfeld, D., Kivity, S., Feierman, E., Topilsky, M. and Kuperman, O. (1985). Effects of *in vitro* colchicine and oral theophylline on suppressor cell function of asthmatic patients. *Clin. Exp. Immunol.*, **61**, 360-7

43. Rocklin, R. E., Pence, H., Kaplan, H. and Evans, R. (1974). Cell-mediated immune reponse of ragweed-sensitive patients to ragweed antigen E. *In vitro* lymphocyte transformation and elaboration of lymphocyte mediators. *J. Clin. Invest.*, **53**, 735-44

44. Maini, R. N., Dumonde, D. C., Faux, J. A., Hargreave, F. E. and Pepys, J. (1971). The production of lymphocyte mitogenic factor and migration inhibition factor by antigen-stimulated lymphocytes of subjects with grass pollen allergy. *Clin. Exp. Immunol.*, **9**, 449-65

45. Gerblich, A. A., Campbell, A. E. and Schuyler, M. R. (1984). Changes in T-lymphocyte subpopulations after antigenic bronchial provocation in asthmatics. *N. Engl. J. Med.*, **310**, 1349-52

46. Gonzalez, C., Diaz, P., Galleguillos, F., Ancic, P. and Kay, A. B. (1986). T helper (T$_H$) and suppressor (T$_S$) cells in bronchoalveolar lavage during antigen-induced late-phase asthmatic reactions. *J. Allergy Clin. Immunol.*, **77**, 244

9
Target Tissues for Mediators in Human Allergic Reactions

R. W. FULLER

INTRODUCTION

Inflammation is a fundamental component of the body's response to trauma and the invasion of foreign material. Although inflammation can occur in all tissues, as the structure of tissue at various sites differs, the response of the tissues are not necessarily the same. It is the purpose of this chapter to review the spectrum of mediators released during human allergic reactions in general, and in three specific target sites for the reaction, i.e. the skin, nose and airway. The effect of the mediators on the target tissues and the evidence for the relative importance for each mediator, or group of mediators, in the production of the reaction at each specific site is also discussed.

THE ALLERGIC REACTION

The primary cells triggering the allergic reactions include mast cells[1], tissue macrophages[2] and the cells comprising the target tissue, i.e. the epithelial[3], endothelial[4] and nerve cells[5] and possibly the smooth muscle[6]. The activation of the inflammatory cells by the interaction of antigen with specific reaginic antibodies (discussed elsewhere) leads to the release of preformed mediators, principally histamine and peptides, as well as newly formed mediators derived from membrane-bound lipids and active oxygen species. These mediators act in the tissues to induce the early inflammatory response, the nature of which will be determined by the combination of mediators released and the structure of the target tissue itself. The initial response may lead to the activation of further mediators from the plasma[7], and the activity of chemotaxins will cause cellular accumulation which results in a late allergic reaction.

The result of allergic inflammation in a particular tissue depends upon both the primary (resident) and secondary (migratory) cells involved in the reaction and, therefore, the cellular structure of the tissue and the mediators released into the tissue. It follows that allergic reactions in the skin should involve altered blood flow, oedema and cellular infiltration, whereas in the airways and gut smooth muscle contraction and altered secretion from glands will also be involved. The target cells for the mediators released by the inflammatory cells are the following: (1) the cells forming the connective tissue, e.g. fibroblasts, resident inflammatory cells and neurones; (2) the blood vessels, principally the vascular smooth muscle, endothelial cells and circulating cells, and (3) the airway smooth muscle, the respiratory and bronchial epithelium and the mucous secreting cells which are found in the respiratory tract.

Allergic responses in the skin

An allergic reaction in the skin can be elicited by intradermal or subcutaneous dosing of the allergen. Intradermal injection of antigen into an atopic subject leads to a Lewis triple response[8] with a dose-dependent weal and flare reaction associated with itching. In some subjects a dose-dependent late reaction will appear 4–6 hours later. This consists of an area of flare and swelling which may persist for 24 hours.

The flare requires an intact nerve supply to the area of the skin, and is due to vasodilatation following the release of neurotransmitters by antidromic stimulation of the sensory nerves[5, 9]. This stimulation of the nerves is also responsible for pain and itch at the site of the injection. The weal is a reflection of local oedema formation caused by an increase in arteriolar blood flow combined with an increase in capillary leakiness and venular-constriction, the alteration in blood flow causing the extravasation of fluid through the leaky capillaries. The late reaction follows the accumulation of inflammatory cells at the site of the oedema. These cells are principally granulocytes with some mononuclear cells[10]. Mediators released from these cells lead to arteriolar dilatation, flare and further oedema formation.

Allergic responses in the nose

The manifestions of allergic responses following topical antigen in the nose are similar to those in the skin, principally due to an alteration in the local blood flow with the added effect of increased glandular secretion. Increase in arterial blood flow and venular tone in the mucosal circulation of the nose is in part due to the direct action of the mediators. There is, however, a neuroreflex component dependent upon the release of acetylcholine, and perhaps neuropeptides, from the nerves supplying the vasculature[11]. This leads to an increase in the thickness of the mucosa and, therefore, limits airflow. Sensory nerve stimulation in the nose and mucosa also leads to a sensation of itch. Altered capillary permeability induces both perivascular oedema and extravasation of plasma into and from the nasal air passage. This coupled with an increased secretion of the goblet cells and mucous glands into the airway leads to rhinorrhoea. As in the skin, the magnitude

242

of the response is dose-dependent, and is associated with cellular accumulation. After 4–6 hours a second phase of nasal airflow limitation occurs and cellular exudation into the lumen of the nose results.

Allergic responses in the airway

The responses in the bronchi to inhaled antigen are more complex than those in the skin or nose due to the larger number of tissue components involved. These different components of the response occur at different times during the response. The initial response consists of bronchial smooth muscle contraction, mucus secretion and reduced mucociliary clearance following the loss of epithelial integrity, mucosal oedema and cellular influx into the mucosa and lumen of the airway.

Smooth muscle contraction is due to the direct stimulation by mediators and alteration of neural tone resulting in an increase in acetylcholine release, and possibly a reduction in the inhibitory tone of neuropeptides[5]. Increased mucus secretion occurs by a direct stimulation of the goblet cells by the mediators as well as a reflex increase in glandular secretion[12, 13]. Altered mucociliary clearance is produced by inhibition of ciliary beats and an increase in both the sol and gel layer of the mucus layer following increased epithelial chloride transport[13] and increased mucus secretion[12]. The increase of the sol and gel layer reduces the efficiency of ciliary action on the gel. The alteration in epithelial function is, in part, due to the released mediators, but may also result from sensory neuropeptide release[5]. The same factors lead to the loss of integrity of the epithelial layer which is characteristic of asthma[14]. Mucosal oedema is the result of a similar process in the feeding blood vessels which results in the oedema of the skin and nose. Likewise cellular accumulation results from the release of chemotaxins from the stimulated inflammatory cells.

Like the responses in the skin and nose, some 4–8 hours after the initial response, a late phase of airflow limitation occurs which is dependent on the accumulation of inflammatory cells, mucus and plasma in the airways. Unlike the other sites discussed in which resolution is complete, the airways show persistent changes which become manifest as increased bronchoconstrictor responses to inhaled stimulants; this is thought to depend on a persistence of the inflammatory responses in the airways.

MEDIATORS

There are many mediators which can be released by inflammatory or other tissue cells or which may be formed from the plasma. They can mediate inflammatory responses in their own right or in combination with other mediators. The mediators released from the various inflammatory cells activated by the interaction of antigen with reaginic antibody have been studied by challenging these cells *in vitro* and are listed in Tables 9.1 and 9.2.

Table 9.1 Classes of mediators released from inflammatory cells and plasma *in vitro* which may be involved in allergic reactions. See also references 90–100

	Cyclo-oxygenase	Lipoxy-genase	Inorganic	Histamine	Peptides	Enzymes	PAF
Mast cells	+	+	+	+	+	+	+
Macrophage	+	+	+	−	+	+	+
Neutrophils	+	+	+	−	+	+	+
Eosinophils	+	+	+	−	+	+	+
Basophils	+	+	+	+	+	+	?
Platelets	+	+	+	−	+	?	?
Epithelial cells	+	+	+	−	+	+	?
Endothelial cells	+	+	?	−	+	+	?
Plasma	−	−	−	−	+	+	?

? = unknown

Table 9.2 Human mast cell and macrophage mediators

Mast cell	Macrophage
Histamine	Superoxide
Heparin	Proteases
Protease	Lysosomal hydrolase
TAME esterase	Complement fractions
Kinogenase	Interferon
$PGD_2/F_{2\alpha}/TXA_2$	Interleukins
LTC_4	TXA_2
PAF	PGD_2, E_2, $F_{2\alpha}$
LTB_4	LTB_4/C_4
5-HETE	PAF
ECFA	5-HETE
NCFA	12-HETE

Mediators and allergic reactions

The mediators involved in allergic reactions have been assessed by three methods: (1) by measurement of mediators in tissue or blood; (2) by challenge of the tissue with the mediators, singly or in combination, to assess whether the mediators mimic allergic reactions, and (3) by using inhibitors either of mediator formation or receptor stimulation.

However, there are problems with these approaches to the assessment of the importance of a particular mediator. First, the measurement of mediators depends on sensitive and specific assays of the very potent mediators which may be present in only small amounts. Assays have, therefore, led to both false positive and false negative results. A further problem is the release of mediators from cells not involved in the response but which are activated during sampling, for example, basophil histamine release[15].

Secondly, the demonstration of a response to a mediator applied to a tissue may also lead to a false impression, as many non-specific or non-physiological effects can occur by the stimulation of cutaneous nerves

244

Table 9.3 Effects of lipid derived mediators in human tissues in vivo unless otherwise stated. Some of the mediators have actions in vivo and in vitro in animal studies which have not been confirmed in man

Mediator	Skin				Airways				Change in airway reactivity		Nasal airflow
	Local flare	Neurogenic flare	Weal	Late response	Broncho-constriction	Mucus hypersecretion[1]	Altered epithelial function	Cough	Immediate	Late	
PGE_2	+	+	N	N	-/+	+	+	+	+	N*	N
$F_{2\alpha}$	+	+	N	N	+	+	+	+	+	N*	N
I_2	+	N	N	N	N	?	?	N	-	N*	-
D_2	?	+	?	N	+	+	?	+	?	N*	?
TXA_2	N	?	N	?	?	?	?	?	?	+	?
LTB_4	N	+	+	N	N	+	?	N	N	N	?
C_4	N	+	+	N	+	+	?	N	N	N	?
D_4	N	+	+	N	+	+	?	N	N	N	?
E_4	?	?	?	?	+	+	+	N	N	N	?
HETES	?	?	?	?	?	?	?	?	?	?	?
HPETES	?	?	?	?	?	?	?	?	?	?	?
Lipoxins	?	?	?	?	?	?	?	?	?	?	?
PAF	N	+	+	+	+	+	+	+	N	+	?

-/+ cyclooxygenase inhibition does not alter antigen induced change in nasal airflow

* Indomethacin reduced antigen increase in airway reactivity

[1] Information from non-human and in vitro studies

N = no effect

? = effect unknown

245

Table 9.4 Effects of neural mediators in human tissues in vivo unless otherwise stated. Some of the mediators have actions in vivo and in vitro in animal studies which have not been confirmed in man

Mediator	Skin				Airways				Change in airway reactivity		Nasal airflow
	Local flare	Neurogenic flare	Weal	Late response	Broncho-constriction	Mucus hypersecretion[1]	Altered epithelial function	Cough	Immediate	Late	
ACh	+	0	?	N	+	+	+	+	N	N	−
NAdr	−	N	−	N	−	+	−	?	N	N	+
SP	N	+	+	N	N	+	+	N	N	N	−
CGRP	+	±	N	N	N	?	?	?	N	N	?
NK	N	+	+	N	N	?	?	?	N	N	?
VIP	+	N	N	N	−	+	+	N	?	?	?

ACh = Acetylcholine
NAdr = Noradrenaline
SP = Substance P
CGRP = Calcitonine gene related peptide
NK = Neurokinin A/B
VIP = Vasoactive intestinal peptide
[1] Information from non-human and in vitro studies
N = no effect
? = effect unknown

Table 9.5 Effects of autocoids on human tissues *in vivo* unless otherwise stated. Some of the mediators have actions *in vivo* and *in vitro* in animal studies which have not been confirmed in man

| Mediator | Skin | | | | Airways | | | | Change in airway reactivity | | Nasal airflow |
	Local flare	Neurogenic flare	Weal	Late response	Broncho-constriction	Mucus hypersecretion[1]	Altered epithelial function[1]	Cough	Immediate	Late	
Adenosine	N	N	N	N	+	+	?	N	N	N	?
AMP	?	?	?	?	+	?	?	N	N	N	?
ATP	N	+	+	N	+	?	?	N	N	N	?
Histamine	N	+	+	N	+	+	+	+	N	N	–
5-HT	+	N	N	N	N	N	?	N	N	N	?

AMP = Adenosine monophosphate
ATP = Adenosine triphosphate
5-HT = 5 Hydroxytryptamine
[1] Information from non-human and *in vitro* studies
N = no effect
? = effect unknown

Table 9.6 Effects of peptides and inorganic chemical mediators in human tissues in vivo unless otherwise stated. Some of the mediators have actions in vivo and in vitro in animal studies which have not been confirmed in man

Mediator	Skin				Airways				Change in airway reactivity		
	Local flare	Neurogenic flare	Weal	Late response	Broncho-constriction	Mucus hypersecretion	Altered epithelial function	Cough	Immediate	Late	Nasal airflow
Kinins	+	N	+	N	+	+	+	+	N	N	?
Complement	?	?	+	?	?	?	?	?	?	?	?
Interferon	?	?	?	?	?	?	?	?	?	?	?
NCFA	?	?	?	?	?	?	?	?	?	?	?
ECFA	?	?	?	?	?	?	?	?	?	?	?
Hydrolases	?	?	?	?	?	?	?	?	?	?	?
Major basic protein	?	?	?	?	+	?	+	+	?	?	?
Interleukins	?	?	?	?	?	?	?	+	?	?	?
Superoxide	?	?	?	?	?	?	+	+	?	?	?

NCFA = Neutrophil chemotactic factor of anaphylaxis
ECFA = Eosinophil chemotactic factor of anaphylaxis
[1] Information from non-human and in vitro studies
N = no effect
? = effect unknown

248

Table 9.7   Combined mediators causing an enhanced effect in man

	Flare	Weal	Bronchoconstriction
PGE_2/Bradykinin	+	+	?
LTB_4, PGE_2/D_2	+	+	N
Histamine/PGD_2	—	—	+
Histamine/$PGF_{2\alpha}$	—	—	+
LTD_4/$PGF_{2\alpha}$	?	?	+
CGRP and SP	N	+ *	?

*Animals, not man
N = no effect
? = effect unknown

possibly caused by the carrier solution or even by mediator release from resident cells by non-receptor mechanisms[16]. Information about local tissue response may be lacking because some mediators are so unstable that their study in man is so far impractical. Thirdly, inhibitors can be non-specific, e.g. ketotifen, which was originally considered to be an antihistamine and antiallergic compound, is also a platelet activating factor (PAF) antagonist[17]. The lack of response of an inhibitor may also be due to the lack of penetration of the tissue by the inhibitor, for example the lack of effect of nafazatrom, a 5-lipoxygenase inhibitor on antigen induced asthma was found to be due to poor bioavailability[18]. Given these problems, what is the evidence for the involvement of various mediators in allergic tissue responses?

Despite these limitations there has been considerable research into the effects of single mediators, but far less into their combined action. Tables 9.3–7 list the mediators and their effects on: (1) vascular tone and capillary integrity which leads to weal and flare; (2) airway smooth muscle and glandular secretion leading to bronchoconstriction and asthma. Table 9.7 lists the known interactions between mediators which have been studied in the skin following intradermal injection and in the airways by inhalation.

From the Tables it can be seen that in man *in vivo* some mediators have their effects primarily upon blood vessels leading to oedema; others on airway smooth muscle and mucus secretion resulting in asthma, while others are potent chemotactic agents causing a late reaction and the altered tissue responsiveness associated with the disease. There are many other mediators which may be released and have been shown to have potent effects in animal studies (complement, interferon, interleukins, etc.) which have not yet been studied in man, and therefore, their importance has not yet been assessed.

Measurements of mediators released during allergic inflammation

Skin

Mediators released by allergic reaction in the skin have been assessed by sampling fluid taken from blisters formed artificially at the site of challenge[12, 19], and by taking blood samples from the veins draining the site of the reaction. Blisters raised in patients who have cold urticaria contain elevated levels of histamine, PGD_2, E_2, $F_{2\alpha}$, 6-oxo-$PGF_{1\alpha}$, TXB_2, LTC_4, D_4, E_4, PAF and kinins[20], however raising the blister itself is associated with mediator release[19]. Blood draining the sites of antigen induced cutaneous reactions has shown elevated levels of histamine and prostaglandin D_2[21], but not leukotrienes. However, preliminary data from our laboratory suggest the LTE_4, as well as histamine and PGD_2[22], may be present in blood draining cold urticaria reactions. Tissue biopsy has also been employed to confirm the presence of various neuropeptides in the tissue[23], and studies with topical capsaicin, which depletes neuropeptides, have implicated their role in neurogenic flare[24].

Nose

Measurement of nasal derived mediators has been performed on fluid obtained from nasal airways following antigen challenge, and by the study of cells or tissue obtained by biopsy of the nose. These techniques have shown the presence of histamine, PGD_2, LTC_4, D_4, kinins and TAME esterase[25-27], a constituent of mast cell granules. However, nasal secretions contain both inflammatory cells and plasma proteins which could lead to ex-vivo generation of the mediators.

Bronchi

Assessment of the mediators involved in antigen induced airway response has been performed by venous sampling, bronchoalveolar lavage and measurement of mediators in sputum. Claims of elevated plasma levels of histamine, leukotrienes[28, 29], neutrophil chemotactic factors of anaphylaxis (NCFA), adenosine, 13,14-dihydro-15-keto $PGF_{2\alpha}$[1] and PAF[30] following antigen challenge have been made. However, histamine may have been released from circulating basophils[15], and NCFA may also be non-specific as it has been measured in the plasma in other pulmonary diseases[31] and may be produced by circulating cells[32]. The results concerning PAF and LTs require confirmation using improved assay techniques. Many laboratories, including our own, have reported that the peptidoleukotrienes may be rapidly metabolized to LTE_4. Few studies have been made using assays which give an integrated amount of mediator release. One such study[33] has shown that histamine is released in the early, but not late, response to antigen induced bronchoconstriction. Bronchoalveolar lavage has been used to show cellular accumulation in the airways[34], and reports suggest that histamine[33], lysosomal hydrolases[35], prostaglandin D_2[36], kinins[37] and, recently from our laboratories, LTC_4, may be released into the airway following inhaled or local antigen challenge. The mediators released during the late phase have yet to be reported, although histamine appears not to be released[33]. Sputum analysis has demonstrated the presence of histamine and leukotriene in asthmatic patients[38, 39]. However, these mediators could have been derived from cells in the sputum following expectoration.

250

Effect of application of mediators to a tissue

Skin

Intradermal injections have been extensively studied as a method for assessing cutaneous responses to various mediators. Four basic responses are observed, neurogenic (distant) flare, local flare, weal and late reaction. Potent mediators of neurogenic flare are substance P (SP)[16], neurokinin A[40], histamine and LTD$_4$[41], PAF[42] and calcitonin gene related peptide (CGRP)[43] are less active. The tachykinin response requires the release of histamine and cyclooxygenase products[40]. Neurokinin B[40] and bradykinin[44] do not release histamine in human skin and do not cause a neurogenic flare. The release of mediators by the tachykinins is not due to classical receptor stimulation but to the physical property of the molecule[16]. The neurostimulant capsaicin causes a neurogenic flare by direct stimulation of cutaneous nerves; this is independent of histamine release[45], suggesting that insufficient tachykinin may be released under normal circumstance in the human skin to stimulate mast cells. Local flare occurs following injection of CGRP[43], PGE$_2$[46], PGD$_2$[47] and 5-hydroxytryptamine[48]. The response to CGRP appears to be direct as it was not inhibited by antihistamines and aspirin[40]. Weal is induced by the tachykinins[40], bradykinin[49], histamine[8], LTD$_4$[41] and PAF[42]. That due to the neuropeptides and bradykinin is not generally inhibited by antihistamine or aspirin. The response to bradykinin is enhanced by treatment with angiotensin converting enzyme inhibitors[49]. Late reactions have been reported after injection of PAF[42, 50] and co-injections of leukotriene B$_4$ with PGE$_2$[41].

Nose

Studies following histamine[51] and substance P[52] installation of potential mediators in the nose have shown that they will cause nasal blockade and sneezing, but no late reactions. The neurostimulant capsaicin[53] also caused blockage, but it is not known if this is by a reflex or tachykinin release. No studies performed with chemotactic mediators have so far been reported in man.

Bronchi

Many mediators when inhaled cause bronchoconstriction, with LTD$_4$[54], PGD$_2$[55], bradykinin[56] and PGF$_{2\alpha}$[57] the most potent, being 250, 10, 5 times more potent than histamine, respectively. The effect of PGE$_2$ is complex as it causes a reflex bronchoconstriction[57] and a direct relaxation of airway smooth muscle[58]. PAF[59], but not LTB$_4$ either alone or with PGD$_2$ (unpublished results from our laboratory), induces bronchohyperresponsiveness. Most have a direct action, however, some, e.g. bradykinin[56] and leukotriene[60], have an additional action which is in part due to airway reflexes. High dose histamine is subject to tachyphylaxis through the release of other mediators, probably prostaglandins[61]. Other potential mediators do not cause bronchoconstriction when inhaled, but access to the site of action may be impaired or may break down rapidly (e.g. substance P)[62]. Combination of prostaglandin with histamine[63], methacholine[64] and leukotrienes[65] has shown exaggerated bronchoconstrictor response. Mucociliary clearance has been studied in man using radiolabelled particles[66] and under direct vision by bronchoscopy[67]. Apart from studies with muscarinic agonists, which stimulate mucociliary clearance, the effects of individual mediators on mucociliary clearance *in vivo* have not been reported. However, the LTD_4 antagonist FPL 55712 inhibited antigen induced[67] changes in mucociliary clearance[68-70], and anticholinergic agents appear to improve mucociliary clearance, suggesting that the release of acetylcholine makes the clearance less efficient[71]. Epithelial permeability is altered by histamine, possibly by an H_2-receptor[72].

Pharmacological intervention

Skin

A number of inhibitor mediator receptors have been studied for their effect on cutaneous reactions to antigen. Some are non-specific, e.g. adrenaline, whereas others have uncertain mechanisms of action, e.g. sodium cromoglycate. Antihistamines have been shown to reduce antigen-induced flare and weal. The inhibition is dose-dependent and less than the effect of the drug on histamine itself, confirming the partial role of histamine in the response[73]. They also reduce the response to cold challenge in cold urticaria[74]. Cyclooxygenase inhibitors have a small inhibitory action on antigen induced reactions, suggesting a limited contribution of prostaglandins in the response[75]. Despite a large potentiation of bradykinin response in the skin[49], following oral enalapril, there was no effect of this drug on antigen-induced weal or flare[76]. Leukotriene receptor antagonists (unpublished results from our laboratory) studied so far have shown only marginal effects on the response to antigen, however, an optimal concentration may not have been reached in the skin.

Nose

Effective reduction of nasal allergic responses has been demonstrated with antihistamines[77] and with topical anticholinergic agents[78], implying a primary role for histamine and acetylcholine in the early response. Cyclooxygenase inhibitors effectively reduce prostaglandin secretion but not symptoms, implying that they have little importance in nasal allergy. Inhibitory responses are also seen with sodium cromoglycate which may inhibit mediator release or neural reflexes[80].

Bronchi

Tissue penetration is a problem in the study of inhibitors of airway responses. However, the development of drugs which are effective by inhalation may help to resolve this. Antihistamines[81], anti-leukotrienes[82] and antimuscarinic agents[83] as well as cyclooxygenase inhibitors[81, 84] have all reduced inhaled antigen responsiveness to varying extents depending upon dose. PAF antagonists have yet to be studied against antigen in man, however BW 52021[85] does inhibit antigen challenge in guinea-pigs. Antihistamine, antimuscarinic agents and antileukotrienes reduce the early response, and cyclooxygenase and thromboxane[86] inhibitors the late response. Indomethacin[87] also appears to reduce bronchial hyperactivity following antigen challenge in a manner similar to that seen following treatment with corticosteroids[88]. Angiotensin converting enzyme inhibition had no effect on histamine sensitivity, however, it did not potentiate the effect of inhaled bradykinin, suggesting that angiotensin converting enzyme may not be important in the metabolism of kinins in the airway[89]. Apart from the effect of anticholinergic agents, studies of anti-mediator drugs on mucociliary clearance have yet to be performed.

CONCLUSION

In order to establish the relative importance of a mediator in the allergic reaction of a specific tissue, evidence is required first of the release of the mediators during the reaction and evidence of the response of a tissue to the inflammatory mediators. The evidence suggests that all three tissues discussed may be exposed to the full spectrum of mediators during the responses to an allergic stimulus. The evidence is stronger for the preformed mediators (histamine and lysosomal hydrolases) and the arachidonic acid derived mediators, probably because they are present in larger amounts and the techniques for their analysis are well established. Is there sufficient evidence from studies of the mediators themselves or from the effects of antagonist, to conclude that different mediators are more important in the reactions of different tissues?

In terms of potency, assessed by the direct application of the mediator to the tissue, there is evidence for histamine and neuropeptides being most potent at mimicking the early response of the skin and nose, whilst prostaglandins, leukotrienes and bradykinin are potent at causing bronchoconstriction. However, as the amount of histamine released into the lung following antigen challenge is large, it may be an important contributing factor to the early bronchoconstriction (despite its lower potency). The release of acetylcholine by the vagus nerve also plays a part in the early bronchial and nasal response. The late response appears to be under the influence of the same chemotactic agents, especially PAF with perhaps the involvement of LTB$_4$ in the skin.

The lack of a difference in the factors leading to cellular accumulation is not surprising while the difference in the early allergic response may be due to the different structures involved and the nervous supply. Whether these apparent differences are artifactual or real is uncertain as there is a lack of adequate studies to assess the question. The responses to inhibition of single mediator groups is disappointing, and if this is not solely due to poor penetration of the inhibitor it implies a lack of a keystone role for the potential mediators. The presence of such keystone mediators in some animal models, even though extrapolation from animal to man may not be justified, suggests that adequate studies with improved techniques should be performed to rule out the presence of such human allergic disease.

However, on present evidence it is not possible to make a strong case for the importance of any particular mediator in the allergic response. It still remains a possibility that the body has adapted its inflammatory reaction to be able to use a fairly small range of mediators, possibly in combination to produce the responses through a number of independent pathways.

References

1. Holgate, S. T. and Kay, A. B. (1985). Mast cells, mediators and asthma. *Clin. Allergy*, **15**, 221–34
2. Takemura, R. and Werb, Z. (1984). Secretory products of macrophages and their physiological functions. *Am. J. Physiol.*, **246** (Cell Physiol.), C1–C9
3. Holtzman, M. J., Aizawa, H., Nadel, J. A. and Goetzl, E. J. (1983). Selective generation of leukotriene B₄ by tracheal epithelial cells from dogs. *Biochem. Biophys. Res. Commun.*, **114**, 1071–6
4. Gorman, R. R., Oglesby, T. D., Bundy, G. L. and Hopkins, N. K. (1985). Evidence for 15-HETE synthesis by human umbilical vein endothelial cells. *Circulation*, **72**, 708–12
5. Barnes, P. J. (1986). Neural control of human airways in health and disease. *Am. Rev. Resp. Dis.*, **134**, 1289–314
6. Shore, S. A., Powell, W. S. and Martin, J. G. (1985). Endogenous prostaglandins modulate histamine-induced contraction in canine tracheal smooth muscle. *J. Appl. Physiol.*, **58**, 859–68
7. Regoli, D. and Barabe, J. (1980). Pharmacology of bradykinin and related kinins. *Pharmacol. Rev.*, **32**, 1–46
8. Lewis, T. (1927). *The Blood Vessels of the Human Skin and their Responses*. (London: Shaw and Sons)
9. Jancso, N., Jancso-Gabor, A. and Szolcsanyi, J. (1968). The role of sensory nerve endings in neurogenic inflammation induced in human skin and in the eye and paw of the rat. *Br. J. Pharmacol. Chemother.*, **32**, 32–41
10. Fowler, II, J. W. and Louvel, F. C. (1966). The accumulation of eosinophils as an allergic response to allergen applied to the denuded skin surface. *J. Allergy Clin. Immunol.*, **37**, 19–28
11. Konno, A., Togawa, K. and Fujiwara, T. (1983). The mechanisms involved in onset of allergic manifestations in the nose. *Eur. J. Resp. Dis.*, **64**, 155–66
12. Richardson, P. S. and Phipps, R. J. (1978). The anatomy, physiology, pharmacology and pathology of tracheobronchial mucus secretion and the use of expectorant drugs in human disease. *Pharmacol. Ther. B.*, **3**, 441–79
13. Marin, M. G. (1986). Pharmacology of airway secretion. *Pharmacol. Rev.*, **38**, 273–89
14. Laitinen, L. A., Heino, M., Laitinen, A., Kava, T. and Haahtela, T. (1985). Damage of the airway epithelium and bronchial reactivity in patients with asthma. *Am. Rev. Resp. Dis.*, **131**, 599–606
15. Morgan, D. J. R., Moodley, I., Phillips, M. J. and Davies, R. J. (1983). Plasma histamine in asthmatic and control subjects following exercise: influence of circulating basophils and different assay techniques. *Thorax*, **38**, 771–7
16. Foreman, J. C., Jordan, C. C., Oehme, P. and Renner, H. (1983). Structure–activity relationships for some substance P-related peptides that cause wheal and flare reactions in human skin. *J. Physiol.*, **335**, 449–65
17. Morley, J., Page, C. P., Mazzoni, L. and Sanjar, S. (1985). Anti-allergic drugs in asthma. *Triangle*, **24**, 59–70
18. Fuller, R. W., Maltby, N., Richmond, R., Dollery, C. T., Taylor, G. W., Ritter, J. R. and Philipp, E. (1987). Oral nafazatrom in man: effect on inhaled antigen challenge. *Br. J. Clin. Pharmacol.*, **23**, 677–81

19. Heavey, D. J., Richmond, R., Turner, N. C., Kobza-Black, A., Taylor, G. W., Chappell, C. G., Barrow, S. E. and Dollery, C. T. (1986). Measurement of leukotrienes C_4 and D_4 in inflammatory fluids. In Piper, P. J. (ed.) *The Leukotrienes: Their Biological Significance*, pp. 185–98. (NY: Raven Press)

20. Dorsch, W., Ring, J., Reimann, H. J. and Geiger, R. (1982). Mediator studies in skin blister fluid from patients with dual skin reactions after intradermal allergen injection. *J. Allergy Clin. Immunol.*, **70**, 236–42

21. Heavey, D. J., Ind, P. W., Miyatake, A., Brown, M. J., MacDermot, J. and Dollery, C. T. (1984). Histamine released locally after intradermal antigen challenge in man. *Br. J. Clin. Pharmacol.*, **18**, 915–19

22. Heavey, D. J., Kobza-Black, A., Barrow, S. E., Chappell, C. G., Greaves, M. W. and Dollery, C. T. (1986). Prostaglandin D_2 and histamine release in cold urticaria. *J. Allergy Clin. Immunol.*, **78**, 458–61

23. Dalsgaard, C.-J., Jonsson, C.-E., Hökfelt, T. and Cuello, A. C. (1983). Localization of substance P-immunoreactive nerve fibers in the human digital skin. *Experientia*, **39**, 1018–20

24. Anand, P., Bloom, S. R. and McGregor, G. P. (1983). Topical capsaicin pretreatment inhibits axon reflex vasodilatation caused by somatostatin and vasoactive intestinal polypeptide in human skin. *Br. J. Pharmacol.*, **67**, 665–9

25. Proud, D., Togias, A., Naclerio, R. M., Crush, S. A., Normal, P. S. and Lichtenstein, L. M. (1983). Kinins are generated *in vivo* following nasal airway challenge of allergic individuals with allergen. *J. Clin. Invest.*, **72**, 1678–85

26. Naclerio, R. M., Proud, D., Peters, S. P., Silber, G., Kagey-Somotka, A., Adkinson, N. F., Jr. and Lichtenstein, L. M. (1986). Inflammatory mediators in nasal secretions during induced rhinitis. *Clin. Allergy*, **16**, 101–10

27. Creticos, P. S., Peters, S. P., Franklin Adkinson, N., Jr., Naclerio, R. M., Hayes, E. C., Normal, P. S. and Lichtenstein, L. M. (1984). Peptide leukotriene release after antigen challenge in patients sensitive to ragweed. *N. Engl. J. Med.*, **310**, 1626–30

28. Shaw, R. J., Fitzharris, P., Wardlaw, A. J., Cromwell, O. and Kay, A. B. Leukotrienes and the upper airways. In Kay, A. B. (ed.) *Asthma. Clinical Pharmacology and Therapeutic Progress*, pp. 205–12. (Oxford: Blackwell Scientific Publications)

29. Zakrzewski, J. T., Barnes, N. C., Piper, P. J. and Costello, J. F. (1985). Measurement of leukotrienes in arterial and venous blood from normal and asthmatic subjects by radioimmunoassay. *Br. J. Clin. Pharmacol.*, **19**, 574P

30. Nakamura, T., Morita, Y., Kuriyama, M., Ishihara, K., Ito, K. and Miyamato, T. (1987). Platelet-activating factor in late asthmatic response. *Int. Arch. Allergy Appl. Immun.*, **82**, 57–61

31. Cundell, D. R., Morgan, D. J. R. and Davies, R. J. (1984). NCF – A mast cell specific chemotactic factor? *Clin. Sci.*, **66**, 50P

32. Cundell, D. R., Morgan, D. J. R. and Davies, R. J. (1985). NCA – Neutrophil chemoattractant activity released by lymphocytes. *Clin. Sci.*, **68**, 53P–54P

33. De Monchy, J. G. R., Keyzer, J. J., Kauffman, H. F., Beaumont, F. and De Vries, K. (1985). Histamine in late asthmatic reactions following house-dust mite inhalation. *Agents Actions*, **16**, 252–5

34. De Monchy, J. G. R., Kauffman, H. F., Venge, P., Koëter, G. H., Jansen, H. M., Sluiter, H. J. and De Vries, K. (1985). Bronchoalveolar eosinophilia during allergen-induced late asthmatic reactions. *Am. Rev. Resp. Dis.*, **131**, 373–6

35. Tonnel, A. B., Joseph, M., Gosset, P. H., Fournier, E. and Capron, A. (1983). Stimulation of alveolar macrophages in asthmatic patients after local provocation test. *Lancet*, **1**, 1406–8

36. Murray, J. J., Tonnel, A. B., Brash, A. R., Roberts, L. J., II, Gosset, P., Workman, R., Capron, A. and Oates, J. A. (1986). Release of prostaglandin D_2 into human airways during acute antigen challenge. *N. Engl. J. Med.*, **315**, 800–4

37. Christiansen, S. C., Proud, D. and Cochrane, C. G. (1987). Detection of tissue kallikrein in bronchoalveolar lavage fluid of asthmatic subjects. *J. Clin. Invest.*, **79**, 188–97

38. Turnbull, L. S., Turnbull, L. W., Leitch, A. G. and Crofton, J. W. (1977). Mediators of immediate-type hypersensitivity in sputum from patients with chronic bronchitis and asthma. *Lancet*, **2**, 526–9

39. Cromwell, O., Walport, M. J., Morris, H. R., Taylor, G. W., Hodson, M. E., Batten, J. and Kay, A. B. (1981). Identification of leukotrienes D and B in sputum from cystic fibrosis patients. *Lancet*, **2**, 164–5

40. Barnes, P. J., Crossman, D. C. and Fuller, R. W. (1987). Cutaneous effects of neuropeptides are dependent upon both histamine and cyclooxygenase products. *Br. J. Pharmacol.*, **90**, 100P

41. Soter, N. A., Lewis, R. A., Corey, E. J. and Austen, K. F. (1983). Local effects of synthetic leukotrienes (LTC_4, LTD_4, LTE_4, and LTB_4) in human skin. *J. Invest. Dermatol.*, **80**, 115–19

42. Basran, G. S., Page, C. P., Paul, W. and Morley, J. (1983). Cromoglycate (DSCG) inhibits responses to platelet-activating factor (PAF-acether) in man: an alternative mode of action for DSCG in asthma? *Eur. J. Pharmacol.*, **86**, 143–4

43. Brain, S. D., Williams, T. J., Tippins, J. R., Morris, H. R. and MacIntyre, I. (1985). Calcitonin gene-related peptide is a potent vasodilator. *Nature*, **313**, 54–6

44. Crossman, D. and Fuller, R. W. (1987). Effect of terfenidine and aspirin on bradykinin-induced wheals. *Clin. Sci.*, **72**, 75P

45. Barnes, P. J., Brown, M. J., Dollery, C. T., Fuller, R. W., Heavey, D. J. and Ind, P. W. (1986). Histamine is released from skin by substance P but does not act as the final vasodilator in the axon reflex. *Br. J. Pharmacol.*, **88**, 741–5

46. Basran, G. S., Morley, J., Paul, W. and Turner-Warwick, M. (1982). Evidence in man of synergistic interaction between putative mediators of acute inflammation and asthma. *Lancet*, **1**, 935–7

47. Barnes, V. F. and Heavey, D. J. (1986). Effect of prostaglandin D_2 on histamine-induced weals in human skin. *Br. J. Pharmacol.*, **87**, 357–60

48. Heavey, D. J., Barnes, V. F., Orwin, J. and Brown, M. J. (1985). Inhibition of 5-HT induced axon reflex flares by MDL 72422. *Br. J. Clin. Pharmacol.*, **21**, 558P

49. Fuller, R. W., Warren, J. B., McCusker, M. and Dollery, C. T. (1987). Effect of enalapril on the skin response to bradykinin in man. *Br. J. Clin. Pharmacol.*, **23**, 88–90

50. Henocq, E. and Vargaftig, B. B. (1986). Accumulation of eosinophils in response to intracutaneous PAF-acether and allergens in man. *Lancet*, **1**, 1378–9

51. Wihl, J.-A. (1983). Methods for assessing nasal reactivity. *Eur. J. Resp. Dis.*, **64**, 175–9

52. Karlsson, G., Pipkorn, V. and Andreasson, L. (1986). Substance P and human nasal mucociliary activity. *Eur. J. Clin. Pharmacol.*, **30**, 355–7

53. Collier, J. G. and Fuller, R. W. (1984). Capsaicin inhalation in man and the effects of sodium cromoglycate. *Br. J. Pharmacol.*, **81**, 113–17

54. Smith, L. J., Greenberger, P. A., Patterson, R., Krell, R. D. and Bernstein, P. R. (1985). The effect of inhaled leukotriene D_4 in humans. *Am. Rev. Resp. Dis.*, **131**, 368–72

55. Hardy, C. C., Robinson, C., Tattersfield, A. E. and Holgate, S. T. (1984). The bronchoconstrictor effect of inhaled prostaglandin D_2 in normal and asthmatic men. *N. Engl. J. Med.*, **311**, 209–13

56. Fuller, R. W., Dixon, C. M. S., Cuss, F. M. and Barnes, P. J. (1987). Bradykinin-induced bronchoconstriction in humans. Mode of action. *Am. Rev. Resp. Dis.*, **135**, 176–80

57. Mathe, A. A. and Hedqvist, P. (1975). Effect of prostaglandins $F_{2\alpha}$ and E_2 on airway conductance in healthy subjects and asthmatic patients. *Am. Rev. Resp. Dis.*, **111**, 313–20

58. Costello, J. F., Dunlop, L. S. and Gardiner, P. J. (1985). Characteristics of prostaglandin induced cough in man. *Br. J. Clin. Pharmac.*, **20**, 355–9

59. Cuss, F. M., Dixon, C. M. S. and Barnes, P. J. (1986). Effects of inhaled platelet activating factor on pulmonary function and bronchial responsiveness in man. *Lancet*, **2**, 189–92

60. Bisgaard, H. and Groth, S. (1987). Bronchial effects of leukotriene D_4 inhalation in normal human lung. *Clin. Sci.*, **72**, 585–92

61. Manning, P. J., Jones, G. L. and O'Byrne, P. M. (1987). Indomethacin prevents histamine tachyphylaxis in asthmatics. *Am. Rev. Resp. Dis.*, **135**, A313

62. Fuller, R. W., Maxwell, D. L., Dixon, C. M. S., McGregor, G. P., Barnes, V. F., Bloom, S. R. and Barnes, P. J. (1987). Effect of substance P on cardiovascular and respiratory function in subjects. *J. Appl. Physiol.*, **62**, 1473–9

63. Walters, E. H., Parrish, R. W., Bevan, C. and Smith, A. P. (1981). Induction of bronchial hypersensitivity: evidence for a role for prostaglandins. *Thorax*, **36**, 571–4

64. Fuller, R. W., Dixon, C. M. S., Dollery, C. T. and Barnes, P. J. (1986). Prostaglandin D_2 potentiates airway responsiveness to histamine and methacholine. *Am. Rev. Resp. Dis.*, **133**, 252–4
65. Barnes, N. C., Piper, P. J. and Costello, J. F. (1984). Actions of inhaled leukotrienes and their interactions with other allergic mediators. *Prostaglandins*, **28**, 629–31
66. Pavia, D., Bateman, J. R. M., Sheahan, N. F., Agnew, J. E., Newman, S. P. and Clarke, S. W. (1980). Techniques for measuring lung mucociliary clearance. *Eur. J. Resp. Dis.*, **61** (Suppl. 110), 157–68
67. Mezey, R. J., Cohn, M. A., Fernandez, R. J., Janusziewicz, A. J. and Wanner, A. (1978). Mucociliary transport in allergic patients with antigen-induced bronchospasm. *Am. Rev. Resp. Dis.*, **118**, 677–84
68. Wanner, A. (1985). Mucociliary and mucus secretory function. *Am. Rev. Resp. Dis.*, **131**, S36–S38
69. Ahmed, T., Greenblatt, D. W., Birch, S., Marchette, B. and Wanner, A. (1980). Mucociliary transport in allergic patients with antigen-induced bronchospasm: role of slow reacting substance of anaphylaxis (SRS-A). *Am. Rev. Resp. Dis.*, **121**, A106
70. Wanner, A., Maurer, D., Abraham, W. M., Szepfalusi, Z. and Sielczak, M. (1983). Effects of chemical mediators of anaphylaxis on ciliary function. *J. Allergy Clin. Immunol.*, **72**, 663–7
71. Pavia, D., Sutton, P. P., Lopez-Vidriero, M. T., Agnew, J. E. and Clarke, S. W. (1983). Drug effects on mucociliary function. *Eur. J. Resp. Dis.*, **64**, 304–17
72. Braude, S., Royston, D., Coe, C. and Barnes, P. J. (1984). Histamine increases lung permeability by an H_2-receptor mechanism. *Lancet*, **2**, 372–4
73. Galant, S. P., Bullock, J., Wong, D. and Maibach, H. I. (1973). The inhibitory effect of antiallergy drugs on allergen and histamine induced wheal and flare response. *J. Allergy Clin. Immunol.*, **51**, 11–21
74. Krause, L. B. and Shuster, S. (1984). H_2-receptor-active histamine not sole cause of chronic idiopathic urticaria. *Lancet*, **2**, 929–30
75. Farr, P. M. and Diffey, B. L. (1985). A quantitative study of the effects of topical indomethacin on cutaneous erythema induced by ultraviolet radiation (UVR). *Br. J. Dermatol.*, **113**, 771–2
76. Warren, J. B., Pixley, F. J., Fuller, R. W. and Dollery, C. T. (1987). Effect of enalapril and terfenadine on skin antigen challenge. *Clin. Sci.*, **73**, 8P
77. Mygind, N., Secher, C. and Kirkegaard, J. (1983). Role of histamine and antihistamines in the nose. *Eur. J. Resp. Dis.*, **64**, 16–20
78. Mygind, N. and Borum, P. (1983). Effect of a cholino-ceptor antagonist in the nose. *Eur. J. Resp. Dis.*, **64**, 167–74
79. Proud, D., Kagey-Sobotka, A., Naclerio, R. M. and Lichtenstein, L. M. (1987). Pharmacology of upper airways challenge. *Int. Arch. Allergy Appl. Immun.*, **82**, 493–7
80. Mygind, N., Hansen, I. B. and Jørgensen, M. B. (1972). Disodium cromoglycate nasal spray in adult patients with perennial rhinitis. *Acta Allergologica*, **27**, 372–80
81. Holgate, S. T., Twentyman, O. P., Rafferty, P., Beasley, R., Hutson, P. A., Robinson, C. and Church, M. K. (1987). Primary and secondary effector cells in the pathogenesis of bronchial asthma. *Int. Arch. Allergy Appl. Immun.*, **82**, 498–506
82. Britton, J., Hanley, S. P. and Tattersfield, A. E. (1987). The effect of an orally active leukotriene D_4 (LTD_4) antagonist L-649, 923 on the airway response to inhaled antigen in asthma. *Thorax*, **42**, 219–20
83. Booij-Noord, H., Quanjer, H. and de Vries, K. (1971). Protektive Wirkung von Berotec bei Provokationstesten mit provozierischer Allergeninhalation und Histamin. *Int. J. Clin. Pharmacol. Ther. Toxicol.*, **4**, 69–72
84. Fairfax, A. J. and Morley, J. (1981). NSAIDs inhibit the late asthmatic response to antigen challenge. *Br. J. Pharmacol.*, **74**, 984P–985P
85. Braquet, P., Etienne, A., Touvay, C., Bourgain, R. H., Lefort, J. and Vargaftig, B. B. (1985). Involvement of platelet activating factor in respiratory anaphylaxis, demonstrated by PAF-acether inhibitor BN 52021. *Lancet*, **1**, 1501
86. Fujimura, M., Sasaki, F., Nakatsumi, Y., Takahashi, Y., Hifumi, S., Taga, K., Mifune, J.-I., Tanaka, T. and Matsuda, T. (1986). Effects of a thromboxane synthetase inhibitor (OKY-046) and a lipoxygenase inhibitor (AA-861) on bronchial responsiveness to acetylcholine in asthmatic subjects. *Thorax*, **41**, 955–9

87. Kirby, F. E., Hargreave, P. M. and O'Byrne, P. M. (1987). Indomethacin inhibits allergen-induced airway hyperresponsiveness but not allergen-induced asthmatic responses. *Am. Rev. Resp. Dis.*, **135**, A312

88. Dahl, R. and Johansson, S.-A. (1982). Importance of duration of treatment with inhaled budesonide on the immediate and late bronchial reaction. *Eur. J. Resp. Dis.*, **63** (Suppl. 122), 167–75

89. Dixon, C. M. S., Fuller, R. W. and Barnes, P. J. (1987). The effect of angiotensin converting enzyme inhibitor, ramipril on bronchial responses to inhaled histamine and bradykinin in asthmatic subjects. *Br. J. Clin. Pharmacol.*, **23**, 91–3

90. Holgate, S. T., Burns, G. B., Robinson, C. and Church, M. K. (1984). Anaphylactic- and calcium-dependent generation of prostaglandin D_2 (PGD_2), thromboxane B_2 and other cyclooxygenase products of arachidonic acid by dispersed human lung cells and relationship to histamine release. *J. Immunol.*, **133**, 2138–44

91. MacDermot, J., Kelsey, C. R., Waddell, K. A., Richmond, R., Knight, R. K., Cole, P. J., Dollery, C. T., Landon, D. N. and Blair, I. A. (1982). Synthesis of leukotriene B_4, and prostanoids by human alveolar macrophages: analysis by gas chromatography/mass spectrometry. *Prostaglandins*, **27**, 163–79

92. Fels, A. O. S. and Cohn, Z. A. (1986). The alveolar macrophage. *J. Appl. Physiol.*, **60**, 353–69

93. Arnoux, B., Simoes Caeiro, M. H., Landes, A., Mathieu, M., Duroux, P. and Benveniste, J. (1982). Alveolar macrophages from asthmatic patients release platelet-activating factor (PAF-acether) and lyso-PAF-acether when stimulated with the specific allergen. *Am. Rev. Resp. Dis.*, **125**, 70

94. Borgeat, P. and Samuelsson, B. (1979). Arachidonic acid metabolism in polymorphonuclear leukocytes: Effects of ionophore A23187. *Proc. Natl. Acad. Sci. USA*, **76**, 2148–52

95. Maurice, P. D. L., Bather, P. C. and Allen, B. R. (1986). Arachidonic acid metabolism by polymorphonuclear leukocytes in psoriasis. *Br. J. Dermatol.*, **114**, 57–64

96. Venge, P., Hakansson, L. and Peterson, C. G. B. (1987). Eosinophil activation in allergic disease. *Int. Arch. Allergy Appl. Immun.*, **82**, 333–7

97. Schleimer, R. P., MacGlashan, D. W., Jr., Peters, S. P., Naclerio, R., Proud, D., Adkinson, N. F., Jr. and Lichtenstein, L. M. (1984). Inflammatory mediators and mechanisms of release from purified human basophils and mast cells. *J. Allergy Clin. Immunol.*, **74**, 473–81

98. Capron, A., Joseph, M., Ameisen, J. C., Capron, M., Pancre, V. and Auriault, C. (1987). Platelets as effectors in immune and hypersensitivity reactions. *Int. Arch. Allergy Appl. Immun.*, **82**, 307–12

99. Knauer, K. A., Lichtenstein, L. M., Adkinson, N. F., Jr. and Fish, J. E. (1981). Platelet activation during antigen-induced airway reactions in asthmatic subjects. *N. Engl. J. Med.*, **304**, 1404–7

100. Morley, J., Sanjar, S. and Page, C. P. (1984). The platelet in asthma. *Lancet*, **2**, 1142–4

10
Modulation of Mast Cell Mediator Secretion by Drugs used in the Treatment of Allergic Diseases

M. K. CHURCH

Mast cells are pivotally involved in many diseases with an allergic basis, e.g. asthma and urticaria. In human airways, mast cells constitute 0.5% of the cells lining the bronchi[1] where they are ideally situated to interact with inhaled allergens. Evidence for mast cell activation, at least in allergen provocation experiments, derives from the detection of elevated mast cell mediators in bronchoalveolar lavage fluid[2] and in blood plasma[3,4]. Similarly, provocation of urticarial reactions with allergen[5] or non-immunological stimuli[6-9] is associated with a local elevation of mast cell mediators. The possible therapeutic benefit of drugs which inhibit mast cell mediator release would, therefore, appear to be great. This chapter describes the effects on mast cells of drugs used in the treatment of allergic diseases.

SODIUM CROMOGLYCATE AND RELATED DRUGS

Sodium cromoglycate (SCG) was first synthesized in 1965 whilst trying to improve upon the biological properties of khellin, a plant extract with bronchodilator and vasodilator properties which had unpleasant side effects[10, 11]. When administered by inhalation to an asthmatic volunteer, it did not have the expected bronchodilator properties but inhibited allergen induced bronchoconstriction[12, 13]. This observation led to the hypothesis that its mechanism of action was to inhibit the release of bronchoconstrictor mediators from mast cells within the bronchial lumen[13]. It is now clear that the ability of SCG to relieve asthma is also dependent on other properties of the drug, e.g. inhibition of neuronal reflexes within the lung[14] and inhibitory actions on leukocyte activation[15, 16]. However, it is its effects upon mast cells which will be considered here.

The concept of SCG as a non-specific mast cell stabilizer is erroneous. It is clear that its ability to suppress mediator release is dependent on the source of the mast cell, both species and tissue site within a single species, and upon the stimulus for mast cell activation.

In the rat, SCG is an effective inhibitor of IgE-dependent mediator release from the so-called connective tissue mast cells of the peritoneal cavity[17-19] and skin[20], whereas it is ineffective in mucosal or atypical mast cells separated from the lamina propria of the small intestine[21,22]. The dependence upon stimulus of mast cell activation for demonstration of SCG activity is exemplified by observations that mediator release induced by IgE-dependent mechanisms[17-19], compound 48/80[18,23], phospholipase A[24], polymixin B[25], dextran plus phosphatidyl serine[25,26] and low concentrations of calcium ionophore A23187[27] are inhibited, whereas release induced by higher concentrations of A23187[28], substance P[29] and IgG-dependent mechanisms[20] are less readily inhibited.

In the mouse, SCG is ineffective regardless of the type of antibody mediating the response[30], and more potent SCG-like drugs are only weakly effective even at high concentrations[31-33]. However, exposure of mouse bone marrow derived mast cells in culture to $10 \mu mol/l$ SCG for 4–7 days has been reported to inhibit IgE-dependent histamine release by 50%[34]. In the guinea pig, IgE-mediated anaphylaxis is partially inhibited by SCG, whereas IgG-dependent anaphylaxis is not[35-37]. The influence of mast cell heterogeneity in this species on SCG activity is exemplified by the observations that brufolin, a compound with 300 times the activity of SCG in rat passive autaneous anaphylaxis (PCA), inhibits anaphylactic bronchoconstriction and histamine release from guinea pig chopped lung, but does not inhibit PCA reactions in guinea pig skin[31,32].

Blockade of the release of histamine and neutrophil chemotactic activity (NCA) into the circulation following allergen provocation of mild asthmatic subjects[38,39] provides in vivo evidence of the ability of SCG to prevent mast cell mediator release in man. In in vitro tests, however, SCG is less effective on human mast cells than it is on rat mast cells. In human lung fragments, SCG has only a partial and extremely variable inhibitory effect on IgE-dependent mediator release[40,41]. However, the variability of the human lung fragment model and the inconsistent responses of lung samples from different donors allows only a gross estimate of drug efficacy to be made[41]. In human dispersed lung mast cells, SCG shows a concentration related inhibition of between 11 and 23% histamine release at $1-1000 \mu mol/l$[42]. Comparison at 20% inhibition of histamine release showed salbutamol to be more than 1000 times more potent in the same experiments. Three other pertinent points arose from this study. First, the efficacy of SCG in suppressing histamine release was inversely related to the intensity of immunological stimulation and, consequently, to histamine release. As, in comparison with in vitro tests, the level of immunological stimulation and consequential histamine release in asthma are low[39], it is likely that SCG would be an effective inhibitor of mast cell mediator release in the clinical situation. The second point is that while SCG at $1000 \mu mol/l$ inhibited histamine release by only 25%, it inhibited the release of prostaglandin (PG) D_2 by 85%. This prostaglandin, which is derived only from mast cells[43], is a potent broncho-constrictor[44] and induces the accumulation of secondary inflammatory cells[45]. The third point is that three other SCG-like compounds, lodoxamide, traxanox and RU31156 showed similar potencies to SCG against human lung mast cells. In the rat PCA test, indicative of activity against rat connective tissue mast cells, the potencies of these drugs differ markedly, lodoxamide, traxanox and RU31156 being respectively, 2500, 8 and 260-fold more potent than SCG[42].

In mast cells recovered from the lung by bronchoalveolar lavage (BAL) SCG appears to be more effective than against mast cells dispersed from human lung tissue by enzymatic digestion[46]. This difference is not due to the effects of the enzymes used for digestion as mast cells dispersed from lung tissue by mechanical methods and those dispersed by the use of enzymes have a similar sensitivity to SCG[42]. The likelihood is, therefore, that BAL mast cells represent a separate sub-population of human mast cells[46]. In contrast, SCG has no inhibitory effect on IgE-dependent histamine release from human basophils or skin mast cells either *in vitro* or *in vivo*[47-49].

One characteristic of the effect of SCG in rat mast cells is the rapid development of tachyphylaxis to its inhibitory effects[50, 51]. This phenomenon is also observed with SCG-like drugs, and cross-tachyphylaxis with SCG is often taken as an indication that the drugs have a similar mechanism of action[52]. Tachyphylaxis has also been observed with SCG in mast cells dispersed from human lung tissue, the inhibitory effect of SCG being negligible following 15 minutes preincubation with cells before challenge[42]. Similar effects have been observed with lodoxamide, traxanox and RU31156, as has cross-tachyphylaxis with SCG[42]. In contrast, studies with BAL mast cells have suggested that tachyphylaxis does not occur, inhibition of IgE-dependent histamine release by 1000 μmol/l SCG being 40% with no preincubation and 50% with 10 minutes preincubation of drug and cells together before challenge[46]. Similarly, no tachyphylaxis to the inhibitory effects of SCG has been reported using human adenoidal mast cells[53].

Possible mechanisms of action of SCG

Although SCG has been investigated in many laboratories over the last 20 years its mechanism of action is still largely obscure. Because SCG is highly ionized at physiological pH (pKa = 2) and, therefore, remains in the extracellular water, suggestions have been made that its ability to sequester cations, particularly calcium, in the extracellular environment leads to the inhibition of mast cell function. This theory of action is, however, unlikely since it does not explain the development of tachyphylaxis or the differences in sensitivity to SCG between different mast cell populations. Furthermore, sequestration of calcium would have profound effects *in vivo*, e.g. a reduction in blood clotting.

A second proposed mechanism, which I feel can be dismissed at this stage, is the proposal that it is related to inhibition of cyclic AMP phosphodiesterase. Clearly in broken cell preparations SCG and related compounds are phosphodiesterase inhibitors in high concentrations[54-56]. However, the acidic nature of SCG would preclude its entry into the cell to have such an effect. Furthermore, the characteristics of the actions of SCG are quite distinct from those of methylxanthine inhibitors of phosphodiesterase[57].

As the effects of SCG are extracellular in nature it is most likely that it would first have to associate with a receptor on the cell membrane. Because SCG is a notoriously poor ligand for affinity studies, the search for an SCG receptor has proved to be difficult. Mazurek *et al.*[58] reported the existence of a specific binding site for SCG on the membrane of rat basophil leukaemia cells (RBL-2H3). Futhermore they suggested that this receptor is linked to a calcium gating mechanism[59]. This mechanism, however, is not readily compatible with the ability of SCG to inhibit histamine release initiated by low concentrations of A23187[27] nor with the fact that RBL-2H3 cells respond very poorly to SCG.

The observation that the inhibitory effect of SCG in rat mast cells is associated with the phosphorylation of a 78 kD protein[60, 61] provides a more likely mechanism. When rat mast cells are activated by antigen or compound 48/80 in the presence of ^{32}P four proteins are phosphorylated[61, 62]. Three of these, with molecular weights of 42, 59 and 68 kD are phosphorylated within 10 seconds and are thought to be involved in the initiation of secretion. The fourth, a 78 kD protein, is not evident for 30–60 seconds after challenge and is thought to be associated with termination of the secretory response. Exposure of cells to SCG, SCG-like drugs and dibutyryl cyclic GMP, but not dibutyryl cyclic AMP, β-adrenoceptor agonists or methylxanthine phosphodiesterase inhibitors, causes phosphorylation of the 78 kD protein in isolation. The observation that the decay of this protein parallels tachyphylaxis to SCG provides strong circumstantial evidence that it is responsible for the intracellular effects of SCG[60, 61].

A further suggestion is that SCG inhibits cell activation by inhibiting the actions of protein kinase C[63], an enzyme which requires calcium and phosphatidylserine for full expression of its activity[64]. The association of SCG with protein kinase C stems from the observation that high extracellular levels of phosphatidylserine overcome the actions of the antiallergic drug[65]. Although the evidence presented by Dr Sagi-Eisenberg is, by her own admission, circumstantial[63], it is supported by the preliminary observations of De Souza and Findlay[66]. More direct evidence of an association between SCG and protein kinase C stems from studies in the skin of the lizard *Anolis carolinensis* in which SCG inhibits enhancement of melanosome dispersion by the phorbol ester, 12-*O*-tetradecanoylphorbol-13-acetate (TPA)[67]. The only obvious loophole in this hypothesis is that it assumes the action of TPA to be solely on protein kinase C. Clearly TPA may also have other effects such as the inhibition of the hydrolysis of phosphoinositides[68, 69].

The increasing volume of evidence linking SCG with protein kinase C and the observations of phosphorylation of a 78 kD protein suggest that they must both play a role in the inhibitory effects of the drug. How they are related and which is the cause of the other must await further research.

β-ADRENOCEPTOR AGONISTS

Agents which elevate intracellular cyclic AMP (cAMP) levels by interacting with cell membrane β-adrenoceptors have been used in the treatment of asthma for over 80 years. The short duration of action and potential cardiotoxicity of adrenaline and isoprenaline, however, have limited their use. These limitations stimulated changes to be made in the chemical structure of the catecholamine molecule to minimize these problems. These changes have resulted in the synthesis of the newer bronchodilator agents such as salbutamol, terbutaline and fenoterol, in which the duration of action has been prolonged by modifying the catechol moiety to protect them from degradation by catechol-o-methyltransferase, and the selectivity for β-receptors has been increased by the introduction of a tertiary butyl group on the terminal amino group[70].

Although β-adrenoceptor agonists were introduced for the treatment of asthma because of their ability to relax bronchial smooth muscle, it is now clear that they are potent inhibitors of mediator secretion from human lung mast cells. This has been demonstrated *in vitro* using human lung fragments and dispersed lung mast cells where concentrations in the nanomolar to micromolar range have been shown to be effective inhibitors of allergen or anti-IgE induced release of histamine and SRS-A leukotrienes[40, 42, 71–75]. A similar action has also been demonstrated *in vivo* where terbutaline and salbutamol have been shown to inhibit the rise of mast cell mediators in the plasma following allergen challenge of mild asthmatic subjects[39, 76]. The results from these experiments indicate that β-adrenoceptor agonists are several thousand times more potent than sodium cromoglycate in inhibiting mast cell mediator release[39, 42].

Dr Benyon has reviewed, in Chapter 7, the evidence for a role of cyclic nucleotides in the coupling of activation to mediator secretion in mast cells. Briefly, there is a body of evidence to suggest a dual function of cAMP; an immediate and transient role in enhancing activation–secretion coupling, and a later more prolonged role to turn off the secretory process. Preincubation of mast cells with agents which elevate intracellular cAMP would, therefore, be expected to initiate the turn off mechanism thereby inhibiting mediator release on subsequent activation. This certainly appears to be the case in human lung mast cells[40, 42, 71–75] and guinea pig lung tissue where β-adrenoceptor stimulants are potent inhibitors of mediator release[77–79]. In rat mast cells, however, β-adrenoceptor stimulants produce inconsistent effects on mediator secretion, the majority of reports showing no inhibition of release[70, 80–83]. This lack of effect cannot be explained by an absence of β-adrenoceptors for these cells have around 4×10^4 binding sites/cell, stimulation of which causes a marked elevation in cAMP levels[83]. The reason for the lack of effectiveness of β-adrenoceptor stimulants may lie in the duration of the cAMP rise. Ishizaka and Ishizaka[84] reported inhibition of histamine release in two rat mast cell preparations where there was a maintained cAMP response, but not in four preparations where the response was smaller and transient.

The effect of β-adrenoceptor stimulants on histamine release from human basophils depends on how the experiments are performed. When basophils are challenged with allergen in the presence of extracellular calcium at 37 °C, inhibition is only observed with isoprenaline concentrations of around $1 \, mmol/l$[85]. If, however, the cells are incubated with isoprenaline and allergen in the absence of extracellular calcium and then the release reaction is initiated by addition of calcium afterwards, then isoprenaline shows good activity[85]. These experiments indicate that β-adrenoceptor stimulation inhibits mast cell activation rather than the subsequent mediator release stages.

That β-adrenoceptor agonists mediate their effects by interaction with β-adrenoceptors rather than a non-specific effect of the drug is evidenced by the observation that their effects are prevented by D,L-propranolol to a greater extent than by D-propranolol[40], the D-enantiomer of the drug having membrane stabilizing effects, but negligible β-blockade[86, 87]. Furthermore, experiments using selective agonists and antagonists have indicated the mast cell receptor to be of the β_2-subtype[72].

Like sodium cromoglycate, the effectiveness of β-adrenoceptor stimulants in inhibiting mast cell mediator release is inversely related to the strength of immunological stimulation and the degree of histamine release[42]. Similar results have been reported in human basophils using agents which elevate intracellular cAMP[88]. Unlike sodium cromoglycate, however, the effect of salbutamol *in vitro* is largely independent of the time of preincubation of cells with drug before challenge. Furthermore, salbutamol is still active in cells made tolerant to the effects of sodium cromoglycate, thus indicating a separate mechanism of action[42].

Experiments *in vivo*[89] and *in vitro*[48] have demonstrated that IgE-dependent histamine release from human skin mast cells is also inhibitable by β-adrenoceptor stimulants. However, recent experiments *in vitro* (Lowman, Benyon and Church, unpublished observations) indicate that histamine release initiated by substance P, the mechanism of which appears to be quite different from IgE-dependent release[90], is not inhibited by β-adrenoceptor stimulants.

The potent ability of β-adrenoceptor agonists to relax bronchial smooth muscle and to prevent mast cell mediator release makes them the ideal type of drug for the treatment of the immediate phase of the asthmatic reaction. However, these drugs do not inhibit the late asthmatic reaction or the increase in bronchial hyperresponsiveness in asthma[91]. From a therapeutic standpoint this means that while the symptoms of asthma may be suppressed the underlying inflammatory process in the bronchi may progress unabated. This may lead to a potentially dangerous situation where a rapid deterioration in symptoms, which are untreatable by β-adrenoceptor agonists, may increase the risk of sudden death[92].

METHYLXANTHINES

Methylxanthines such as theophylline have been used for the treatment of asthma for over a century. The efficacy of theophylline, however, is restricted to a narrow therapeutic range, 55–110 μmol/l[93]. Below this concentration it is ineffective. Above this concentration it causes nausea, vomiting, headache, diarrhoea, irritability and insomnia, whilst at higher concentrations still cardiac arrhythmias, seizures and death may occur.

Following the report by Butcher and Sutherland in 1962[94] that theophylline was a cAMP phosphodiesterase inhibitor, the majority of studies aimed at elucidating the mechanism of action of methylxanthines have focused on their ability to inhibit cAMP phosphodiesterase[95]. The early observations that relaxation of bronchial smooth muscle and mast cell mediator secretion were significantly correlated with the ability of theophylline to elevate intracellular cAMP levels[81, 96–99] added impetus to this theory. However, the relevance to the clinical situation must be questioned as the concentrations of theophylline required for effective inhibition of both cAMP and cGMP phosphodiesterase are in the region of 10^{-4}–10^{-2} mol/l[100–102], i.e. in the toxic range rather than the therapeutic range.

Although the concentration range of theophylline for inhibition of cAMP phosphodiesterase is consistent with that necessary to inhibit mast cell mediator release, inconsistencies have been reported in this relationship with other phosphodiesterase inhibitors. For example, it has been shown that although theophylline, isobutylmethylxanthine, ICI 63197 and Ro20-1724 all elevate mast cell cAMP levels to a similar degree, only the first two drugs inhibit histamine release[103]. Also, the β-adrenoceptor agonist isoprenaline, while synergizing with isobutylmethylxanthine in elevating mast cell cAMP levels, does not synergize in inhibiting histamine release[104]. Moreover, in some strains of rat, isobutylmethylxanthine enhances rather than inhibits mast cell histamine release[105].

The recent observation that theophylline may reduce histamine release into the nose during pollen-induced rhinitis[106] suggests an alternative mechanism of action of theophylline on mast cells which occurs at therapeutic concentrations. One possible mechanism is the inhibition of the effects of adenosine, an action which occurs at concentrations within the therapeutic range[107].

The observation that adenosine and its immediate precursor adenosine 5′-monophosphate(AMP) cause bronchoconstriction in asthmatic and allergic, but not in normal, subjects[108, 109], and that this effect is inhibited by the prior administration of sodium cromoglycate[110, 111] or histamine H_1-receptor antagonists[112, 113] has led us to suggest that adenosine release in asthma[114] may enhance mast cell mediator release. Support for this theory has been obtained *in vitro* using human lung mast cells[115], human basophils[116] and rodent mast cells[117, 118]. Theophylline reduces both adenosine-induced bronchoconstriction *in vivo*[119, 120] and enhancement of IgE-dependent histamine release from human mast cells[115] and basophils[116]. Enprofylline (3-propylxanthine), an anti-asthmatic xanthine which does not have adenosine antagonist properties[121, 122], does not block adenosine-induced bronchoconstriction[123] illustrating that this is not the only mechanism of action of methylxanthines. Other mechanisms of action such as a reduction in the levels of free calcium in the cytosol[124], inhibition of prostaglandin generation[125], effects on diaphragmatic contractility[126] and elevation of circulating catecholamine levels[127] must also be considered. Furthermore, the recent observation that an infusion of theophylline reduced the late asthmatic reaction but had only a weak effect on the early reaction[128] suggest that the major effect of this drug in asthma may be on inflammatory cells other than the mast cell.

ANTIHISTAMINES (H_1 AND H_2-RECEPTOR ANTAGONISTS)

The effects of histamine at its effector site follow its interaction with one of two distinctly separate receptors, H_1 and H_2[129]. H_1-receptors are stimulated preferentially with 2-methylhistamine and blocked by H_1-receptor antagonists or classical antihistamines such as chlorpheniramine, promethazine, terfenadine or astemizole. H_1-receptor mediated events are normally associated with the pro-inflammatory effects of histamine such as oedema, vasodilation, bronchospasm and increased leukocyte chemotaxis. H_2-receptors are stimulated preferentially by 4-methyl histamine and blocked by specific H_2-receptor antagonists such as cimetidine and ranitidine. These actions of histamine, in addition to increasing gastric acid secretion, are generally anti-inflammatory, in that they are inhibitory to leukocyte chemotaxis and activation. Recently, a further subtype of histamine receptor has been tentatively identified. This receptor, termed H_3, has been suggested as having a negative feedback role in histamine secreting nerves[130].

H_1-RECEPTOR ANTAGONISTS

Although H_1-receptor antagonists have poor efficacy in the treatment of asthma[131], they are among the frontline drugs used for rhinitis and urticaria. The advent of newer non-sedating H_1-antagonists such as terfenadine[132] and astemizole[133] has revolutionized antihistamine therapy by allowing more effective doses to be given without the problems of drowsiness.

Besides antagonizing the end-organ effects of histamine, claims have also been made that H_1-antagonists and related compounds may prevent mast cell mediator release[134]. The original reports of this activity were made by Arunlakshana in 1953[135] and by Mota and Dias da Silva in 1960[136], the latter workers demonstrating that at higher concentrations the drugs may also induce histamine release. It is clear from a number of studies that this property is unrelated to histamine H_1-receptor blockade[137-141]. Seeman[142] suggested that both mast cell stabilization and drug induced release were consequent upon the lipophilic nature of the drugs. At low concentrations, membrane expansion causes stabilization, whereas at higher concentrations the membrane is no longer able to maintain its structural integrity and disruption occurs. Evidence in support of this derives from experiments in which hypotonic lysis and compound 48/80-induced mediator release were blocked equally by chlorpromazine[143]. If both mast cell stabilization and histamine release were both directly attributable to the lipophilicity of the drugs then it would be expected that a correlation between the two actions would be observed. The finding that they are not[138] implicates additional mechanisms.

An interference with the ability of calcium to associate with the cell membrane has been suggested from the observation that cationic amphiphilic drugs replace calcium from lipid monolayers in the same concentrations as those which inhibit histamine release[144, 145]. Evidence to support this derives from experiments using human lung fragments in which chlorpromazine and lanthanum, which has an ionic radius similar to that of calcium and is able to diplace it from superficial sites on cell membranes[146], are both more effective inhibitors when the external calcium concentration is lowered[143].

The ability of antihistamines to prevent the mobilization of intracellular calcium has also been suggested from experiments in which rat mast cells were stimulated with substance P in the absence of extracellular calcium[29]. That this may be the predominant effect is suggested from the observation that antihistamines are significantly more effective in inhibiting substance P-induced histamine release from rat mast cells in the absence of extracellular calcium than they are against antigen-induced release in its presence (De Vos, personal communication). An intracellular action would also explain why the onset of action is slow in developing[40].

A pertinent question which still needs to be answered satisfactorily is whether mast cell stabilization by antihistamines contributes to their activity in the treatment of human allergic diseases. Local administration of antihistamines to the nose has provided evidence of both stabilization and drug induced mediator release[147], as has inhalation of large concentrations of antihistamines[148]. However, concentrations likely to be achieved after systemic administration are much lower than those required to demonstrate effects on mast cells *in vitro*. In asthma, astemizole does not block the rise in plasma histamine levels following allergen provocation[149]. Similarly, terfenadine, whilst blocking the bronchoconstrictor effects of allergen-induced histamine release, does not block the PGD_2 component of the reaction, indicating that mast cell mediator release was unimpeded[150, 151]. In systemic mastocytosis, chlorpheniramine does not reduce the raised systemic histamine levels[152]. In contrast, Ting *et al.*[153] reported that oral hydroxyzine inhibited both the rise in histamine levels in skin chamber fluid and mast cell degranulation, as evidenced by microscopic analysis of biopsies, following local allergen challenge. Whether this is a direct effect of the drug or consequent upon the reduction by the H_1-antagonist of the histamine-induced vasodilation and oedema, thereby reducing the dispersion of the allergen, is not known. Certainly *in vitro* experiments would suggest that human skin mast cells do not show a special sensitivity to the inhibitory effects of hydroxyzine (Lowman, Benyon and Church, unpublished observations).

H_2-receptor antagonists

Leukocyte membranes have H_2-receptors, stimulation of which by histamine leads to an elevation of intracellular cAMP levels and a reduction of the response to activation[154, 155]. In human basophils this leads to a negative feedback loop which limits histamine secretion. Blockade of H_2-receptors leads to an enhancement of histamine release which is more obvious at low levels of stimulation[154, 156, 157].

Although H_2-receptor antagonists have been reported to enhance histamine release from guinea pig[157] and primate lung[158], neither human[159] nor rat mast cells[160] appear to possess H_2-receptors.

It is noteworthy that, despite the ability of histamine H_2-antagonists to enhance histamine release from human basophils *in vitro* and also reduce histamine metabolism[161], there have been no reports of them exacerbating allergic reactions in man *in vivo*. One can infer from this that either the drugs are not present in sufficient concentrations to inhibit the histamine negative feedback mechanism or, more likely, that the local concentrations of histamine attained *in vivo* are insufficient to cause feedback inhibition on the H_2-receptor.

CALCIUM ANTAGONISTS

Stimulation of contractile and secretory cells results in an increase of free intracellular calcium which is necessary for the activation of calcium-dependent coupling. The dependency of mast cell mediator secretion on an adequate supply of extracellular calcium[43, 90, 146] suggests that an increase in the permeability of the cell membrane to calcium ions is an essential event in cell activation. That inhibition of membrane calcium transport would block mast cell activation and mediator secretion is, therefore, an attractive hypothesis.

Calcium antagonists such as verapamil and nifedipine have been developed to inhibit the action-potential stimulated influx of calcium into cardiac and vascular smooth muscle. However, their ability to reduce the intensity of allergen-[162] and exercise-[163-166] induced bronchoconstriction has stimulated interest in their potential use in allergic disease.

In vivo, sublingual nifedipine reduces the rise in plasma levels of histamine following exercise provocation of patients with asthma[164], suggesting an ability of the drug to inhibit mast cell mediator release. *In vitro*, calcium antagonists reduce histamine secretion from rat mast cells[167-171], from human basophils[172-174] and from human lung and tonsillar mast cells[175-178]. However, in human lung mast cells, the IgE-dependent generation of SRS-leukotrienes is inhibited more effectively than is the release of preformed mediators such as histamine[175-177].

The concentrations of calcium antagonist ($10 \mu mol/l$) required to inhibit mast cell or basophil histamine release[168, 172, 174, 178] are considerably higher than the nanomolar concentrations necessary to inhibit the voltage dependent entrance of calcium into vascular smooth muscle[179]. Histamine secretion from human lung mast cells induced by calcium ionophore A23187, which bypasses physiological calcium channels by inserting calcium directly through the cell membrane[146], is blocked by similar concentrations of calcium antagonists to those effective against IgE-dependent release[178]. Furthermore, inhibition is not reversed by increasing the extracellular concentration of calcium[178]. These results indicate that the effect of calcium antagonists in inhibiting mast cell mediator secretion may not be due to blockade of calcium channel function but rather to other effects of these drugs which include Na^+, K^+, Cl^- channel blockade, local anaesthetic activity, membrane stabilization, α- and β-adrenoceptor blockade, antihistaminic activity, antimuscarinic activity, and inhibition of phosphodiesterases, calmodulin and oxidative phosphorylation[179]. Of these, phosphodiesterase inhibition may have particular relevance, for the concentrations of nifedipine which inhibit cAMP phosphodiesterase, $5-13 \mu mol/l$[180] are similar to those which inhibit mast cell mediator release[168, 172, 174, 178].

Although calcium antagonists have been shown to be of benefit against allergen[162] and exercise[163–166]-induced asthma, the weak effects against mast cell mediator release at clinically relevant concentrations suggest an action on the contractile components of the lung. This is supported by the inhibitory effects of calcium antagonists against bronchoconstriction in man induced by histamine[181–183], methacholine[182] and hyperventilation[184, 185], and in the dog induced by citric acid and methacholine[186]. Also, calcium antagonists reverse the contraction of human and animal airways smooth muscle preparations at concentrations below those required for inhibition of mast cell mediator release[162, 175, 187]. Even so, the selectivity of current calcium antagonists for vascular and cardiac smooth muscle rather than airways smooth muscle or mast cells indicates that they are unlikely to provide effective anti-asthmatic therapy without considerable chemical modification.

CORTICOSTEROIDS

Glucocorticosteroids have long been the drugs of choice for the treatment of chronic severe allergic diseases in the lung, nose and skin. The actions of corticosteroids against immediate hypersensitivity reactions in man are, however, controversial. Booij Noord and co-workers[188] and Pepys and co-workers[189] reported no effect of corticosteroids on the immediate reaction following allergen provocation. In contrast, Martin and co-workers[76] reported that prednisolone given over a 36 hour period before challenge reduced the immediate response to challenge in parallel with suppressed rises in plasma histamine and neutrophil chemotactic activity. In rodents, administration of corticosteroids 24 hours before challenge inhibits the immediate reaction to allergen challenge[190].

In vitro studies have demonstrated that the human mast cell is refractory to the effects of corticosteroids. Incubation of human lung fragments for up to 24 hours with high concentrations of dexamethasone fails to inhibit IgE-dependent histamine release[191, 192]. Also, in purified human lung mast cells, corticosteroids do not block the release of histamine, SRS-A leukotrienes or prostaglandin D_2[193]. The generation of prostaglandins, other than prostaglandin D_2, is suppressed when lung fragments are incubated with glucocorticoids, suggesting that release of newly generated mediators from other cells secondary to mast cell activation is steroid susceptible[193–195].

Although anaphylactic bronchoconstriction in rats is blocked by dexamethasone[190], histamine release from lung tissue taken from rats in the same series of experiments was not reduced[193]. A similar insensitivity of rodent mast cells to glucocorticoids has been reported from experiments measuring prostaglandin D_2 release[194]. The anomaly of the ability of glucocorticoids to suppress immediate hypersensitivity and yet not block allergen induced mast cell mediator release may be explained by the capacity of the drugs to cause involution of rodent mucosal mast cells[195]. Retrospective analysis of the histamine release studies from the lungs of steroid treated rats has revealed that, although histamine release expressed in percentage terms was not reduced, the initial histamine content of the lung was dramatically reduced. Hence histamine release expressed in absolute terms was markedly lower in test animals when compared with untreated controls[193].

In man also, corticosteroid treatment has been shown to inhibit the accumulation of mast cells in the nasal mucosa of allergic rhinitis sufferers during the pollen season[196]. However, mast cells normally resident within the skin are less sensitive, requiring high concentrations of glucocorticoids for long periods to cause their disappearance[197]. It is tempting to speculate that, as in the rodent, there are two sub-populations of mast cells in man of which only one is steroid sensitive, probably the T-cell dependent tryptase-only containing mast cell (see Chapter 4).

Unlike mast cells, basophils do appear to be sensitive to corticosteroids. Incubation of human basophils for 24 hours with dexamethasone causes a marked reduction in the release of both histamine and leukotriene[198, 199]. Studies in rat basophilic leukaemia cells have demonstrated that this corticosteroid inhibits receptor-activated phosphoinositide breakdown[200], thereby inhibiting histamine release and decreasing the availability of arachidonic acid for the synthesis of newly generated mediators. Whether or not this effect of corticosteroids is consequential upon the generation and effects of lipocortin[201] is not known.

Thus corticosteroids may modulate the immediate reaction by decreasing the number of mast cells at mucosal surfaces, by inhibiting the release of prostaglandins and leukotrienes from accessory cells and by inhibiting basophil mediator release. The effects on the late reaction are likely to be due to effects on the accumulation of leukocytes.

CONCLUSION

This chapter has surveyed the effect on mast cells of drugs used in the treatment of human allergic diseases. It is of interest to point out that, with the exception of sodium cromoglycate and its analogues, the inhibitory effects of drugs on mast cells is serendipitous rather than designed by drug developers. With the increasing knowledge of the biochemistry of the mast cell it is hoped that new drugs which are more effective and more specific will be developed in the near future. Only then can we fully understand the role of the mast cell in allergic diseases and the benefits of mast cell stabilizers in their treatment.

References

1. Lamb, D. and Lumsden, A. (1982). Intra-epithelial mast cells in human airway epithelium – evidence for smoking-induced changes in their frequency. *Thorax*, **37**, 334–42
2. Murray, J. J., Tonel, A. B., Brash, A. R., Roberts, L. J., Gosset, P., Workman, R., Capron, A. and Oates, J. A. (1986). Release of prostaglandin D2 into human airways during acute antigen challenge. *N. Engl. J. Med.*, **315**, 800–4
3. Howarth, P. H., Durham, S. R., Kay, A. B. and Holgate, S. T. (1987). The relationship between mast cell mediator release and bronchial reactivity in allergic asthma. *J. Allergy Clin. Immunol.*, **80**, 703–11
4. Bhat, K. W., Arroyave, C. M., Marney, S. R., Stevenson, D. D. and Tan, E. M. (1976). Plasma histamine changes during provoked bronchoconstriction in asthmatic patients. *J. Allergy Clin. Immunol.*, **58**, 647–56

5. Heavey, D. J., Kobza-Black, A., Barrow, S. E., Chappell, C. G., Greaves, M. W. and Dollery, C. T. (1986). Prostaglandin D2 and histamine release in cold urticaria. *J. Allergy Clin. Immunol.*, **78**, 458–61

6. Soter, N. A., Wasserman, S. I. and Austen, K. F. (1976). Cold urticaria: release of histamine and ECF-A during cold challenge. *N. Engl. J. Med.*, **294**, 687–90

7. Atkins, P. C. and Zweiman, B. (1981). Mediator release in local heat urticaria. *J. Allergy Clin. Immunol.*, **68**, 286–9

8. Brunet, C., Bedard, P. M., Pelletier, G., Borgeat, P. and Herbert, J. (1986). Profile of histamine and leucotriene (LTC4) release in urticaria. *J. Allergy Clin. Immunol.*, **77** (Suppl.), 227 (Abstr.)

9. Heavey, D. J., Ind, P. W., Myatake, A., Brown, M. J., MacDermot, J. and Dollery, C. T. (1985). Histamine release locally after intradermal antigen challenge in man. *Br. J. Clin. Pharmacol.*, **18**, 915–19

10. Anrep, G. V., Barsoum, G. S., Kenawy M. R. and Misrahy, G. (1947). Therapeutic uses of khellin. *Lancet*, **1**, 557–8

11. Bagouri, M. M. (1949). The coronary vasodilator action of the crystalline principles of *Ammi visnaga*. *J. Pharm. Pharmacol.*, **1**, 177–80

12. Cox, J. S. G. (1967). Disodium cromoglycate (FPL 670, Intal): a specific inhibitor of reaginic antibody–antigen mechanisms. *Nature*, **216**, 1328–9

13. Cox J. S. G. and Altounyan, R. E. C. (1970). Nature and modes of action of disodium cromoglycate (Lomudal). *Respiration*, **27** (Suppl.), 292–309

14. Dixon, M., Jackson, D. M. and Richards, I. M. The action of sodium cromoglycate on 'C' fibre endings in the dog lung. *Br. J. Pharmacol.*, **70**, 11–13

15. Moqbel, R., Walsh, G. M., Macdonald, A. J. and Kay, A. B. (1986). Effect of disodium cromoglycate on activation of human eosinophils and neutrophils following reversed (anti-IgE) anaphylaxis. *Clin. Allergy*, **16**, 73–83

16. Moqbel, R., Walsh, G. M. and Kay, A. B. (1986). Inhibition of human granulocyte activation by nedocromil sodium. *Eur. J. Resp. Dis.*, **69** (Suppl. 147), 227–9

17. Fullarton, J., Martin, L. E. and Vardey, C. J. (1973). Studies on the inhibition of cellular anaphylaxis. *Int. Arch. Allergy Appl. Immunol.*, **45**, 84–6

18. Garland, L. G. (1973). Effect of cromoglycate on anaphylactic histamine release from rat peritoneal mast cells. *Br. J. Pharmacol.*, **49**, 128–30

19. Johnson, H. G. and Van Hout, C. A. (1975). The enhanced efficacy of disodium cromoglycate (DSCG) in DSCG predosed rats. *Proc. Soc. Exp. Biol. Med.*, **143**, 427–9

20. Goose, J. and Blair, A. M. J. N. (1969). Passive cutaneous anaphylaxis in the rat induced by two homologous reagin-like antibody sera and its specific inhibition with disodium cromoglycate. *Immunology*, **16**, 749–60

21. Leung, K. B. P., Barrett, K. E. and Pearce, F. L. (1984). Differential effects of anti-allergic compounds on peritoneal mast cells of the rat mouse and hamster. *Agents Actions*, **14**, 461–7

22. Pearce, F. L., Befus, A. D., Gauldie, J. and Bienenstock, J. (1982). Mucosal mast cells. II. Effects of anti-allergic compounds on histamine secretion by isolated intestinal mast cells. *J. Immunol.*, **128**, 2481–6

23. Orr, T. S. C., Hall, D. E., Gwilliam, J. M. and Cox, J. S. G. (1971). Effect of disodium cromoglycate on the release of histamine and degranulation of mast cells induced by compound 48/80. *Life Sci.*, **10**, 805–12

24. Orr, T. S. C. and Cox, J. S. G. (1969). Disodium cromoglycate, an inhibition of mast cell degranulation and histamine release induced by phospholipase A. *Nature*, **233**, 197–8

25. Orr, T. S. C. (1975). Recent developments concerning the mast cell and the mode of action of disodium cromoglycate. *Acta Allergol.*, **12** (Suppl.), 13–29

26. Marshall, R. (1972). Protective effect of disodium cromoglycate on rat peritoneal mast cells. *Thorax*, **27**, 38–43

27. Johnson, H. G. and Bach, M. K. (1975). Prevention of calcium ionophore-induced release of histamine in rat mast cells by disodium cromoglycate. *J. Immunol.*, **114**, 514–16

28. Foreman, J. C., Hallett, M. B. and Mongar, J. L. (1977). Site of action of the antiallergic drugs cromoglycate and doxantiazole. *Br. J. Pharmacol.*, **59**, 473P–4P

29. Tasaka, K. (1985). Intracellular calcium release provoked by certain histamine releasers and its prevention by some antiallergic drugs. *J. Allergy Clin. Immunol.*, **75** (Suppl.) 124

30. Miller, P. (1976). Pinnal anaphylaxis in the mouse *PhD Thesis*. London: Council for National Academic Awards, 127–32
31. Evans, D. P., Gilman, D. J., Thomson, D. S. and Waring, W. S. (1974). Inhibition of allergic reactions by a novel phenanthroline, ICI-74917. *Nature*, **250**, 592–3
32. Evans, D. P. and Thomson, D. S. (1975). Inhibition of immediate hypersensitivity reactions in laboratory animals by a phenanthroline salt (ICI-74917). *Br. Pharmacol.*, **53**, 409–18
33. Miller, P. and James, G. W. L. (1978). Inhibition of immediate hypersensitivity reactions by a novel xanthone, RU-31,156. *Arch. Int. Pharmacodyn. Ther.*, **231**, 328–39
34. Marquardt, D. L., Walker, L. L. and Wasserman, S. I. (1986). Cromolyn inhibition of mediator release in mast cells derived from bone marrow. *Am. Rev. Resp. Dis.*, **133**, 1105–9
35. Taylor, W. A. and Roitt, I. M. (1973). Effect of disodium cromoglycate on various types of anaphylactic reactions in the guinea pig. *Int. Arch. Allergy Appl. Immunol.*, **45**, 795–807
36. Carney, I. F. (1976). IgE-mediated anaphylactic bronchoconstriction in the guinea pig and effect of DSCG. *Int. Arch. Allergy Appl. Immunol.*, **50**, 322–8
37. Andersson, P. (1980). Antigen-induced bronchial anaphylaxis in actively sensitized guinea-pigs. Antianaphylactic effects of sodium cromoglycate and aminophylline. *Br. J. Pharmacol.*, **69**, 467–72
38. Atkins, P. C., Norman, M. E. and Zwieman, B. (1978). Antigen-induced neutrophil chemotactic activity in man: correlation with bronchospasm and inhibition by disodium cromoglycate. *J. Allergy Clin. Immunol.*, **62**, 149–55
39. Howarth, P. H., Durham, S. R., Lee, T. H., Kay, A. B., Church, M. K. and Holgate, S. T. (1985). Influence of albuterol, cromolyn sodium and ipratropium bromide on the airway and circulating mediator responses to antigen bronchial provocation in asthma. *Am. Rev. Resp. Dis.*, **132**, 986–92
40. Church, M. K. and Young, K. D. (1983). The characteristics of inhibition of histamine release from human lung fragments by sodium cromoglycate, salbutamol and chlorpromazine. *Br. J. Pharmacol.*, **78**, 671–9
41. Young, K. D. and Church, M. K. (1983). Passive anaphylaxis in human lung fragments as a model for testing anti-allergic drugs: its variability and constraints. *Int. Arch. Allergy Appl. Immunol.*, **70**, 138–42
42. Church, M. K. and Hiroi, J. (1987). Inhibition of IgE-dependent histamine release from human dispersed lung mast cells by anti-allergic drugs and salbutamol. *Br. J. Pharmacol.*, **90**, 421–9
43. Church, M. K., Pao, G. J.-K. and Holgate, S. T. (1982). Characterization of histamine secretion from dispersed human lung mast cells: effects of anti-IgE, calcium ionophore A23187, compound 48/80 and basic polypeptides. *J. Immunol.*, **129**, 2116–21
44. Hardy, C. C., Robinson, C., Tattersfield, A. E. and Holgate, S. T. (1984). The bronchoconstrictor effect of inhaled prostaglandin D2 in normal and asthmatic men. *N. Engl. J. Med.*, **311**, 209–13
45. Soter, N. A., Lewis, R. A., Corey, E. J. and Austen, K. F. (1983). Local effects of synthetic leukotrienes (LTC4, LTD4, LTE4 and LTB4) in human skin. *J. Invest. Dermatol.*, **80**, 115–19
46. Flint, K. C., Leung, K. B. P., Pearce, F. L., Hudspith, B. N., Brostoff, J. and Johnson, N. McI. (1985). Human mast cells recovered from bronchoalveolar lavage: their morphology, histamine release and effects of sodium cromoglycate. *Clin. Sci.*, **68**, 427–32
47. Church, M. K. (1982). The role of basophils in asthma: 1; Sodium cromoglycate on histamine release and content. *Clin. Allergy*, **12**, 223–8
48. Benyon, R. C., Church, M. K., Clegg, L. S. and Holgate, S. T. (1986). Dispersion and characterization of mast cells from human skin. *Int. Arch. Allergy Appl. Immunol.*, **79**, 332–4
49. Ting, S., Zweiman, B. and Lavker, R. M. (1983). Cromolyn does not modulate human allergic skin reactions *in vivo*. *J. Allergy Clin. Immunol.*, **71**, 12–17
50. Sung, C. P., Saunders, H. L., Krell, R. D. and Chakrin, L. W. (1977). Studies on the mechanism of tachyphylaxis to disodium cromoglycate. *Int. Arch. Allergy Appl. Immunol.*, **55**, 374–84

51. Sung, C. P., Saunders, H. L., Lenhardt, E. and Chakrin, L. W. (1977). Further studies on the tachyphylaxis to disodium cromoglycate: the effects of concentration and temperature. *Int. Arch. Allergy Appl. Immunol.*, **55**, 385–94
52. Marshall, P. W., Thomson, D. S. and Evans, D. P. (1976). The mechanism of tachyphylaxis to ICI 74,917 and disodium cromoglycate. *Int. Arch. Allergy Appl. Immunol.*, **51**, 274–83
53. Schmutzler, W., Delmich, K., Eichelberg, D., Gluck, S., Greven, T., Jurgensen, H. and Riesener, K. P. (1985). The human adenoidal mast cell. Susceptibility to different secretagogues and secretion inhibitors. *Int. Arch. Allergy Appl. Immunol.*, **77**, 177–8
54. Roy, A. C. and Warren, B. T. (1974). Inhibition of cAMP phosphodiesterase by disodium cromoglycate. *Biochem. Pharmacol.*, **23**, 917–20
55. Tateson, J. E. and Trist, D. G. (1976). Inhibition of adenosine 3'5'-cyclic monophosphate phosphodiesterase by potential anti-allergic compounds. *Life Sci.*, **18**, 153–62
56. Lavin, N., Rachelefsky, G. S. and Kaplan, S. A. (1976). An action of disodium cromoglycate: Inhibition of cyclic 3',5'-AMP phosphodiesterase. *J. Allergy Clin. Immunol.*, **57**, 80–8
57. Church, M. K. (1985). The biochemical basis of pulmonary and anti-allergic drugs. In Devlin J. P. (ed.) *Pulmonary and Anti-allergic Drugs*, pp. 43–121. (NY: Wiley)
58. Mazurek, N., Berger, G. and Pecht, I. (1980). A binding site on mast cells and basophils for the antiallergic drug cromolyn. *Nature*, **286**, 722–3
59. Mazurek, N., Baskin, P., Loyter, A. and Pecht, I. (1983). Restoration of the calcium influx and degranulation capacity of variant RBL-2H3 cells upon implantation of isolated cromolyn binding protein. *Proc. Natl. Acad. Sci. USA*, **80**, 6014–18
60. Theoharides, T. C., Seighart, W., Greengard, P. and Douglas, W. W. (1980). Antiallergic drug cromolyn may inhibit secretion by regulating phosphorylation of a mast cell protein. *Science*, **207**, 80–2
61. Wells, E. and Mann, J. (1983). Phosphorylation of a mast cell protein in response to treatment with anti-allergic compounds. Implications for the mode of action of sodium cromoglycate. *Biochem. Pharmacol.*, **32**, 837–42
62. Seighart, W., Theoharides, T. C., Alper, S. L., Douglas, W. W. and Greengard, P. (1978). Calcium dependent protein phosphorylation during secretion by exocytosis in the mast cell. *Nature*, **275**, 329–31
63. Sagi-Eisenberg, R. (1985). Possible role for a calcium-activated, phospholipid-dependent protein kinase in mode of action of DSCG. *Trends Pharmacol. Sci.*, **6**, 198–200
64. Kikkawa, U., Takai, Y., Minakuchi, R., Inohara, S. and Nishizuka, Y. (1982). Calcium-activated, phospholipid-dependent protein kinase from rat brain: Subcellular distribution, purification and properties. *J. Biol. Chem.*, **257**, 13341–8
65. Garland, L. G. and Mongar, J. L. (1974). Inhibition by cromoglycate of histamine release from rat peritoneal mast cells induced by mixtures of dextran, phosphatidylserine and calcium ions. *Br. J. Pharmacol.*, **50**, 137–43
66. DeSouza, R. N. and Findlay, J. B. C. *cited in* Kay, A. B. (1987). The mode of action of anti-allergic drugs. Report of a meeting of the Section of Clinical Immunology and Allergy, Royal Society of Medicine, London, February, 1986. *Clin. Allergy*, **17**, 153–64
67. Lucas, A. M. and Schuster, S. (1987). Cromolyn inhibition of protein kinase C activity. *Biochem. Pharmacol.*, **36**, 562–5
68. Watson, S. P. and Lapetina, E. G. (1985). 1,2 Diacylglycerol and phorbol esters inhibit agonist-induced formation of inositol phosphates in human platelets: possible implications for negative feedback regulation of inositol phospholipid hydrolysis. *Proc. Natl. Acad. Sci. USA*, **82**, 2623–6
69. Orellana, S. A., Solski, P. A. and Brown, J. H. (1985). Phorbol ester inhibits phosphoinositide hydrolysis and calcium mobilization in cultured astrocytoma cells. *J. Biol. Chem.*, **260**, 5236–9
70. Shenfield, G. M., Brogden, R. N. and Ward, A. (1984). Pharmacology of bronchodilators. In Clarke, T. J. H. and Cochrane, C. McL. (eds.) *Bronchodilator Therapy*, pp. 17–46. (New Zealand: ADIS)
71. Butchers, P. R., Fullerton, J. R., Skidmore, I. F., Thomson, L. E., Vardey, C. J. and Wheeldon, A. (1979). A comparison of the anti-anaphylactic activities of salbutamol and disodium cromoglycate in the rat, the rat mast cell and in human lung tissue. *Br. J. Pharmacol.*, **67**, 23–32

72. Butchers, P. R., Skidmore, I. F., Vardey, C. J. and Wheeldon, A. (1980). Characterization of the receptor mediating the anti-anaphylactic effects of β-adrenoceptor agonsts in human lung tissue *in vitro*. *Br. J. Pharmacol.*, **71**, 663–7
73. Assem, E. S. K. and Schild, H. O. (1969). Inhibition by sympathomimetic amines of histamine release induced by antigen in passively sensitized human lung. *Nature*, **224**, 1028–9
74. Strandberg, K., Pegelow, K. O., Persson, C. G. A. and Sorenby, L. (1979). Anti-anaphylactic and bronchodilating action of a beta-adrenergic stimulator, KWD 2131 in human lung tissue. *Allergy*, **34**, 221–4
75. Schulman, E. S., MacGlashan, D. W., Peters, S. P., Schleimer, R. P., Newball, H. H. and Lichtenstein, L. M. (1982). Human lung mast cells: purification and characterization. *J. Immunol.*, **129**, 2662–7
76. Martin, G. L., Atkins, P. C., Dunsky, E. H. and Zwieman, B. (1980). Effects of theophylline, terbutaline and prednisolone on antigen-induced bronchospasm and mediator release. *J. Allergy Clin. Immunol.*, **66**, 204–12
77. Assem, E. S. K. and Richter, A. W. (1971). Comparison of *in vivo* and *in vitro* inhibition of the anaphylactic mechanism by β-adrenergic stimulants and disodium cromoglycate. *Immunology*, **21**, 729–39
78. Malta, E. and Raper, C. (1975). Beta-adrenoceptors involved in inhibition of histamine release from sensitized guinea-pig lung. *Eur. J. Pharmacol.*, **30**, 79–85
79. Forsberg, K. and Sorenby, L. (1979). Release of slow reacting substance from anaphylactic lung tissue and its modification by beta-sympathomimetics. *Int. Arch. Allergy Appl. Immunol.*, **58**, 430–5
80. Johnson, A. R. and Moran, N. C. (1970). Inhibition of the release of histamine from rat mast cells: the effect of cold and adrenergic drugs on release of histamine by compound 48/80 and antigen. *J. Pharmacol. Exp. Ther.*, **175**, 632–40
81. Sullivan, T. J., Parker, K. L., Eisen, S. A. and Parker, C. W. (1975). Modulation of cyclic AMP in purified rat mast cells. II Studies on the relationship between intracellular cyclic AMP concentrations and histamine release. *J. Immunol.*, **114**, 1480–5
82. Donlon, M., Hunt, W. A., Catravas, G. N. and Kalmer, M. (1982). A characterization of beta-adrenergic receptors on cellular and perigranular membranes of rat peritoneal mast cells. *Life Sci.*, **31**, 411–16
83. Marquardt, D. L. and Wasserman, S. I. (1982). Characterization of rat mast cell beta-adrenergic receptor in resting and stimulated cells by radio-ligand binding. *J. Immunol.*, **129**, 2122–7
84. Ishizaka, T. and Ishizaka, K. (1984). Activation of mast cells for mediator release through IgE receptors. *Prog. Allergy*, **34**, 188–235
85. Lichtenstein, L. M. and DeBarnardo, R. (1971). The immediate allergic response: *in vitro* action of cyclic AMP-active and other drugs on the two stages of histamine release. *J. Immunol.*, **107**, 1131–6
86. Howe, R. and Shanks, R. G. (1969). Optical isomers of propranolol. *Nature*, **210**, 1336–8
87. Kalsner, S. (1980). The effects of (+) and (−) propranolol on 3H-transmitter efflux in guinea pig atria and the beta-adrenoceptor hypothesis. *Br. J. Pharmacol.*, **70**, 491–8
88. Tung, R. and Lichtenstein, L. M. (1981). cAMP agonist inhibition increases at low levels of histamine release from human basophils. *J. Pharmacol. Exp. Ther.*, **218**, 642–6
89. Ting, S., Zweiman, B. and Lavker, R. M. (1983). Terbutaline modulation of human allergic skin reactions. *J. Allergy Clin. Immunol.*, **71**, 437–41
90. Benyon, R. C., Lowman, M. A. and Church, M. K. (1987). Human skin mast cells: their dispersion, purification and secretory characterization. *J. Immunol.*, **138**, 861–7
91. Cockcroft, D. W. and Murdock, K. Y. (1986). Protective effect of inhaled albuterol, cromolyn, beclomethasone and placebo on allergen-induced early asthmatic response (EAR), late asthmatic response (LAR) and allergen-induced increases in bronchial responsiveness to inhaled histamine. *J. Allergy Clin. Immunol.*, **77** (Suppl.), 122 (Abstr.)
92. Cochrane, G. M. and Clark, T. J. H. (1975). A survey of asthma mortality between the ages of 35 and 64 in the Greater London Hospitals in 1971. *Thorax*, **30**, 300–5
93. Weinberger, M. (1978). Theophylline for treatment of asthma. *J. Pediatr.*, **92**, 1–7
94. Butcher, R. E. and Sutherland, E. W. (1968). Some aspects of the biological role of adenosine 3′,5′-monophosphate (cyclic AMP). *Circulation*, **37**, 279–306

95. Cushley, M. J. and Holgate, S. T. (1984). The development of theophylline preparations. In Smith, H. and Buckle, D. R. (eds.). *New Development of Anti-Asthmatic Drugs*, pp. 205–23. (Edinburgh: Butterworth)
96. Kaliner, M. and Austen, K. F. (1974). Cyclic AMP, ATP and anaphylactic histamine release from rat mast cells. *J. Immunol.*, **112**, 664–74
97. Newman, D. J., Colella, D. F., Spainhour, C. B., Brann, E. G., Zabko Potapovich, B. and Wardell, J. R. (1978). cAMP-phosphodiesterase inhibitors and tracheal smooth muscle relaxation. *Biochem. Pharmacol.*, **27**, 729–32
98. Hayaski, H., Ichikawa, K., Saito, T. and Tomita, K. (1976). Inhibitory role of cyclic adenosine 3′,5′-monophosphate in histamine release from rat peritoneal mast cells *in vitro*. *Biochem. Pharmacol.*, **25**, 1907–13
99. Winslow, C. M. and Austen, K. F. (1984). Role of cyclic nucleotides in the activation response. *Prog. Allergy*, **34**, 236–70
100. Bergstrand, H., Kristoffersson, J., Lundquist, B. and Schurmann, A. (1977). Effects of anti-allergic compounds, compound 48/80 and some reference inhibitors on the activity of partially purified human lung tissue cyclic 3′,5′-monophosphate phosphodiesterases and guanosine 3′,5′-monophosphate phosphodiesterases. *Mol. Pharmacol.*, **13**, 38–43
101. Bergstrand, H. (1980). Phosphodiesterase inhibition and theophylline. *Eur. J. Resp. Dis.*, **61** (Suppl. 109), 37–44
102. Polson, J. B., Krzanowski, J. J., Goldman, A. L. and Szentivanyi, A. (1978). Inhibition of human pulmonary phosphodiesterase activity by therapeutic levels of theophylline. *Clin. Exp. Pharmacol. Physiol.*, **5**, 535–9
103. Sydbom, A. and Fredholm, B. B. (1982). On the mechanism by which theophylline inhibits histamine release from rat mast cells. *Acta Physiol. Scand.*, **114**, 243–51
104. Norn, S., Geisler, A., Stahl Skov, P. and Klysner, R. (1979). Differentiation between cyclic AMP level and allergic histamine release in rat mast cells. *Agents Actions*, **9**, 64–5
105. Norn, S., Geisler, A., Stahl Skov, P. and Klysner, R. (1977). Cyclic AMP and allergic histamine release. Influence of methylxanthines on rat mast cells. *Acta Allergol.*, **32**, 183–91
106. Naclerio, R. M., Bartenfelder, D., Proud, D., Togias, A. G., Meyers, D. A., Kagey-Sobokta, A., Norman, P. S. and Lichtenstein, L. M. (1986). Theophylline reduces histamine release during pollen-induced rhinitis. *J. Allergy Clin. Immunol.*, **78**, 874–6
107. Fredholm, B. B. (1980). Theophylline actions on adenosine receptors. *Eur. J. Pharmacol.*, **61** (Suppl. 109), 29–36
108. Cushley, M. J., Tattersfield, A. E. and Holgate, S. T. (1983). Inhaled adenosine and guanosine on airway resistance in normal and asthmatic subjects. *Br. J. Clin. Pharmacol.*, **15**, 161–5
109. Church, M. K., Featherstone, R. L., Cushley, M. J., Mann, J. S. and Holgate, S. T. (1986). Relationship between adenosine, cyclic nucleotides and xanthines in asthma. *J. Allergy Clin. Immunol.*, **78**, 670–6
110. Cushley, M. J. and Holgate, S. T. (1985). Adenosine induced bronchoconstriction in asthma: role of mast cell mediator release. *J. Allergy Clin. Immunol.*, **75**, 272–8
111. Crimi, N., Palermo, F., Oliveri, R., Cacopardo, B., Vancheri, C. and Mistretta, A. (1986). Adenosine-induced bronchoconstriction: comparison between nedocromil and sodium cromoglycate. *Eur. J. Resp. Dis.*, **69** (Suppl. 147), 158–62
112. Rafferty, P., Beasley, R. and Holgate, S. T. (1987). The inhibitory effect of terfenadine on bronchoconstriction induced by adenosine monophosphate and antigen (Abstr.). *Thorax.* (In press)
113. Rafferty, P., Beasley, C. R. and Holgate, S. T. (1987). The contribution of histamine to bronchoconstriction produced by inhaled allergen and adenosine 5′-monophosphate in asthma. *Am. Rev. Resp. Dis.*, **136**, 369–73
114. Mann, J. S., Holgate, S. T., Renwick, A. G. and Cushley, M. J. (1986). Airway effects of purine nucleosides and nucleotides and release with bronchial provocation in asthma. *J. Appl. Physiol.*, **61**, 1667–76
115. Hughes, P. J., Holgate, S. T. and Church, M. K. (1984). Adenosine inhibits and potentiates IgE-dependent histamine release from human lung mast cells by an A2-purinoceptor mediated mechanism. *Biochem. Pharmacol.*, **33**, 3847–52

116. Church, M. K., Holgate, S. T. and Hughes, P. J. (1983). Adenosine inhibits and potentiates IgE-dependent histamine release from human basophils by an A2-receptor mediated mechanism. *Br. J. Pharmacol.*, **80**, 719–26
117. Church, M. K., Hughes, P. J. and Vardey, C. J. (1986). Studies on the receptor mediating cyclic AMP-independent enhancement by adenosine of IgE-dependent mediator release from rat mast cells. *Br. J. Pharmacol.*, **87**, 233–42
118. Marquardt, D. L., Parker, C. W. and Sullivan, T. J. (1978). Potentiation of mast cell mediator release by adenosine. *J. Immunol.*, **120**, 871–8
119. Mann, J. S. and Holgate, S. T. (1985). Specific antagonism of adenosine induced bronchoconstriction in asthma by oral theophylline. *Br. J. Clin. Pharmacol.*, **19**, 685–92
120. Mann, J. S., Cushley, M. J. and Holgate, S. T. (1985). Adenosine induced bronchoconstriction in asthma and its antagonism by theophylline. *Prog. Resp. Res.*, **16**, 102–5
121. Persson, C. G. A. and Kjellin, G. (1981). Enprofylline, a principally new anti-asthmatic xanthine. *Acta Pharmacol. Toxicol. (Copenh.)*, **49**, 313–16
122. Persson, C. G. A., Karlsson, J. A. and Erjefalt, J. (1982). Differentiation between bronchodilation and universal adenosine antagonism amongst xanthine derivatives. *Life Sci.*, **30**, 2181–9
123. Holgate, S. T., Mann, J. S., Church, M. K. and Cushley, M. J. (1987). Mechanisms and significance of adenosine induced bronchoconstriction in asthma. *Allergy*, **42**, 727–30
124. Kolbeck, R. C., Speir, W. A., Carrier, G. O. and Bransome, E. D. (1979). Apparent irrelevance of cyclic nucleotides to the relaxation of tracheal smooth muscle induced by theophylline. *Lung*, **156**, 173–83
125. Horrobin, D. F., Manku, M. S., Franks, D. J. and Hamet, P. (1977). Methylxanthine phosphodiesterase inhibitors behave as prostaglandin antagonists in a perfused mesenteric preparation. *Prostaglandins*, **13**, 33–40
126. Aubier, M., DeTroyer, A., Sampson, M., Macklem, P. T. and Roussos, C. (1981). Aminophylline improves diaphragmatic contractility. *N. Engl. J. Med.*, **305**, 249–52
127. Higbee, M. D., Kumar, M. and Galant, S. P. (1982). Stimulation of endogenous catecholamine release by theophylline: a proposed additional mechanism of action for theophylline effects. *J. Allergy Clin. Immunol.*, **70**, 377–82
128. Pauwels, R., Vanrenterghem, D., Van der Straeten, M., Johannesson, N. and Persson, C. G. A. (1985). The effect of theophylline and enprofylline on allergen-induced bronchoconstriction. *J. Allergy Clin. Immunol.*, **76**, 583–90
129. Black, J. W., Duncan, W. A. M., Durant, C. J., Ganellin, C. R. and Parsons, E. M. (1972). Definition and antagonism of histamine H2-receptors. *Nature*, **236**, 385–90
130. Arrang, J. M., Garbag, M., Lancelot, J. C., Lecomte, J. M., Pollard, H., Robba, M., Schunack, W. and Schwartz, J. C. (1987). Highly potent and selective ligands for histamine H3-receptors. *Nature*, **327**, 117–23
131. Annotation (1955). Anti-histamines and asthma. *Lancet*, **2**, 1182
132. Brandon, M. L. and Weiner, M. (1980). Clinical investigation of terfenadine, a non-sedating anti-histamine. *Ann. Allergy*, **44**, 71–5
133. Holgate, S. T. and Howarth, P. H. (1984). Astemizole in seasonal allergic rhinitis and conjunctivitis. In *Astemizole, A New Non-Sedative Long Acting H1-Antagonist*, pp. 69–77. (Oxford: Medicine Publ. Foundation)
134. Craps, L., Greenwood, C. and Radielovic P. (1978). Clinical investigation of agents with prophylactic anti-allergic effects in bronchial asthma. *Clin. Allergy*, **8**, 373–82
135. Arunlakshana, O. and Schild, H. O. (1953). Histamine release by antihistamines. *J. Physiol.*, **119**, 47P–48P
136. Mota, I. and Dias Da Silva, W. (1966). The antianaphylactic and histamine releasing properties of the anti-histamines: their effect on mast cells. *Br. J. Pharmacol.*, **15**, 396–404
137. Guschin, I. S., Deryugin, I. L. and Kaminka, M. E. (1978). Histamine liberating action of antihistamines on isolated rat mast cells. *Bull. Exp. Biol. Med.*, **85**, 352–5
138. Church, M. K. and Gradidge, C. F. (1980). Inhibition of histamine release from human lung *in vitro* by antihistamines and related drugs. *Br. J. Pharmacol.*, **69**, 663–7
139. Frisk Holmberg, M. and Van der Kleijn (1972). The relationship between the lipophilic nature of tricyclic neuroleptics and anti-depressants and histamine release. *Eur. J. Pharmacol.*, **18**, 139–47

140. Johnson, A. G. and Miller, M. D. (1979). Inhibition of histamine release and ionophore-induced calcium flux in rat mast cells by lidocaine and chlorpromazine. *Agents Actions*, **9**, 239–43

141. Kazimierczak, W., Peret, M. and Maslinski, C. (1976). The action of local anaesthetics on histamine release. *Biochem. Pharmacol.*, **25**, 1747–50

142. Seeman, P. (1972). The membrane actions of anaesthetics and tranquillizers. *Pharmacol. Rev.*, **24**, 583–655

143. Young, K. D. (1982). Pharmacological antagonism of mast cell secretion in human lung tissue. *PhD Thesis*. University of Southampton.

144. Kwant, W. O. and Seeman, P. (1969). The displacement of membrane calcium by a local anaesthetic (chlorpromazine). *Biochim. Biophys. Acta*, **193**, 338–49

145. Lullmann, H., Plosch, H. and Ziegler, A. (1980). Calcium replacement by cationic amphiphillic drugs from lipid monolayers. *Biochem. Pharmacol.*, **29**, 2969–74

146. Pearce, F. L. (1982). Calcium and histamine secretion from mast cells. *Prog. Med. Chem.*, **19**, 59–109

147. Charlier, R. and Philippot, E. (1949). Modifications pharmacologique du volume pulmonaire chez l'homme sain. *Arch. Int. Pharmacodyn. Ther.*, **219**, 1–12

148. Herxheimer, H. *The Management of Bronchial Asthma: A Guide to Treatment.* p. 56. (London: Butterworth)

149. Holgate, S. T., Emanuel, M. B. and Howarth, P. H. (1985). Astemizole and other H1-antihistamine drug treatment of asthma. *J. Allergy Clin. Immunol.*, **76**, 375–82

150. Curzen, N., Rafferty, P. and Holgate, S T. (1987). Cyclooxygenase inhibition and H1-histamine receptor antagonism alone and in combination on allergen-induced bronchoconstriction in man. *Thorax*. (Submitted)

151. Rafferty, P., Beasley, C. R. and Holgate, S. T. (1987). The contribution of histamine to bronchoconstriction produced by inhaled allergen and adenosine 5'-monophosphate in asthma. *Am. Rev. Resp. Dis.* (In press)

152. Frieri, M., Alling, D. W. and Metcalfe, D. D. (1985). Comparison of the therapeutic efficacy of cromolyn sodium with that of combined chlorpheniramine and cimetidine in systemic mastocytosis. *Am. J. Med.*, **78**, 9–14

153. Ting, S., Rauls, D. O. and Reiman, B. E. F. (1985). Inhibitory effect of hydroxyzine on antigen-induced histamine release *in vivo*. *J. Allergy Clin. Immunol.*, **75**, 63–6

154. Lichtenstein, L. M. and Gillespie, E. (1972). The effects of the H1 and H2 antihistamines on 'allergic' histamine release and its inhibition by histamine. *J. Pharmacol. Exp. Ther.*, **192**, 441–50

155. Bourne, H. R., Lichtenstein, L. M., Melmon, K. L., Henney, C. S., Weinstein, Y. and Shearer, G. M. (1974). Modulation of inflammation and immunity by cyclic AMP. *Science*, **184**, 19–28

156. Tung, R., Kagey-Sobotka, A., Plaut, M. and Lichtenstein, L. M. (1982). H2 anti-histamines augment antigen-induced histamine release from human basophils *in vitro*. *J. Immunol.*, **129**, 2113–15

157. Dulabh, R. and Vickers, M. R. (1978). The effect of H2-receptor blockers on anaphylaxis in the guinea pig. *Agents Actions*, **8**, 559–65

158. Krell, R. D. and Chakrin, L. W. (1977). The effect of metiamide in *in vitro* and *in vivo* canine models of type 1 hypersensitivity reactions. *Eur. J. Pharmacol.*, **44**, 35–44

159. Platshon, L. F. and Kaliner, M. (1978). The effects of the immunological release of histamine upon human lung cyclic nucleotide levels and prostaglandin generation. *J. Clin. Invest.*, **62**, 1113–21

160. Lichtenstein, L. M., Foreman, J. C., Conroy, M. C., Marone, G. and Newball, H. H. (1979). Differences between histamine release from rat mast cells and human basophils and mast cells. In Pepys, J. and Edwards, A. M. (eds.). *The Mast Cell: Its Role in Health and Disease*, pp. 83–96. (London: Pitman)

161. Barth, H., Niemeyer, I. and Lorenz, W. (1973). Studies on the mode of action of histamine H1- and H2-receptor antagonists on gastric histamine methyltransferase. *Agents Actions*, **3**, 138–47

162. Henderson, A. F., Heaton, R. W., Dunlop, L. S. and Costello, L. S. (1983). Effects of nifedipine on antigen-induced bronchoconstriction. *Am. Rev. Resp. Dis.*, **127**, 549–53

163. Cerrina, J., Denjean, A., Alexandre, G., Lockhart, A. and Duroux, P. (1981). Inhibition of exercise induced asthma by a calcium antagonist, nifedipine. *Am. Rev. Resp. Dis.*, **123**, 156–60

164. Barnes, P. J., Wilson, N. M. and Brown, M. J. (1981). A calcium antagonist, nifedipine, modifies exercise induced asthma. *Thorax*, **36**, 726–30

165. Patel, K. R. (1981). The effect of a calcium antagonist, nifedipine, in exercise-induced asthma. *Clin. Allergy*, **11**, 429–32

166. Patel, K. R. (1981). Calcium antagonists in exercise-induced asthma. *Br. Med. J.*, **282**, 932–3

167. Suzuki, T., Mori, K. and Uchida, M. (1982). Inhibition by calcium antagonists of histamine release and calcium influx of rat mast cells: differences between induction of histamine release by concanavalin A and compound 48/80. *Eur. J. Pharmacol.*, **85**, 155–61

168. Tanizaki, Y., Akagi, K., Lee, K. N. and Townley, R. G. (1987). Inhibitory effect of nifedipine and cromolyn sodium on skin reactions and ^{45}Ca uptake and histamine release in rat mast cells induced by various stimulating agents. *Int. Arch. Allergy Appl. Immunol.*, **72**, 102–9

169. Legrand, A., Cerrina, J., Bonne, C., Lockhart, A. and Benveniste, J. (1984). Inhibition of rat mast cell degranulation by verapamil. *Agents Actions*, **14**, 153–6

170. Ennis, M., Ind, P. W., Pearce, F. L. and Dollery, C. T. (1983). Calcium antagonists and histamine secretion from rat peritoneal mast cells. *Agents Actions*, **13**, 144–8

171. Chand, N., Diamantis, W., Pillar, J. and Sofia, R. D. (1984). Inhibition of allergic and non-allergic histamine secretion from rat peritoneal mast cells by calcium antagonists. *Br. J. Pharmacol.*, **83**, 899–902

172. Jensen, C., Stahl Skov, P. and Norn, S. (1983). Inhibitory effects of calcium antagonists on histamine release from human leucocytes. *Allergy*, **38**, 233–7

173. Atkins, F., Middleton, E., Triggle, D. and Drzewiecki, G. (1981). Effects of calcium antagonists on human basophil histamine release. *J. Allergy Clin. Immunol.*, **68**, 28

174. Bedard, R. M. and Busse W. W. (1983). Nifedipine inhibition of human basophil histamine release (Abstr.). *Am. Rev. Resp. Dis.*, **129**, A9

175. Butchers, P. R., Skidmore, I. F., Vardey, C. J. and Wheeldon, A. (1982). Calcium antagonists in exercise induced asthma. *Br. Med. J.*, **282**, 1792

176. Cerrina, J., Hadji, L., Marche, E., Duroux, P. and Benveniste, J. (1982). Effects of the calcium antagonist nifedipine on histamine and SRS release from human lung tissue. *Am. Rev. Resp. Dis.*, **125**, 64

177. Lee, V. Y., Hughes, J. M., Seale, J. P. and Temple, D. M. (1983). Verapamil inhibits mediator release from human lung in vitro. *Thorax*, **38**, 386–7

178. Kim, Y. Y., Holgate, S. T. and Church, M. K. (1985). Inhibition of histamine release from dispersed human lung and tonsillar mast cells by nicardipine and nifedipine. *Br. J. Clin. Pharmacol.*, **19**, 631–8

179. Kazda, S., Knorr, A. and Towart, R. (1983). Common properties and differences between various calcium antagonists. *Prog. Pharmacol.*, **5**, 83–116

180. Nishikori, K., Takenaka, T. and Maeno, H. (1981). A possible mechanism for relaxation of rat uterine smooth muscle by nicardipine hydrochloride (YC-93), a new potent vasodilator. *Jpn. J. Pharm.*, **31**, 701–9

181. Williams, D. O., Barnes, P. J., Vickers, H. P. and Rudolph, M. (1981). Effect of nifedipine on bronchomotor tone and histamine reactivity in asthma. *Br. Med. J.*, **283**, 348

182. Malik, S., O'Reilly, J. and Sudlow, M. F. (1982). The effects of sublingual nifedipine on inhaled histamine- and methacholine-induced bronchoconstriction in asthmatic subjects. *Thorax*, **32**, 230

183. Corris, P. A., Nariman, S. and Gibson, G. J. (1983). Nifedipine in the prevention of asthma induced by exercise and histamine. *Am. Rev. Resp. Dis.*, **128**, 991–2

184. Rolla, G., Bucca, C., Polizzi, S., Maina, A., Giachino, O. and Salvini, P. (1982). Nifedipine inhibits deep inspiration-induced bronchoconstriction in asthmatics. *Lancet*, **1**, 1305–6

185. Henderson, A. F., Heaton, R. W. and Costello, L. S. (1983). The effect of nifedipine in bronchoconstriction induced by cold air. *Thorax*, **38**, 506–11

186. Brugman, T. M., Darnell, M. L. and Hirshman, C. A. (1983). Nifedipine aerosol attenuates airway constriction in dogs with hyperreactive airways. *Am. Rev. Resp. Dis.*, **128**, 14–17

187. Fanta, C. H., Venugopulan, C. S., Lascouture, P. G. and Drazen, J. M. (1982). Inhibition of bronchoconstriction in the guinea pig by a calcium channel blocker, nifedipine. *Am. Rev. Resp. Dis.*, **125**, 61–6
188. Booij Noord, H., Orie, N. G. M. and de Vries, K. (1971). Immediate and late bronchial obstructive reactions to inhalation of house dust and protective effects of disodium cromoglycate and prednisolone. *J. Allergy Clin. Immunol.*, **48**, 344–54
189. Pepys, J., Davies, R. J., Breslin, A. B. X., Hendrick, D. J. and Hutchcroft, C. A. (1974). The effect of inhaled beclomethasone dipropionate (Becotide) and sodium cromoglycate on asthmatic reactions to provocation tests. *Clin. Allergy*, **4**, 13–24
190. Church, M. K., Collier, H. O. J. and James, G. W. L. (1972). The inhibition by dexamethasone and disodium cromoglycate of anaphylactic bronchoconstriction in the rat. *Br. J. Pharmacol.*, **46**, 56–65
191. Schleimer, R. P., Schulman, E. S., MacGlashan, D. W., Peters, S. P., Hayes, E. C., Adams, G. K., Lichtenstein, L. M. and Adkinson, N. F. (1983). Effects of dexamethasone on mediator release from human lung fragments and purified human lung mast cells. *J. Clin. Invest.*, **71**, 1830–5
192. Schleimer, R. P., Davidson, D. A., Lichtenstein, L. M. and Adkinson, N. F. (1986). Selective inhibition of archidonic acid metabolite release from human lung tissue by anti-inflammatory steroids. *J. Immunol.*, **136**, 3006–11
193. Church, M. K. (1970). Inhibition of the anaphylactic response. *PhD Thesis*, London: Council for National Academic Awards
194. Robin, J. L., Seldin, D., Austen, K. F. and Lewis, R. A. (1985). Regulation of mediator release from mouse bone marrow-derived mast cells by glucocorticoids. *J. Immunol.*, **135**, 2719–26
195. King, S. J., Miller, H. R., Newlands, G. F. and Woodbury, R. G. (1985). Depletion of mucosal mast cell protease by glucocorticosteroids: effect on intestinal anaphylaxis in the rat. *Proc. Natl. Acad. Sci. USA*, **82**, 1214–18
196. Otsuka, H., Denburg, J. A., Befus, A. D., Hitch, D., Lapp, P., Rajan, R. S., Bienenstock, J. A. and Dolovich, J. (1986). Effect of beclomethasone dipropionate on nasal metachromatic sub-populations. *Clin. Allergy*, **16**, 589–95
197. Lavaker, R. M. and Schechter, N. M. (1985). Cutaneous mast cell depletion results from topical corticosteroid usage. *J. Immunol.*, **135**, 2368–73
198. Schleimer, R. P., Lichtenstein, L. M. and Gillespie, E. (1981). Inhibition of basophil histamine release by anti-inflammatory steroids. *Nature*, **292**, 454–5
199. Schleimer, R. P., Davidson, D. A., Peters, S. P. and Lichtenstein, L. M. (1985). Inhibition of basophil leukotriene release by anti-inflammatory steroids. *Int. Arch. Allergy Appl. Immunol.*, **77**, 241–3
200. Berenstein, E. H., Garcia-Gil, M. and Siraganian, R. P. (1987). Dexamethasone inhibits receptor-activated phosphoinositide breakdown in rat basophilic leukemia (RBL-2H3) cells. *J. Immunol.*, **138**, 1914–18
201. Flower, R. J. (1985). The lipocortins and their role in controlling defence reactions. *Adv. Prostaglandin Thromboxane Leukotriene Res.*, **15**, 201–3

Index